Cardiac Arrhythmias

Cardiac Arrhythmias

Current Diagnosis and Practical Management

Roger A. Winkle, M.D.
Associate Professor of Medicine
Stanford University School of Medicine
Stanford, California

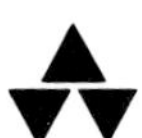

ADDISON-WESLEY PUBLISHING COMPANY
Medical Division • Menlo Park, California
Reading, Massachusetts • London • Amsterdam
Don Mills, Ontario • Sydney

To Lynn, Brooke, and Bryce

Sponsoring Editor: Richard W. Mixter
Production Coordinator: Susan Harrington
Copyeditor: Dorilee Bingham
Cover and Book Design: Michael A. Rogondino

Library of Congress Cataloging in Publication Data
Main entry under title:

Cardiac arrhythmias.

Bibliography: p.
Includes index.
1. Arrhythmia. I. Winkle, Roger A. [DNLM:
1. Arrhythmia--Diagnosis. 2. Arrhythmia--Therapy.
WG 330 C26715]
RC685.A65C2727 1983 616.1'28 83-9968
ISBN 0-201-08280-2

ISBN 0-201-08280-2

ABCDEFGHIJ-MA-89876543

The authors and publishers have exerted every effort to ensure that drug selection and dosage formulations and composition of formulas set forth in this text are in accord with current recommendations and practice at the time of publication. However, in view of ongoing research, changes in government regulations, the reformulation of nutritional products, and the constant flow of information relating to drug therapy and drug reactions, the reader is urged to check product information on composition or the package insert for each drug for any change in indications of dosage and for added warnings and precautions. This is particularly important where the recommended agent is a new and/or infrequently employed drug.

The paper in this book meets the guidelines for permanence and durability of the Committee on Production Guidelines for Book Longevity of the Council on Library Resources.

Addison-Wesley Publishing Company
Medical Division
2725 Sand Hill Road
Menlo Park, California 94025

Contributors

Jeffrey L. Anderson, M.D.
Associate Professor of Internal Medicine (Cardiology)
University of Utah School of Medicine
Salt Lake City, Utah

Ronald W. F. Campbell, M.D.
Honorary Consultant Cardiologist
The University of Newcastle-upon-Tyne
Newcastle-upon-Tyne, England

Robert F. DeBusk, M.D.
Associate Professor Clinical Medicine
Stanford University School of Medicine
Stanford, California

Michael Eliastam, M.P.P.
Assistant Professor of Medicine and Surgery
Stanford University School of Medicine
Stanford, California

Jerry C. Griffin, M.D.
Director of Pacing Programs
Baylor College of Medicine and The Methodist Hospital
Houston, Texas

Roger J. Hall, M.D., M.R.C.P.
Consultant Cardiologist and Physician
Royal Victoria Infirmary
Queen Victoria Road
Newcastle-upon-Tyne, England

Jay W. Mason, M.D.
Chief, Cardiology Division
University of Utah Medical Center
Salt Lake City, Utah

David L. Ross, M.B., F.R.A.C.P.
Staff Specialist (Cardiology)
Cardiology Unit
Westmead Hospital
Westmead, Australia

Edward B. Stinson, M.D.
Professor of Cardiovascular Surgery
Stanford University School of Medicine
Stanford, California

Roger A. Winkle, M.D.
Associate Professor of Medicine
Stanford University School of Medicine
Stanford, California

Preface

The diagnosis and management of cardiac arrhythmias have changed drastically during the past ten years. Electrophysiologic studies have progressed from a research test for measuring HV intervals to a complex and clinically useful diagnostic and therapeutic tool. There has also been a marked increase in our understanding of the mechanism of many cardiac arrhythmias. The widespread application of surgical techniques to the management of cardiac arrhythmias, as well as the introduction of a large number of new antiarrhythmic drugs, sophisticated pacemakers, and other implantable antiarrhythmic devices, have provided new therapeutic modalities for the treatment of difficult arrhythmia cases. The advances have occurred so rapidly that there has been little time to summarize them in a form usable to the practicing physician, who may not have the time or inclination to delve deeply into the many books and articles on these subjects.

This book has been written to give the practicing physician a readable compilation of recent advances in the diagnosis and management of cardiac arrhythmias and to permit integration of this knowledge into his or her daily practice. The first chapter summarizes the current knowledge of the cellular basis of cardiac arrhythmias. Subsequent chapters describe individual diagnostic tests, such as ambulatory ECG recordings, exercise treadmill ECGs, and electrophysiologic studies, and their indications and limitations for the diagnosis and management of cardiac arrhythmias. Chapter 3, Antiarrhythmic Therapy, summarizes the principles of clinical pharmacology and the specific clinical pharmacology, side effects, and therapeutic uses of antiarrhythmic drugs that are currently available or under investigation. Chapter 7 summarizes current pacemaker terminology and discusses the advantages and disadvantages of dual chamber and antitachycardia pacing. Chapter 11 provides information on the various types of cardiac surgery for treatment of cardiac arrhythmias. Finally, a series of chapters describes current diagnosis and management of a variety of commonly encountered arrhythmias. Each chapter integrates the application of electrophysiologic testing and other diagnostic and therapeutic modalities as appropriate.

Most of the authors contributing to this text have been or are currently associated with the Cardiac Arrhythmia Study Unit at Stanford Medical Center. Our common experience, coupled with extensive editing, has minimized many of the problems that can occur in multi-authored textbooks and helps to provide a coherent approach to patient management. We have minimized the duplication of information in different chapters and attempted to avoid major gaps in subjects covered. Throughout the text, references are made to other chapters where pertinent additional information may be found. We have attempted to be certain that the information provided is current at the time of printing and that specified drug doses are accurate. However, the clinician is urged to check drug doses carefully with manufacturers' information or current medical literature prior to use.

It would be impossible to thank everyone who contributed to the publication of this book. However, several people deserve special recognition. I would like to thank Drs. William Clusin and Robert Kates, who provided input for Chapters 1 and 3, respectively. A special note of thanks is due to Dr. Jay Mason, who not only contributed several chapters, but whose ideas and knowledge over the years have influenced many of the other authors. I would also like to thank Richard Mixter and Susan Harrington of Addison-Wesley Publishing Company, whose efforts markedly improved the book's quality, and Glenda Rhodes, for her tireless secretarial support. Finally, I would like to thank my wife, Lynn, and my children, Brooke and Bryce, whose encouragement and understanding made this book possible.

Roger A. Winkle, M.D.

Contents

1 Cellular Basis of Cardiac Arrhythmias

Roger A. Winkle, M.D.

Associate Professor of Medicine
Stanford University School of Medicine
Stanford, California

ANATOMY OF THE CARDIAC CONDUCTION SYSTEM

The normal spread of excitation over the heart follows an organized and repetitive sequence (Figure 1-1). This permits the proper efficient and sequential contraction of atrial and ventricular muscle.

Sinus Node

The sinus node is situated at the anterolateral junction of the superior vena cava and the right atrium. It receives its blood supply from the sinus node artery, which is a branch of the right coronary artery in approximately 60% of patients and the left circumflex coronary artery in the remaining 40% of patients. Microscopic studies indicate that the sinus node is made up of P cells (pale staining with hematoxylin and eosin) and transitional (or T) cells. The P cells are the normal pacemaker cells of the sinus node. They have no contractile function and connect only to other P or T cells (Bigger, 1980). The T cells are present in greater numbers than the P cells and serve as a bridge between the P cells and working atrial muscle or specialized internodal tracts.

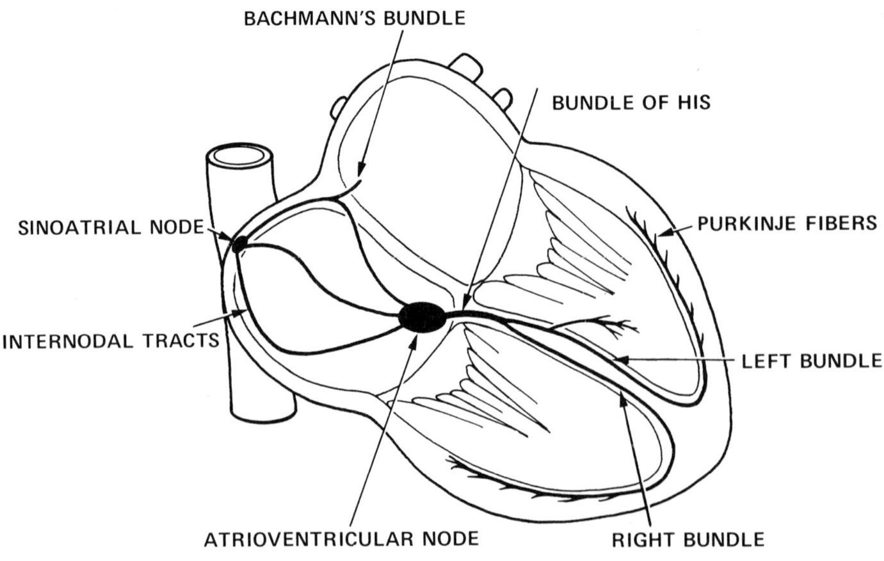

Figure 1-1 The anatomy of the cardiac conduction system.

Internodal and Interatrial Tracts

Some investigators believe that there are three anatomically discrete pathways containing Purkinje-like cells that connect the sinus node to the atrioventricular (AV) node (James, 1963; James and Sherf, 1971). These pathways are known as the anterior, middle, and posterior internodal tracts. Other researchers have argued that anatomically separate tracts connecting the nodes do not actually exist (Becker and Anderson, 1976). Studies have shown that these pathways of conduction from the sinoatrial (SA) node to the AV node are different from normal atrial muscle cells in that they remain functional at potassium concentrations that render working atrial muscle inactive (Holsinger, et al., 1968). The functional role of the internodal tracts during normal cardiac conduction remains unclear. The anterior internodal tract gives rise to Bachmann's bundle, which is the primary pathway for impulses to traverse from the right atrium to the left atrium.

The Atrioventricular Node

The atrioventricular node is a right atrial subendocardial structure that is situated just anterior to the ostium of the coronary sinus. It lies just above the septal leaflet of the tricuspid valve and wraps around the mitral valve annulus. The AV node has multiple inputs from the internodal tracts and atrial muscle fibers and receives its blood supply from the AV nodal artery, which courses from the crux of the heart (see Chapter 6). In approximately 90% of patients this is a branch of the right coronary artery; in the 10% of patients who have dominant left coronary artery systems the left circumflex gives off this branch. The cells of the AV node follow multiple directions and have multiple interconnections in the mid-portion but become more linear as they approach the exit that lies in the region of the His bundle. These AV nodal cells have been divided functionally into the proximal, or AN cells, the mid-portion, or N cells, and the distal, or NH cells (Janse, et al., 1976). Although the majority of conduction delay occurs in the AN portion of the AV node, Wenckebach block of impulses usually occurs in the N portion.

The His-Purkinje System

The bundle of His emerges from the distal end of the AV node and consists of a bundle of muscle fibers that penetrate the central fibrous body of the heart. The His bundle proceeds approximately 12-15 mm and reaches the muscular interventricular septum. This region receives its blood supply from both the left anterior and posterior descending coronary arteries via their septal branches. The His bundle divides into the right bundle branch, which courses along the right interventricular septum fairly directly to the right ventricular apex, and the left bundle branch, which divides into a number of not necessarily discrete (Massing and James, 1976) branches, including septal branches and groups that have been termed the anterior and posterior fascicles. These fascicles cause early activation of the anterior and posterior papillary muscle regions. The bundle branches and fascicles branch into the fine Purkinje fiber network on the endocardial surface of the right and left ventricles. These fibers penetrate a short distance into working muscle cells and activate the ventricular muscle cells. Because of their subendocardial position, these fibers may survive and remain functional following transmural myocardial infarction (Friedman, et al., 1973a; Friedman, et al., 1973b; Lazzara, et al., 1973).

CELLULAR ELECTROPHYSIOLOGY

Considerable knowledge has been amassed through the use of microelectrodes regarding the cellular basis of cardiac arrhythmias. These microelectrodes are small electrolyte-filled glass capillary tubes that are used to penetrate individual cells and record intracellular potentials. These recordings indicate that there is a negative intracellular resting membrane potential, which for Purkinje cells is approximately −90 millivolts. When a cardiac cell is disturbed by depolarization of other surrounding cells or external stimuli, its membrane may be sufficiently depolarized to reach a threshold potential. Once the threshold potential is reached an all-or-none action potential occurs. The cardiac action potential is displayed as a graph of intracellular potential measured by the microelectrode against time. The action potential in a given cell depolarizes nearby cells and, therefore, will propagate through cardiac tissue.

For Purkinje fibers the action potential has been divided into five distinct phases (Figure 1-2). Phase 0 is the initial, and usually rapid, depolarization of the membrane, which is often called the upstroke phase. Phase 1, often called the overshoot phase, is a brief period of early rapid repolarization. However, repolarization during phase 1 does not return the cell to the resting membrane potential. Phase 2 is the relatively prolonged plateau phase that often lasts for 100-200 milliseconds. Phase 3 is the period of late repolarization when the cell returns to its resting membrane potential, and phase 4 is the period of electrical diastole. There may be important differences in resting membrane potential and the morphology of the action potential, depending on the type of cardiac tissue studied (such as the SA node, AV node, or Purkinje fibers) (Figure 1-3), the presence of disease states, and changes in local membrane conditions caused by drugs, an electrolyte imbalance or hypoxia, or changes in the autonomic nervous system.

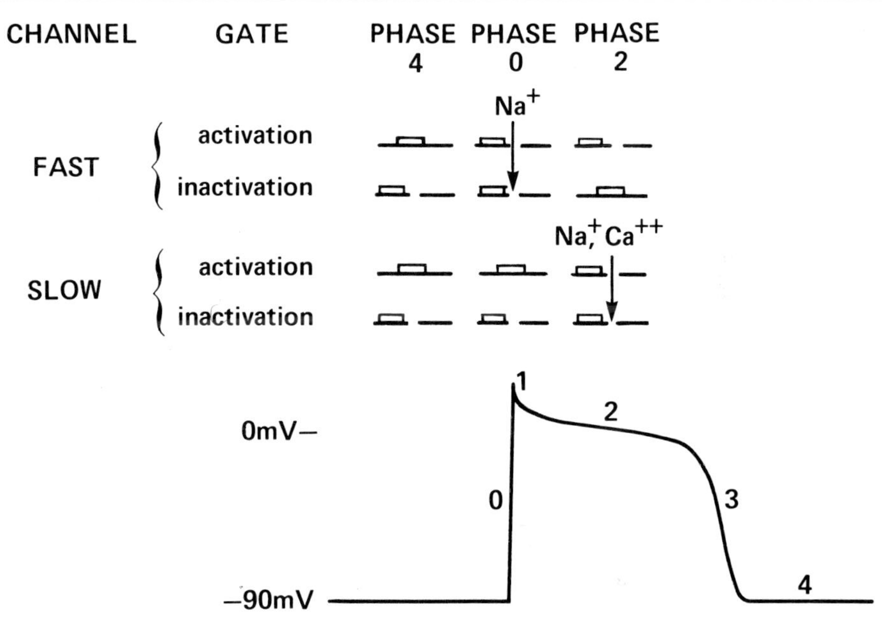

Figure 1-2 Characteristic action potential for Purkinje cells. During Phase 4 the resting diastolic intracellular potential is maintained at approximately −90 millivolts. During this phase the fast and slow activation gates are closed and the fast and slow inactivation gates are open. During Phase 0 (rapid depolarization phase) the fast sodium activation gates open and sodium rapidly enters the cell. This rapid upstroke usually lasts from 1 to 2 milliseconds. As the fast channel activation gate opens the fast inactivation gate begins to close. This closing of the fast inactivation gate ends Phase 0. Phase 1 is the period of early repolarization, which is slowed by the opening of the slow channel activation gates. During Phase 2 the fast inactivation gates remain closed; however, sodium and calcium enter the cell through the slow channels. During Phase 3, or late repolarization, the slow channels are inactivated, an outward potassium current is activated, and the cell returns to its resting diastolic membrane potential.

IONIC EVENTS

In the resting state the intracellular concentration of sodium is considerably lower than that of extracellular sodium, and for potassium the converse is true. The changes in potential recorded by microelectrodes are caused by ion fluxes across the cell membrane. These ion fluxes have been studied in great detail through voltage clamp experiments in which the transmembrane potential can be stepped to specified levels while the ionic composition of the perfusate is varied or specific ionic channel blocking agents are introduced. Normal Purkinje fibers from several species

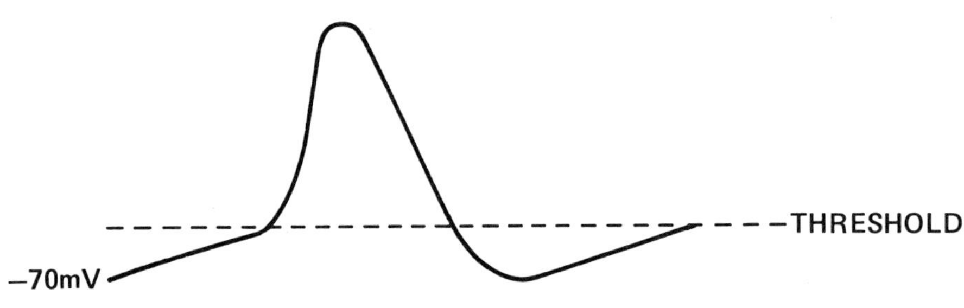

Figure 1-3 Intracellular action potential for a SA nodal cell. Note the differences between this action potential and that for Purkinje fibers shown in Figure 1-2. The maximum diastolic membrane potential is −70 millivolts, as opposed to −90 millivolts. There is a spontaneous Phase 4 depolarization, and the initial upstroke velocity here is considerably slower than in the Purkinje fiber. In SA nodal cells the Phase 0 upstroke is dependent on the slow calcium channel rather than the fast sodium channel.

have been the most extensively studied; recently, however, there has been considerable interest in studying SA nodal and AV nodal cells, as well as diseased Purkinje fibers and atrial and ventricular muscle.

Phase 0—Rapid Depolarization

When local membrane changes cause a sufficient increase in intracellular potential, an all-or-none depolarization of the cell occurs. In Purkinje fibers and healthy atrial and ventricular muscle sodium ions pass rapidly into the cell, flowing down an electrochemical gradient and causing the intracellular potential to rise rapidly to a positive value of approximately +20 to +30 millivolts. The rate of rise (often called Vmax) is related to the rapidity with which (and the total number of) sodium ions enter the cell. The ionic theory of excitation proposes that there are specific sodium channels with activation gates and inactivation gates (Hodgkin and Huxley, 1952). In the resting state the inactivation gates are open and the activation gates are closed (Figure 1-2). During depolarization the activation gates open, allowing a rapid inward flow of sodium ions. In healthy tissues this lasts approximately 1-2 milliseconds. Depolarization also initiates closure of the inactivation gates, which ultimately curtails the rapid sodium influx. The fast sodium channels may be blocked by tetrodotoxin.

Phase 1—Early Repolarization

Early repolarization begins when the sodium channel inactivation gates close. This results in an initial rapid return toward the resting membrane potential. However, at approximately 0 millivolts this rapid return slows markedly. This slowing of repolarization is caused by the opening of a second inward current channel, called the slow channel (Beeler and Reuter, 1970; Reuter, 1967). The slow channel is also sensitive to membrane voltage but differs from the fast channel in several respects. Both sodium *and* calcium ions enter the cardiac cell through the slow channel (Figure 1-2). The maximum ionic conductance of the slow channels is relatively small, which prevents them from mediating such rapid changes in membrane potential as do the fast channels. The slow channels are thought to undergo inactivation over a period 50 to 100 times longer than the 1-2 milliseconds required for fast channel inactivation. The slow channels may be blocked by lanthanum, manganese, or calcium influx-blocking drugs, such as D600 or verapamil (Zipes, 1976) (Table 1-1).

Table 1-1 Distinguishing features of the fast and slow currents.

Electrophysiologic property	Rapid current	Slow current
Activation and inactivation kinetics	Rapid	Slow
Dependent on extracellular ion concentration of:	Sodium	Calcium
Abolished by:	Tetrodotoxin	Manganese, cobalt, nickel, lanthanum, verapamil, D600
Threshold of activation	−60 to −70 mV	−30 to −40 mV
Resting membrane potential	−80 to −95 mV	−40 to −70 mV
Conduction velocity	0.5-3.0 m/s	0.01-0.1 m/s
Overshoot	+20 to +35 mV	0 to +15 mV
Rate of rise (dV/dt) of action potential upstroke	200-1000 V/s	1-10 V/s
Action potential amplitude	100-130 mV	35-75 mV
Response stimulus	All-or-none	Affected by characteristics of stimulus
Safety factor for conduction	High	Low
Recovery of excitability	Prompt, ends with repolarization	Delayed, outlasts full repolarization

Source: Zipes, D. P. 1976. Recent observations supporting the role of slow current in cardiac electrophysiology. In *The conduction system of the heart: structure, function, and clinical implications.* H. J. J. Wellens; K. I. Lie; and M. J. Janse, editors. Philadelphia: Lea & Febiger.

Phase 3—Late Repolarization

Late repolarization is probably caused by inactivation of the slow channels, as well as activation of an outward potassium current. During this phase the cell returns to the resting membrane potential.

Phase 4—Resting Membrane Potential

In the resting state the electrochemical gradient favors a slow influx of sodium ions and a corresponding loss of intracellular potassium. An active ATP-using sodium-potassium pump must be used to maintain the ionic asymmetries that give rise to the resting membrane potential.

Voltage Dependence of Depolarization

The previous discussion of depolarization assumes that a cell begins depolarization from a normal resting membrane potential of −90 millivolts. It has been demonstrated, however, that the ability of the fast and slow channels to open and close is significantly affected by the level of the resting membrane potential of the cell. The voltage range over which the fast channels normally activate is approximately −60 to −70 millivolts. If the resting membrane potential is in this range, the sodium conductance that is subsequently achievable is reduced because of partial closure of the inactivation gates. This results in a diminished rate of rise (Vmax) of depolarization, which translates into a slowing of conduction through the cardiac tissue (Purkinje fibers) from its normal value of approximately 2-4 m/s. Action potentials with slowed upstrokes caused by elevated membrane potentials are commonly referred to as *depressed fast responses* (Wit and Rosen, 1981a; Wit and Rosen, 1981b) (Figure 1-4).

At resting membrane potentials of approximately −50 millivolts or higher the inactivation gates of the fast sodium channel remain closed and a normal Purkinje cell is completely refractory and cannot be excited. Slow channel activation occurs over a voltage range of approximately −30 to −40 millivolts. While the normal resting membrane potential of Purkinje fibers and atrial and ventricular muscle is approximately −90 millivolts, the normal cells of the SA and AV nodes depend primarily on the slow channels for the upstroke of their action potentials, and have a resting membrane potential of only approximately −70 millivolts. When normal Purkinje fibers are treated with tetrodotoxin in the presence of high potassium concentrations and catecholamines, they also exhibit a slow channel response (Figure 1-4).

Automaticity

Working atrial and ventricular muscle cells have a flat phase 4. Thus, when the cell is in a resting state it will remain so until disturbed either by an

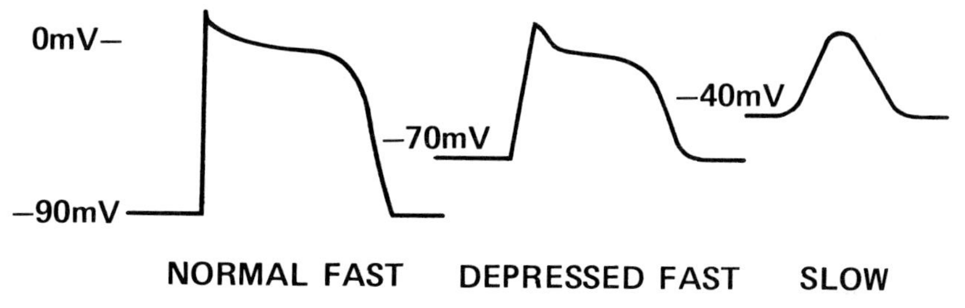

Figure 1-4 Voltage dependence of depolarization. The action potential on the left is typical for normal Purkinje fibers. If the resting membrane potential is increased to −70 millivolts (the center action potential), the rate of rise of the Phase 0 upstroke is significantly reduced. This is because of a partial inactivation of the fast sodium channel that diminishes the rapid entry of sodium into the cell. This is referred to as a depressed fast response. In the right-hand action potential the resting membrane potential is only −40 millivolts. This occurs in experimental preparations and in certain diseased Purkinje fibers. At this level of resting membrane potentials the fast sodium channels are completely inactivated and the upstroke of the action potential is dependent on the slow channel response.

external stimulus or by a response propagated from nearby cells. However, the P cells of the sinus node and certain cells of the atrium and AV nodal region, as well as normal Purkinje fibers, possess the property of automaticity. Automatic cells show a slow spontaneous depolarization during phase 4 (Figure 1-5), which is caused by a progressive decline in the selective permeability of the membrane to potassium ions. The permeability changes that mediate spontaneous depolarization in the normal sinus node and AV node and in some diseased tissues may also be significantly dependent on calcium ion fluxes because calcium channel blocking agents can alter automaticity in these cells; however, the exact role of calcium ions is imperfectly understood. When the intracellular potential of Purkinje fibers spontaneously increases to approximately −70 millivolts or when the sinus node and AV node intracellular potentials increase to approximately −40 millivolts, voltage-dependent sodium and calcium channels are activated, resulting in an action potential.

In the normal situation the sinus node discharge rate is faster than that of AV nodal junctional tissue or Purkinje fibers. Thus, the sinus node is the dominant pacemaker, and each of the subsidiary pacemakers are reset to their maximum negative resting membrane potential each time they are depolarized as a result of a propagated action potential.

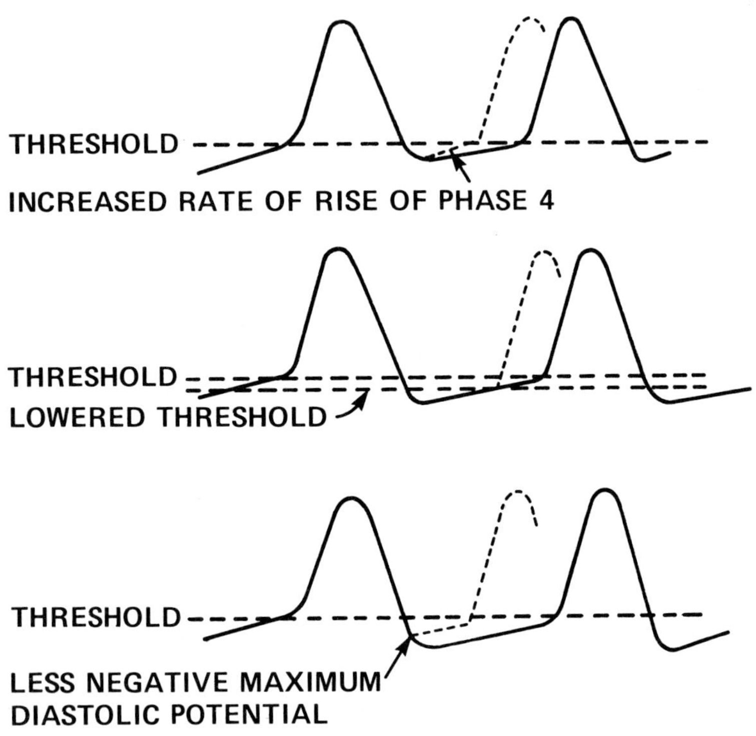

Figure 1-5 This figure shows the action potential for a typical SA nodal cell demonstrating spontaneous automaticity. Note that during Phase 4 a spontaneous depolarization occurs that reaches the threshold potential and results in another action potential. In the top panel the dotted lines show an increased rate of rise of Phase 4 depolarization that causes the cell to reach threshold earlier, which results in an earlier-occurring action potential (corresponding to an increase in rate). The middle panel illustrates that an increase in rate can also be accomplished if the threshold potential is lowered so that Phase 4 depolarization reaches threshold earlier. The bottom panel demonstrates that an increase in rate may also occur if a cell achieves a less negative maximum diastolic potential.

MECHANISM OF ARRHYTHMIAS

Abnormalities of Automaticity

Factors influencing phase 4 automaticity Changes in the maximum diastolic membrane potential, the threshold potential, or the rate of spontaneous diastolic depolarization will cause a change in the rate of discharge of a cell exhibiting automaticity (Figure 1-5). Normally automatic cardiac tissue, such as the sinus node, responds to a variety of autonomic and external influences. Sympathetic stimulation or infusion of systemic catecholamines will increase the rate of discharge of most pacemaker cells, whereas vagal stimulation via the parasympathetic nerves will slow the rate of discharge of most supraventricular pacemaker cells. Factors such as catecholamines, stretch, and hypokalemia can all depolarize the cell membrane and thus enhance automaticity. Excessive slowing of the sinus discharge rate may result in escape of a low or subsidiary pacemaker. Typical clinical examples of this are sinus node disease or excessive vagal tone. Likewise, enhancement of automaticity of lower pacemakers to a rate exceeding that of the sinus node discharge will result in emergence of ectopic pacemakers. These may occur either as isolated individual premature beats or as a sustained automatic tachycardia.

In a variety of disease states myocardial fibers, which normally do not exhibit diastolic depolarization, may acquire automaticity. During ischemic states the resting potential of ventricular muscle cells may decrease from a normal value of about −90 millivolts to approximately −60 millivolts. This may cause spontaneous diastolic depolarization, leading to abnormal slow channel action potentials. These responses may have exceedingly long refractory periods that markedly outlast action potential duration.

Triggered automaticity *Early after-depolarization* During conditions of low potassium levels, catecholamine stimulation, digitalis intoxication, hypoxia, and stretch an abnormal secondary depolarization of the membrane can occur at the end of the plateau phase (phase 2) or during early phase 3 repolarization (Cranefield, 1977) (Figure 1-6). This abnormal depolarization may lead to a second action potential, which, if propagated, may result in a premature beat. These second action potentials are dependent on the slow calcium channel responses because at these higher membrane potentials the fast sodium channels remain inactive. The second slow channel action potential may also be followed by another early after-depolarization, which may also reach threshold. If the sequence continues to repeat itself a self-sustaining tachycardia may occur.

Delayed after-depolarizations In many of the same experimental situations where early after-depolarizations can occur (such as digitalis toxicity and excessive catecholamine stimulation) an unexpected increase in membrane potential may occur after the membrane reaches its normal maximum diastolic potential (early in phase 4) (Ferrier, et al., 1973) (Figure 1-7). These increases in membrane potential are of low amplitude, but they increase in amplitude following premature beats, during catecholamine stimulation, or during stimulation at faster rates. If a beat is sufficiently premature or if the pacing rate is sufficiently rapid, these late afterpotentials may reach threshold and initiate a single premature beat or a sustained tachycardia (Wit and Cranefield, 1977) in a manner

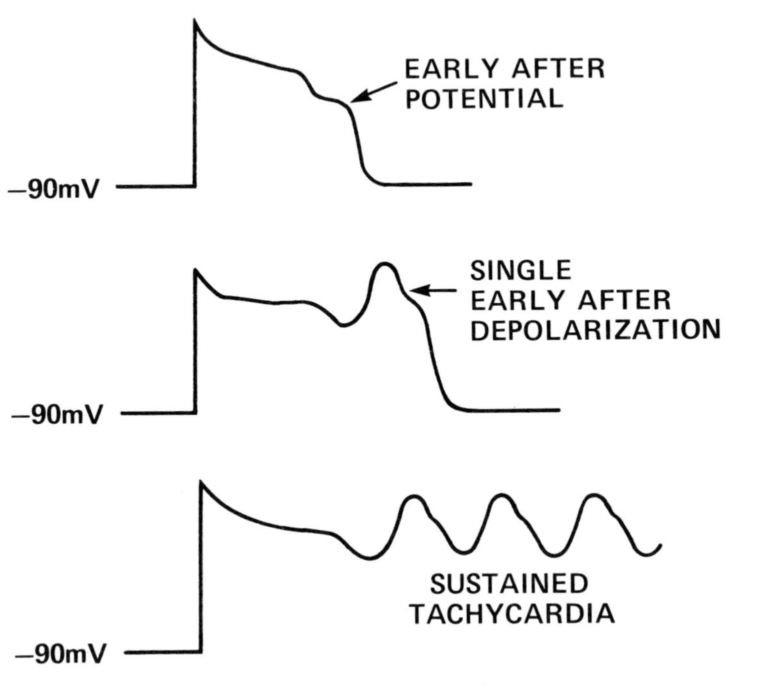

Figure 1-6 Arrhythmias caused by early afterpotentials. The top panel illustrates an early afterpotential that can occur at the end of Phase 2 or early in Phase 3 in situations of catecholamine stimulation, digitalis intoxication, hypoxia, and other abnormal conditions. In the middle panel the early after-depolarization has reached the threshold for activation of the slow channels, and a second depolarization occurs. This would correspond clinically to the occurrence of a single premature beat. Note that this second action potential may also have an early afterpotential. The bottom panel shows that this second early afterpotential may also reach threshold and result in a third depolarization. The process may become self-sustaining and result in a sustained tachycardia.

analogous to those caused by early after-depolarizations (Figure 1-7). These late afterpotentials may also be dependent on slow channel calcium currents (Ferrier and Moe, 1973), and verapamil decreases their amplitude or abolishes them altogether (Wit and Cranefield, 1976). Although some controversy still exists as to their clinical significance (Rosen, et al., 1980), one would expect arrhythmias caused by after-depolarization to be initiated by either a single premature beat or an increase in the pacing rate (Wyndham, et al., 1980). As opposed to the typical situation in a reentrant arrhythmia, where the shorter the coupling interval of the initiating beat the longer the initial return cycle of the sustained

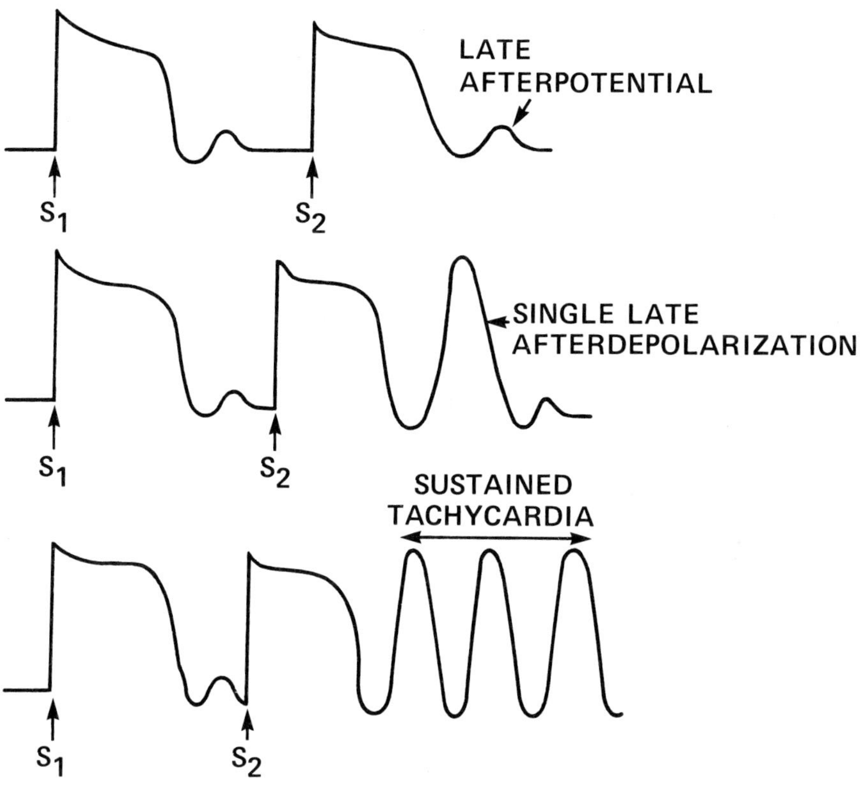

Figure 1-7 Arrhythmias caused by late afterpotentials. Many of the same experimental situations that result in early afterpotentials can also cause late afterpotentials. These afterpotentials reflect unexpected increases in the intracellular potential that occur after the cell has achieved a maximum diastolic potential. The top panel shows a late afterpotential. If the second normal action potential occurs earlier, corresponding to a shortening of the S1-S2 coupling interval, the late afterpotential will increase in amplitude and may reach threshold, which results in a single extra depolarization, as shown in the middle panel. Clinically, this would correspond to a single extra beat. Note that this late after-depolarization may also be followed by a small afterpotential. If this afterpotential also reaches threshold, a third depolarization may occur, and in a manner analogous to Figure 1-6 a sustained tachycardia may result.

tachycardia, in triggered automaticity the earlier the initiating premature beat the shorter the first cycle of the tachycardia should be (Wellens, et al., 1981).

Arrhythmias Caused by Reentry

Reentry occurs when an action potential that has traversed a region of cardiac tissue is able to reexcite the same region by propagating over a circuit (Mines, 1913; Schmitt and Erlanger, 1928). For reentry to occur an appropriate anatomic or functional tissue loop must exist. As long as the wavelength (the conduction velocity times the refractory period) of the propagated signal is shorter than the length of the pathway, the action potential will continue to propagate. In reality this loop may involve many different tissues and structures with multiple refractory periods and conduction velocities. However, as long as the propagating wavefront does not encounter refractory tissue the reentry will persist.

For reentry to begin, a block must exist in one portion of the loop and conduction must be slow enough through the rest of the loop to permit recovery of the block area, thus fulfilling the criterion of unidirectional block (Figure 1-8). In normal sinus node or atrial ventricular nodal tissue conduction is slow enough to allow reentry in nondiseased tissue. To achieve critical block and conduction delay in these structures a premature beat is usually required to initiate reentry because premature beats are more likely to encounter refractory tissue and are propagated with a much slower conduction velocity. It is more difficult for reentry to occur in healthy atrial and ventricular muscle. For ventricular muscle the refractory period is approximately 250 milliseconds and the conduction velocity is at least 2 m/s. To sustain reentry the circuit would have to be at least 0.5 m long. A circuit of this length obviously could not exist in a human ventricle.

For reentry to occur in human ventricular muscle a significant shortening of the refractory period or a decrease in the conduction velocity must occur. If cells are stimulated late in the repolarization phase (phase 3), before there has been a complete return to the resting potential, some of the fast sodium channels will be inactivated, thus reducing peak sodium conductance during the upstroke. The result is a marked decrease in Vmax and a slowing of conduction. Cardiac disease may reduce the resting membrane potential, resulting in depressed fast responses that may also be conducted extremely slowly. In the extreme state sufficient reduction of the resting membrane potential may occur to completely inactivate the sodium channels, allowing only slow channel responses to develop and propagate (Cranefield, et al., 1972). Premature beats occurring in diseased tissues may result in conduction slow enough to permit reentry in areas as small as 0.5-1 cm (Cranefield, et al., 1971).

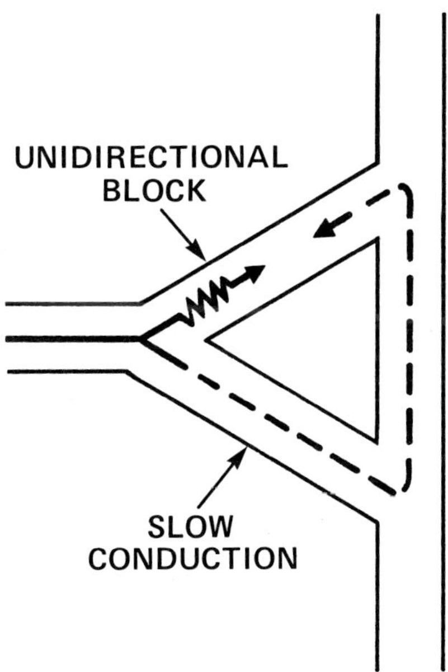

Figure 1-8 The classical model of reentry. Note that for reentry to occur there must be a functional or anatomic loop. A conducted impulse must be blocked in one limb of this loop and be conducted slowly through the remaining portion of the loop. If conduction is slow enough, the blocked area may have recovered sufficiently to allow retrograde conduction across the area of unidirectional block. If this occurs, the conditions of reentry have been satisfied and either single extra beats or sustained tachycardias may result.

In diseased hearts a variety of anatomic and functional situations may exist in which areas of conduction block and slowed conduction may coexist. If an impulse encounters such an area, it may be delayed until the surrounding tissue has become responsive and may emerge as a single premature beat (Wit, et al., 1972a; Wit, et al., 1972b). A sustained tachycardia may result if the reentry loop continues to be completed by the premature beat. If the area of reentry is small enough, it may even appear to be a localized focus, and the remainder of the myocardium may be activated from this small reentry circuit. Large reentry circuits may occur, utilizing anatomic structures or barriers such as the vena cavae (atrial flutter), an accessory pathway (AV reciprocating tachycardia), or an aneurysm (ventricular tachycardia in a patient with coronary heart disease) (Mason, et al., 1981) (Figure 1-9).

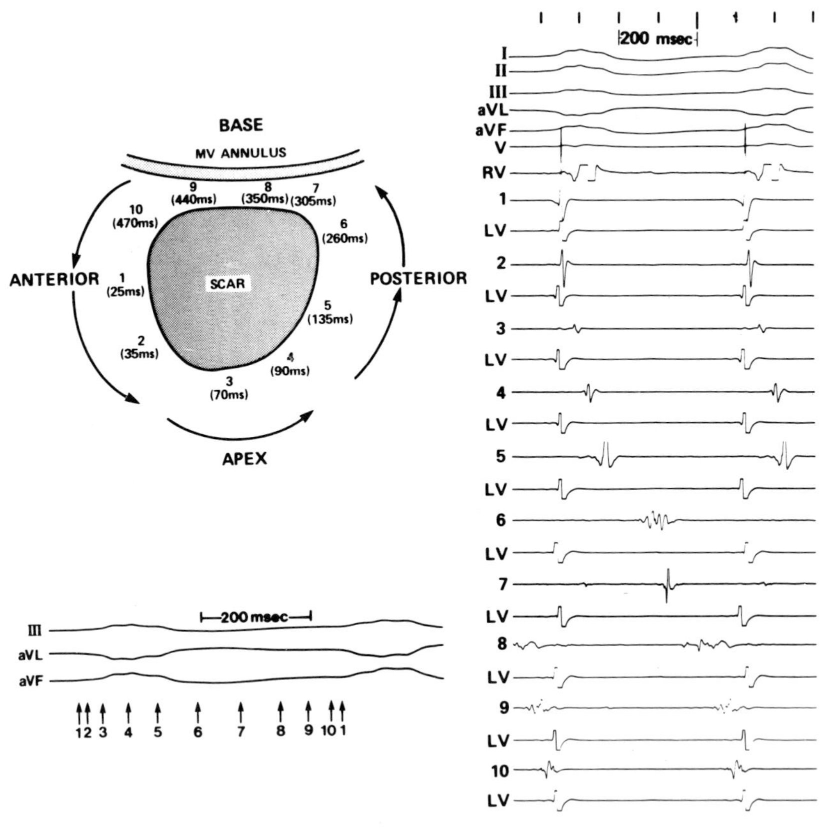

Figure 1-9 Reentrant ventricular tachycardia utilizing a macroreentry circuit around a ventricular aneurysm. This figure shows the intraoperative activation sequence mapped from a patient with recurrent sustained ventricular tachycardia. The diagram on the left shows the position of the posterolateral aneurysm (stippled area) in proximity to the mitral valve annulus. The positions of the 10 electrical recording sites around the scar are numbered in reference to the electrical tracings shown on the right. The time of activation after the onset of the QRS complex is indicated for each site, and the position during the cardiac cycle of each site's timing is shown below the diagram. The cycle length of tachycardia was approximately 480 milliseconds. In the recording on the right there are six surface ECG leads, as well as right and left ventricular electrograms and moving probe electrograms for sites 1 through 10 that correspond to the sites labelled on the left-hand diagrams. Discrete electrical activity at these 10 sites effectively spans the cardiac cycle. In this case the arrhythmia was caused by macroreentry with circus movement around the scar. (*Source:* Mason, J. W.; Stinson, E. B.; Winkle, R. A., et al. 1981. Mechanisms of ventricular tachycardia: wide complex ignorance. *Am. Heart J.* 102:1083-1087.)

REFERENCES

Becker, A. E.; and Anderson, R. H. 1976. Morphology of the human atrioventricular junctional area. In *The conduction system of the heart: structure, function, and clinical implications.* H. J. J. Wellens; K. I. Lie; and M. J. Janse, editors. Philadelphia: Lea & Febiger.

Beeler, G. W., Jr.; and Reuter, H. 1970. Membrane calcium current in ventricular myocardial fibers. *J. Physiol.* 207:191-209.

Bigger, J. T., Jr. 1980. Anatomical considerations. In *Heart disease: a textbook of cardiovascular medicine.* E. Braunwald, editor. Philadelphia: W. B. Saunders Co. pp. 631.

Cranefield, P. F. 1977. Action potentials, afterpotentials, and arrhythmias. *Circ. Res.* 41:415-423.

Cranefield, P. F.; Klein, H. O.; and Hoffman, B. F. 1971. Conduction of the cardiac impulse. I. Delay, block, and one-way block in depressed Purkinje fibers. *Circ. Res.* 28:199-219.

Cranefield, P. F.; Wit, A. L.; and Hoffman, B. F. 1972. Conduction of the cardiac impulse: III. Characteristics of very slow conduction. *J. Gen. Physiol.* 59:227-246.

Ferrier, G. R.; and Moe, G. K. 1973. Effect of calcium on acetylstrophanthidin-induced transient depolarizations in canine Purkinje tissue. *Circ. Res.* 33:508-515.

Ferrier, G. R.; Saunders, J. H.; and Mendez, C. 1973. A cellular mechanism for the generation of ventricular arrhythmias by acetylstrophanthidin. *Circ. Res.* 32:600-609.

Friedman, P. L.; Stewart, J. R.; Fenoglio, J. J., Jr., et al. 1973a. Survival of subendocardial Purkinje fibers after extensive myocardial infarction in dogs. *Circ. Res.* 33:597-611.

Friedman, P. L.; Stewart, J. R.; and Wit, A. L. 1973b. Spontaneous and induced cardiac arrhythmias in subendocardial Purkinje fibers surviving extensive myocardial infarction in dogs. *Circ. Res.* 33:612-626.

Hodgkin, A. L.; and Huxley, A. F. 1952. A quantitative description of membrane current and its application to conduction and excitation in nerve. *J. Physiol.* 117:500-544.

Holsinger, J. W., Jr.; Wallace, A. G.; and Sealy, W. C. 1968. The identification and surgical significance of the atrial internodal conduction tracts. *Ann. Surg.* 167:447-453.

James, T. N. 1963. The connecting pathways between the sinus node and the A-V node and between the right and the left atrium in the human heart. *Am. Heart J.* 66:498-508.

James, T. N.; and Sherf, L. 1971. Specialized tissues and preferential conduction in the atria of the heart. *Am. J. Cardiol.* 28:414-427.

Janse, M. J.; Van Capelle, F. J. L.; Anderson, R. H., et al. 1976. Electrophysiology and structure of the atrioventricular node of the isolated rabbit heart. In *The conduction system of the heart: structure, function, and clinical implications.* H. J. J. Wellens; K. I. Lie; and M. J. Janse, editors. Philadelphia: Lea & Febiger.

Lazzara, R.; El-Sherif, N.; and Scherlag, B. J. 1973. Electrophysiological properties of canine Purkinje cells in one-day-old myocardial infarction. *Circ. Res.* 33:722-734.

Mason, J. W.; Stinson, E. B.; Winkle, R. A., et al. 1981. Mechanisms of ventricular tachycardia: wide complex ignorance. *Am. Heart J.* 102: 1083-1087.

Massing, G. K.; and James, T. N. 1976. Anatomical configuration of the His bundle and bundle branches in the human heart. *Circulation* 53:609-621.

Mines, G. R. 1913. On dynamic equilibrium in the heart. *J. Physiol.* 46: 349-383.

Reuter, H. 1967. The dependence of slow inward current in Purkinje fibers on the extracellular calcium-concentration. *J. Physiol.* 192:479-492.

Rosen, M. R.; Fisch, C.; Hoffman, B. F., et al. 1980. Can accelerated atrioventricular junctional escape rhythms be explained by delayed afterdepolarizations? *Am. J. Cardiol.* 45:1272-1284.

Schmitt, F. O.; and Erlanger, J. 1928. Directional differences in the conduction of the impulse through heart muscle and their possible relation to extrasystolic and fibrillary contractions. *Am. J. Physiol.* 87:326-347.

Wellens, H. J. J.; Brugada, P.; Vanagt, E. J. D. M., et al. 1981. New studies with triggered automaticity. In *Cardiac arrhythmias: a decade of progress.* D. C. Harrison, editor. Boston: G. K. Hall Medical Publishers.

Wit, A. L.; and Cranefield, P. F. 1976. Triggered activity in cardiac muscle fibers of the simian mitral valve. *Circ. Res.* 38:85-98.

Wit, A. L.; and Cranefield, P. F. 1977. Triggered and automatic activity in the canine coronary sinus. *Circ. Res.* 41:435-445.

Wit, A. L.; Hoffman, B. F.; and Cranefield, P. F. 1972a. Slow conduction and reentry in the ventricular conducting system. I. Return extrasystole in canine Purkinje fibers. *Circ. Res.* 30:1-10.

Wit, A. L.; Cranefield, P. F.; and Hoffman, B. F. 1972b. Slow conduction and reentry in the ventricular conducting system. II. Single and sustained circus movement in networks of canine and bovine Purkinje fibers. *Circ. Res.* 30:11-22.

Wit, A. L.; and Rosen, M. R. 1981a. Cellular electrophysiology of cardiac arrhythmias. Part I. Arrhythmias caused by abnormal impulse generation. *Mod. Concepts Cardiovasc. Dis.* 50:1-6.

Wit, A. L.; and Rosen, M. R. 1981b. Cellular electrophysiology of cardiac arrhythmias. Part II. Arrhythmias caused by abnormal impulse conduction. *Mod. Concepts Cardiovasc. Dis.* 50:7-12.

Wyndham, C. R. C.; Arnsdorf, M. F.; Levitsky, S., et al. 1980. Successful surgical excision of focal paroxysmal atrial tachycardia: observations in vivo and in vitro. *Circulation* 62:1365-1372.

Zipes, D. P. 1976. Recent observations supporting the role of slow current in cardiac electrophysiology. In *The conduction system of the heart: structure, function, and clinical implications.* H. J. J. Wellens; K. I. Lie; and M. J. Janse, editors. Philadelphia: Lea & Febiger.

2 Intracardiac Electrophysiologic Studies: Techniques and Indications

Jay W. Mason, M.D.

Chief, Cardiology Division
University of Utah Medical Center
Salt Lake City, Utah

This chapter is designed to introduce the reader to the concepts behind and the methods of performing cardiac electrophysiologic studies and to establish a set of indications for these studies. Direct recordings of electrical activity arising from the bundle of His were obtained in isolated animal hearts in 1958 (Alanis, et al., 1958) and in intact animals using catheters in 1968 (Scherlag, et al., 1968). The catheter technique was first used in humans in 1969 (Scherlag, et al., 1969); serendipitously, however, catheter-recorded His bundle potentials in humans had been unwittingly illustrated in the literature as early as 1950 (Kossman, et al., 1950). Since these initial His bundle recordings in man, recording and pacing techniques have undergone tremendous developments. The result of all these refinements is that the original purpose for performing an electrophysiologic study, measuring the HV interval, has become an infrequent primary indication. Physicians unfamiliar with the technique of intracardiac electrophysiologic studies are often bewildered by the procedures and electronics involved. In fact, the techniques are simple and straightforward, and, conceptually, the electronics are far from sophisticated.

INTRACARDIAC ELECTROPHYSIOLOGIC STUDY TECHNIQUES

Electronics and Recording Methods

Electrical signals recorded from bipolar platinum electrodes with 1 cm interpolar spacing vary from less than 100 microvolts (a low amplitude His bundle potential) to greater han 20 millivolts (the ventricular myocardium). The principal frequencies of the majority of these signals lie between 5 and 1000 Hz. Amplification and filtration are necessary to display and record these signals for diagnostic purposes. The signals of larger amplitude, if amplified to a sufficient size, often require no filtration. The smaller signals, such as the His bundle potential, do require filtration to be detected. The majority of the frequencies produced by depolarization of the His bundle lie between 50 and 200 Hz. Fortunately, most cardiac electrical activity occurring concomitantly with the His bundle depolarization, and of sufficient amplitude to contaminate the His bundle recording, is composed of frequencies well below 50 and above 200 Hz. Thus, a clear His bundle deflection can usually be reliably obtained, after proper catheter positioning, by filtering out signals with frequencies below 30-40 Hz and above 500 Hz. Figure 2-1 illustrates three different systems for amplifying and conditioning electrical signals for intracardiac electrophysiologic studies. Note that each amplifier system has adjustments for gain or amplification of the signal and for upper and lower filter frequency cutoffs.

Intracardiac electrical signals are usually obtained with multipolar electrode catheters. Although virtually any type of electrode catheter

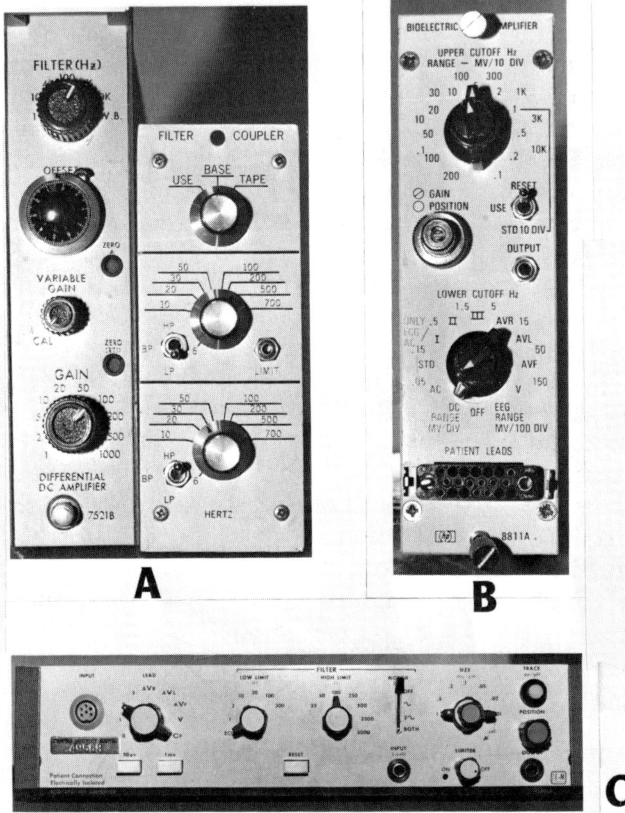

Figure 2-1 Three systems for electronic amplification and filtration of intracardiac electrical signals. In panel A the amplifying component on the left and the filtering component on the right are physically separated. The component on the left is used to adjust the amplification of the signal (gain and variable gain) and to position it on the recording paper (offset). An upper filter cutoff is also included. The component on the right provides continuous filtering capabilities between 10 and 700 Hz. The adjustment at the bottom is used to set the lower limit of filtration. The upper adjustment sets the upper filtration limit. In this instance electrical signals with frequencies below 30 and above 500 Hz will be filtered out of the recorded signals. Panel B shows an amplifier from another recording system. Both amplification and filtration components are included in the single unit. This amplifier can be used both for ECG and for intracardiac electrogram recordings. The amplifier includes upper and lower filter settings and gain and position settings. Panel C shows a third amplifier system. This amplifier is also capable of ECG or intracardiac recordings. It provides step amplification settings and upper and lower filter settings. A notch filter is also included for specific rejection of 60 and 180 cycle noise. The systems in panels A and C also have clipping circuitry to limit the size of especially large signals. This capability is especially useful when high gains are required to obtain recordable His bundle potentials. The clipping circuits can be used to cut the tops and bottoms off of the much larger atrial and ventricular signals so that those signals do not overlap paper recordings from other channels.

can be custom-made, the ones that are commonly available have from two to eight platinum electrodes with 0.5-1 cm interpolar spacing. These electrode catheters vary in diameter from 4 French (the thickness of a pencil lead) to 8 French (slightly smaller than the thickness of intravenous delivery tubing). A 6 French quadripolar electrode catheter is shown in Figure 2-2. Note that it has four pins at its proximal end for connection to recording and stimulating apparatus.

From one to six of these electrode catheters are used in electrophysiologic studies, depending on the information sought. Catheters are usually placed percutaneously by the Seldinger technique but may also be inserted by standard cutdown into peripheral veins or arteries for passage to a variety of intracardiac positions. The femoral, basilic, internal jugular, and subclavian veins and the femoral and brachial arteries are the vascular structures that are most commonly used for catheter insertion. Figure 2-3 shows the typical catheter positioning for electrophysiologic study of a patient with Wolff-Parkinson-White syndrome. The three most commonly used catheter positions for intracardiac electrophysiologic studies are the high right atrium, the His bundle position, and the right

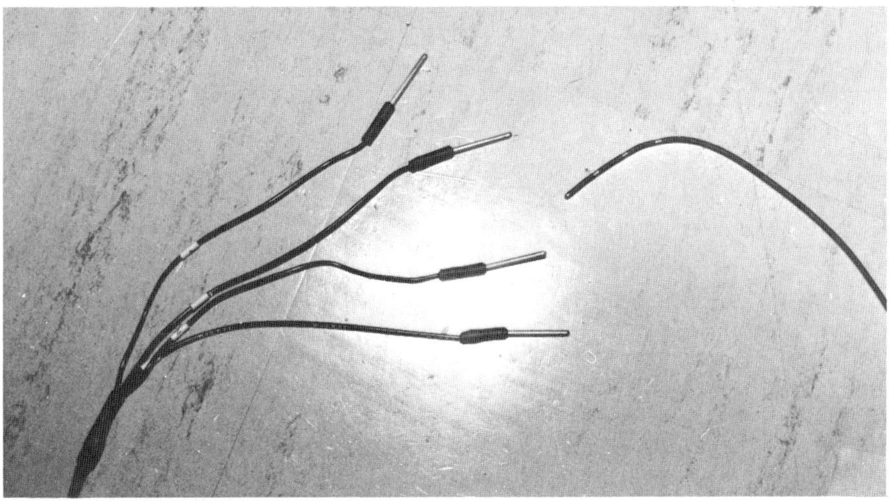

Figure 2-2 The proximal and distal ends of a 6 French quadripolar electrode catheter. Individual insulated wires from the four platinum poles on the tip of the catheter terminate in the four connectors on the proximal end. These connectors can record unipolar signals from any of the four poles or bipolar signals from any pair of poles. Unipolar or bipolar stimulation can also be performed through any single or pair of electrodes.

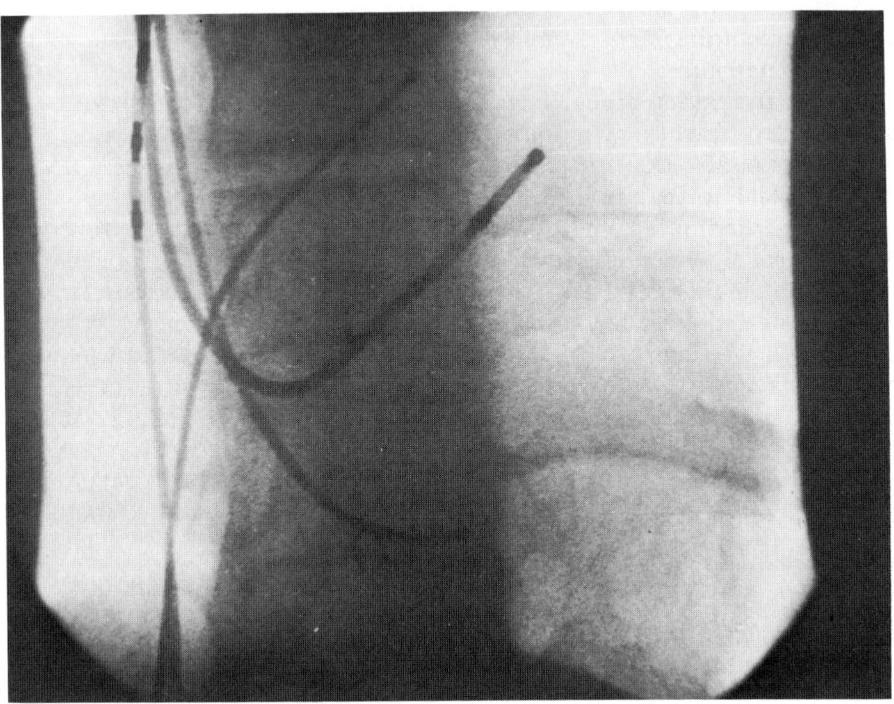

Figure 2-3 Four quadripolar electrode catheters positioned in the heart. Two catheters are directed from a femoral vein through the inferior vena cava; one of these catheters is positioned in the high right atrium, and the other is just across the tricuspid valve in the His bundle recording position. Two other catheters enter the heart from the superior vena cava. The lowest of these two catheters was introduced through the right basilic vein and advanced to the right ventricle. The catheter above it was inserted through the right internal jugular to the coronary sinus. These catheter positions are typical for the majority of recordings in patients with the Wolff-Parkinson-White syndrome and supraventricular tachyarrhythmias of other etiologies.

ventricular apex. Atrial recording and stimulating is usually done from the high right atrium in the region of the sinus node, which is identified fluoroscopically as the junction of the inferior vena cava and the right atrium. The right ventricular apex is usually chosen for ventricular stimulation and recording because it provides stable catheter positioning. The His bundle electrogram is obtained by passing the recording electrodes just across the tricuspid valve. The catheter should be in the most cephalad aspect of the tricuspid annulus, and the recording electrodes must be rotated to a septal position. With experience and the availability of a variety of catheter types, a His bundle potential can be obtained from 99% of patients without congenital heart defects, and stable His bundle potential recording through the entire electrophysiologic study is possible in 95% of patients.

After the catheters have been positioned the electrode pins are inserted into a junction box that delivers the electrical signals to the amplification-filtration system. A variety of junction boxes are commercially available or can be homemade easily (Figure 2-4). After the electrical signals have been properly conditioned they are usually displayed stimultaneously with several surface electrocardiographic leads on a cathode-ray oscilloscope. Most recorders today use light galvanometer or ink-jet systems. Other recording systems, such as electrostatic printing or digitization of the analog signals for subsequent ink and paper printout, have recently been developed or improved because of the high cost of photographic recording paper. The majority of electrophysiologic recordings are made at 50, 100, and 200 mm/s paper speeds. For most clinical studies speeds of 100 mm/s are adequate and accurate to within 5 milliseconds as long as a precise time signal is recorded along with the

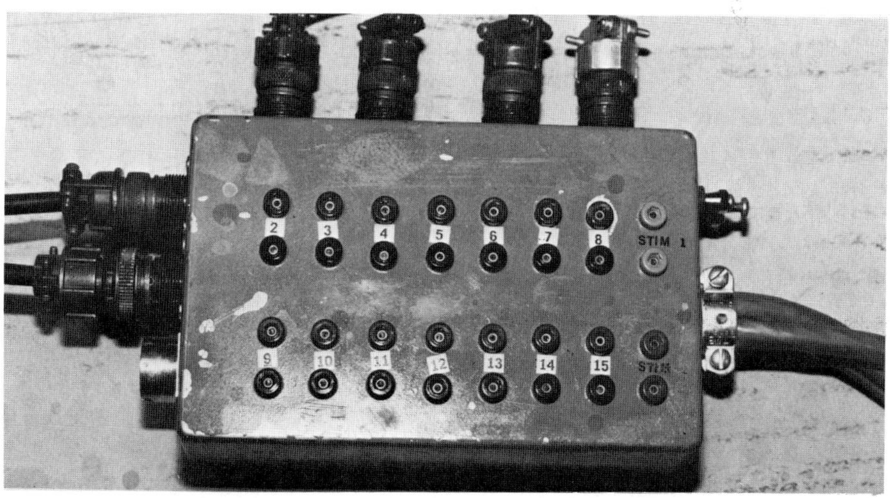

Figure 2-4 A homemade junction box that receives six ECG leads, a pressure signal, and 14 intracardiac electrograms. In addition, two stimulation outputs are included on the right-hand side of the junction box. All connections to the patient are made at this single junction box and lead to the recording and stimulating devices via a single cable (on the right side of the box). Switching capabilities, to direct recordings or stimuli to different electrodes, can be incorporated into junction boxes of this sort but leakage currents are increased.

electrophysiologic data. For research studies and activation sequence mapping studies, where differences of a few milliseconds are important, recording speeds of 200 mm/s or faster are employed.

Patients undergoing electrophysiologic study are asked to refrain from eating solid food for 6 hours prior to the procedure. Only mild sedation is given because the cardiac autonomic nervous system is affected by heavy sedation, which may significantly influence the findings. During electrophysiologic study heparin is utilized when more than two catheters are passed through the inferior vena cava or when the left ventricle is entered.

Cardiac Stimulation and Electrophysiologic Study Techniques

In most laboratories cardiac stimulation is achieved using bipolar pacing with square wave stimuli lasting 1-3 milliseconds. Complete electrophysiologic investigations require programmable stimulators capable of sensing spontaneous and paced rhythm. The stimulator should be capable of delivering during spontaneous or paced rhythm one, two, or three successive extrastimuli followed by a pause before straight pacing is resumed. The stimulator should provide the capacity to program the timing of the extrastimuli with perfect accuracy by 5 milliseconds or smaller time steps. The stimuli should be delivered through optical isolators to protect the patient from the wall current that is used to run the stimulator. Figures 2-5A and 2-5B show two of the many stimulators available for programmed cardiac stimulation.

Evaluation of the sinus node The typical electrophysiologic study in our laboratory proceeds as follows:

1. Baseline recordings.
2. Sinus node recovery time determinations.
3. Rapid atrial pacing for Wenckebach cycle length determination.
4. Programmed atrial extrastimulation to measure conduction system refractory periods.
5. Rapid ventricular pacing to evaluate V-A conduction and block.

Figures 2-5A and 2-5B Two programmable cardiac stimulators. The stimulator in Figure 2-5A has a control module on top that regulates the sequence of firing of the individual pulse modules below it. Each pulse module can be set to deliver basic drive stimuli or appropriately timed early stimuli. Two optically isolated stimulus sources at the bottom of the stimulator deliver the programmed pulses.

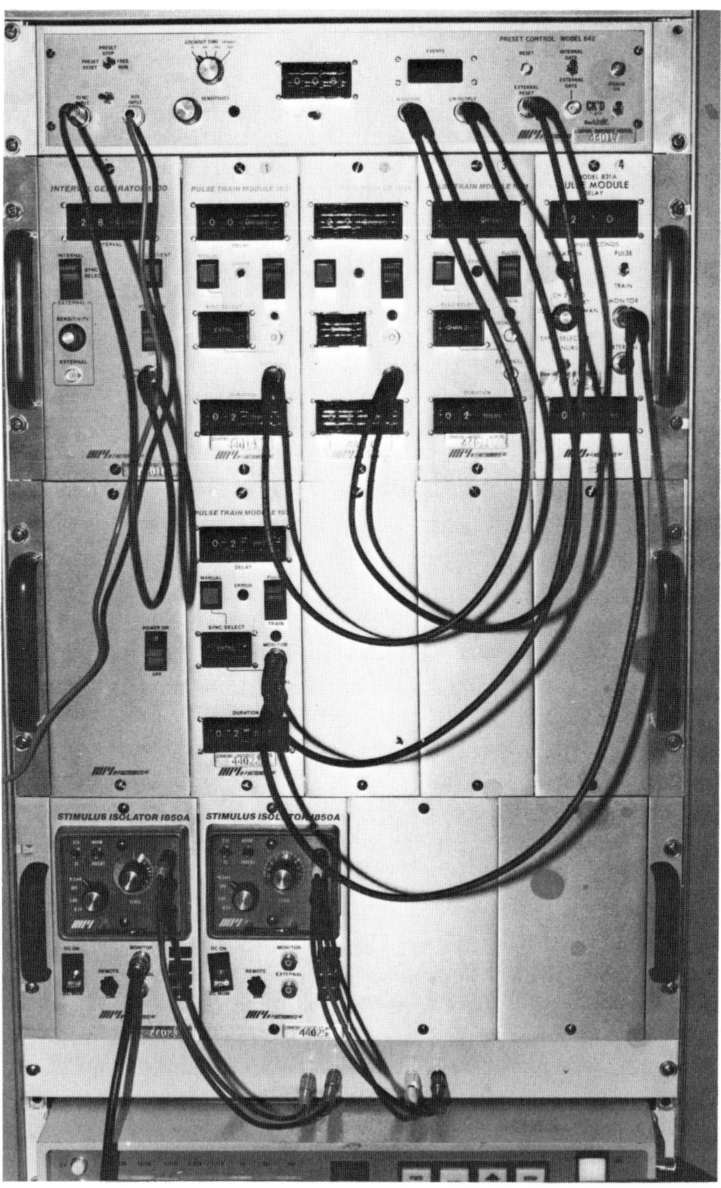

The stimulator in Figure 2-5B functions in a similar manner. The left-hand side of the stimulator is used to control the overall stimulus program. The columns of dials labeled S_1, S_2, and S_3 are used to adjust the intervals for basic pacing and premature stimuli. Modification of the duration and amplitude of the stimuli is achieved with the controls on the right side of the stimulator.

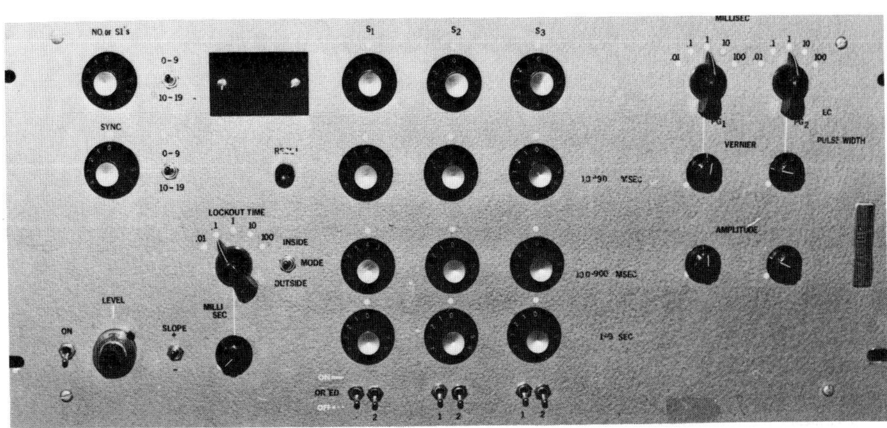

6. Programmed ventricular stimulation to determine V-A and ventricular refractory periods.
7. Atrial or ventricular arrhythmia induction, manipulation, and termination.
8. Atrial or ventricular endocardial mapping.
9. Drug interventions.
10. Repeat of 1-9 as indicated.

After the appropriate catheters are positioned, baseline recordings, including the PR, QRS, QT, PA, AH, HV, and RR intervals (Figure 2-6) and the blood pressure, are obtained. Sinus node recovery times are then determined. The sinus node recovery time is defined as the time required for the sinus node to form an impulse after a period of overdrive atrial pacing. The sinus node recovery time is measured from the last stimulated atrial complex to the first spontaneous atrial beat. In those cases where the first recovery beat is a nonsinus escape beat (Figure 2-6) the actual sinus node recovery time may be underestimated if atrial capture is produced by the escape beat. In evaluating sinus node recovery, it is wise to assess at least the first five cycles after cessation of pacing because any one of them may be longer than the initial or primary pause. It is also essential to drive the atrium at a variety of cycle lengths between 80 and 160 beats/min. Fifteen seconds may be an adequate duration of overdrive pacing, but we commonly pace the atrium for a full minute at each cycle length.

The sinus node recovery time can be expressed in a number of ways. The raw recovery time should always be recorded. This can then be normalized for the spontaneous cardiac rate by dividing it by the average

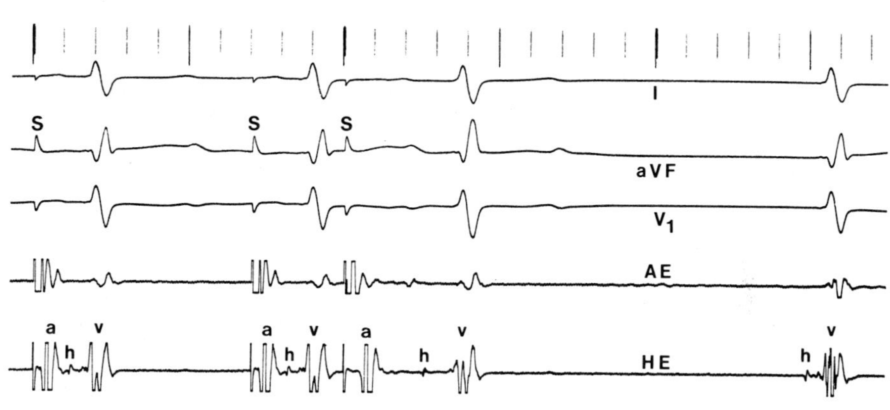

Figure 2-6 Recordings from an electrophysiologic study. Surface ECG leads I, aVF, and V_1 are simultaneously recorded with an atrial electrogram (AE) and a His bundle electrogram (HE). The bold time lines at the top of the page indicate 1-second intervals, and the subdivisions show 100-millisecond intervals. The atrium is being paced at a basic drive cycle length of 700 milliseconds (86 beats/min). Pacing stimuli are indicated by the letter S. In the His bundle electrogram recording the stimulus artifact is followed by an atrial electrogram (a), a His bundle electrogram (h), and a ventricular electrogram (v). During basic drive (the first two beats) the AH interval is 100 milliseconds, and the HV interval is 60 milliseconds. The third beat is an atrial extrastimulus delivered during programmed premature stimulation. This stimulus follows 300 milliseconds after the previous atrial stimulus. With this extrastimulus the stimulus to the QRS interval is increased from the 190-millisecond interval seen during basic drive to 375 milliseconds, indicating AV conduction delay. Examination of the His bundle electrogram reveals that this conduction delay is caused by slowed conduction both in the AV node and in the His-Purkinje system: The AH interval is increased to 200 milliseconds and the HV interval is increased to 105 milliseconds. Note that with the cessation of pacing, sinus node automaticity is abnormally suppressed. After the last atrial paced beat no spontaneous atrial activity is seen for the subsequent 1.8 seconds that are displayed. The recovery beat results from junctional automaticity, which produces a His bundle electrogram and ventricular depolarization not preceded by atrial activity.

spontaneous cycle length, which is determined prior to atrial pacing. The normalized sinus node recovery time (SNRT/SCL, where SNRT = sinus node recovery time and SCL = spontaneous cycle length in milliseconds) is usually less than 1.25. Values in excess of 1.50 are abnormal. The corrected sinus node recovery time (CSNRT) is determined by subtracting the spontaneous cycle length from the raw sinus node recovery time. The normal corrected sinus node recovery time is usually less than 300 mllliseconds. Corrected sinus node recovery times in excess of 500 milliseconds are abnormal. Because the sinus node recovery time is evaluated at multiple atrial drive rates, a variety of sinus node recovery times will be determined in each patient. As a result of autonomic nervous system influences (Mason, 1980) and possibly because of SA nodal entrance block, the longest sinus node recovery time may not be recorded at the fastest pacing rates. It is common practice to use the maximum normalized or corrected sinus node recovery time as the index value.

Pharmacologic interventions are also used to assess the integrity of sinus node function. Bolus administration of small doses of isoproterenol has been studied in normal subjects (George, et al., 1972). Thus, the responsiveness of the sinus node to specific isoproterenol doses can be used as an indicator of sinus node function. In addition, the ability of the sinus node to accelerate in response to vagal blockade by atropine should be determined. The normal patient will develop a sinus rate above 90 beats/min within 90 seconds of receiving a bolus dose of 1 mg/m^2 of atropine intravenously. In addition, perhaps by removing SA nodal entrance block, atropine may paradoxically produce longer postpacing pauses than are seen during sinus node recovery time determinations taken prior to atropine administration (Bashour, et al., 1973). Obviously, drug interventions such as these should be withheld until the end of the electrophysiologic study so that other aspects of the study are not influenced by the pharmacologic alterations in autonomic nervous system status (see also Chapter 6).

Evaluation of the atrioventricular (AV) node After the sinus node has been evaluated the AV node should be assessed. Three basic determinations are made: measurement of the basal conduction velocity, determination of the atrial pacing rate at which Wenckebach AV nodal block appears, and measurement of the AV nodal refractory periods by means of programmed atrial extrastimulation. Basal conduction velocity of the AV node is estimated by measuring the AH interval. The AH interval is defined as the time, in milliseconds, from the onset of atrial depolarization to the onset of His bundle depolarization (Figure 2-6). Atrial depolarization can be measured from anywhere in the atrium for this determination, as long as a consistent policy is used; however, most investigators measure atrial depolarization from the atrial electrogram that is obtained from the catheter used to record His bundle activity. This site is chosen because atrial activity recorded at the His bundle region occurs, presumably, just before entry of the electrical wavefront into the AV node. Likewise, the His bundle deflection should represent the moment at which the impulse exits from the AV node (see Figure 2-6). The electrograms are conventionally measured from the isoelectric crossing of their first rapid deflection. The normal AH interval ranges from 60 milliseconds to 140 milliseconds. During regular sinus rhythm, beat to beat variation of 5-10 milliseconds in the AH interval is not unusual.

In our laboratory the Wenckebach cycle length, that is, the pacing cycle length at which AV nodal Wenckebach block first appears, is determined by incremental atrial pacing. It is essential to use a standardized protocol for determining the Wenckebach cycle length because tremendous variation in this value will be obtained by different protocols. We begin atrial pacing at a rate just above the spontaneous atrial rate and decrease the atrial pacing cycle length by 10-millisecond decrements every 10 seconds until Wenckebach block occurs. This protocol may underestimate Wenckebach cycle length somewhat because it may take longer than 10 seconds for a long Wenckebach period to be completed. However, we feel that 10-second pacing intervals provide a reasonable compromise between accuracy, time consumption, and patient comfort. Tremendous variability in the Wenckebach cycle length exists, not only from patient to patient but even in a single patient, whose autonomic tone may vary from moment to moment. Despite this variability, it is probably valid to consider the appearance of Wenckebach block at pacing rates slower than 130 beats/min abnormal (if arrived at as detailed above). Patients who maintain 1:1 conduction at pacing rates above 250 beats/min usually have enhanced AV nodal conduction; they will usually also have short AH intervals, minimal increases in AH conduction time during rapid pacing, and short AV nodal refractory periods.

The relative, functional, and effective refractory periods of the AV node are determined by programmed atrial extrastimulation. Programmed atrial extrastimulation is performed using a pacing current that is twice the diastolic atrial capture threshold. During spontaneous sinus rhythm or during straight atrial pacing (atrial drive rhythm) single premature atrial depolarizations are introduced after every eighth to twelfth atrial beat using a programmable stimulator as previously described. The first extrastimulus is delivered just prior to the next expected atrial depolarization. The stimulus is then brought progressively closer to the preceding beat by 10-millisecond decrements in the premature interval until the atrium is no longer captured. Table 2-1 gives the nomenclature of drive stimuli and extrastimuli that will be used in the remainder of this chapter.

Table 2-2 gives the definitions of AV nodal refractory periods, as well as atrial, His-Purkinje system, and ventricular refractory periods. The reader must examine this table carefully to appreciate what is being done during programmed extrastimulation for study of the cardiac conduction system. Unfortunately, reliable normal values related to age for the refractory periods do not exist for the adult population. However, approximate guidelines have been given so that the physician can differentiate between those values that are probably normal and those that are probably abnormal. There may be no reasonable upper limit for the relative refractory period of the AV node. However, it is distinctly unusual to see increases of greater than 5 milliseconds in the AH interval resulting from atrial extrastimuli with coupling intervals greater than

Table 2-1 Nomenclature for pacing stimuli

Stimulus	Definition
S_1	Any atrial or ventricular basic drive stimulus. The S_1-S_1 interval refers to the pacing cycle length
S_2	The first extrastimulus delivered during spontaneous or driven rhythm. S_1-S_2 refers to the delay between the last basic drive stimulus and the first early extrastimulus
S_3	The second extrastimulus. S_4, S_5, and so on refer to subsequent extrastimuli. The S_2-S_3 interval refers to the delay between the first and second extrastimuli, and so on
A_1	This may refer either to spontaneous sinus beats, to driven atrial beats, or to the atrial drive stimulus itself
$A_2 A_3$, etc.	The first and subsequent extrastimulated atrial beats or the stimuli themselves
$V_1 V_2 V_3$, etc.	Ventricular beats or stimulation, as defined for the atrium above. Thus, $V_1 V_2 V_3 V_4$ stimulation refers to ventricular drive (V_1) with three ventricular extrastimuli (V_2, V_3, V_4)
H_1	A His electrogram resulting from spontaneous sinus rhythm or during atrial or ventricular drive rhythm
H_2	The His electrogram resulting from a single atrial or ventricular extrastimulus
$H_3 H_4$, etc.	His electrograms resulting from subsequent extrastimuli

800 milliseconds. The functional refractory period of the AV node can be considered abnormal when it exceeds 500 milliseconds, and the effective refractory period is abnormal when it exceeds 400 milliseconds in an adult.

It is worth noting that, for the majority of clinical situations, refractory period determination is not of great importance. It is a rare situation in which a refractory period determination will lead to a specific clinical decision. For example, knowing that the effective refractory period of the AV node was 420 milliseconds in a given patient is not likely to lead to a recommendation for a pacemaker. Although the determination of AV nodal refractory periods by programmed atrial extrastimulation is not of major clinical importance, other data obtained while performing the extrastimulation program are valuable. The presence of dual AV nodal pathways, AV nodal bypass physiology, and inducible supraventricular tachycardia can be discovered during atrial extrastimulation.

Pharmacologic interventions can also be applied to the study of the AV node. Administration of atropine may help in differentiating between AV nodal dysfunction resulting from structural AV nodal disease and

Table 2-2 Refractory period definitions

Refractory period	Definition
AERP	The longest A_1S_2 interval that fails to result in atrial capture by S_2
AVN ERP	The longest A_1A_2 interval that fails to traverse the AV node to produce a His bundle electrogram
AVN FRP	The shortest H_1H_2 interval achieved during atrial extrastimulation
AVN RRP	The A_1A_2 interval at which A_2H_2 first lengthens compared to A_1H_1
HPS ERP	The longest H_1H_2 interval at which H_2 fails to conduct through the His-Purkinje system to produce V_2
HPS FRP	The shortest V_1V_2 interval achieved during atrial extrastimulation or direct His bundle stimulation
HPS RRP	The H_1H_2 interval at which H_2V_2 first increases compared to H_1V_1 or at which the QRS of V_2 first shows aberration
VERP	The longest V_1S_2 interval at which S_2 fails to capture the ventricle

Legend: A = atrial; HPS = His-Purkinje system; V = ventricle; S, A, H, V with subscripts as defined in Table 2-1; ERP = effective refractory period; FRP = functional refractory period; RRP = relative refractory period.

apparent AV nodal disease resulting from excessive vagotonia. With regard to this latter point, one should realize that an absolute differentiation between the influence of autonomic stimuli and structural AV nodal disease can never be made, because structural problems might lead to excessive sensitivity of the AV node to normal vagal traffic (see also Chapter 6).

Evaluation of the His-Purkinje system Much as is the case with the AV node, conduction velocity, the occurrence of pacing-induced block, and the refractory periods of the His-Purkinje system are routinely determined during electrophysiologic study. Early in the use of His bundle electrocardiography, determination of the HV interval (Figure 2-6) was thought to be of potentially great value, especially for the identification of those patients at risk of developing infranodal block. Greatest attention has centered on measurement of the HV interval in patients with bifascicular conduction disease (right bundle branch block with left anterior or posterior hemiblock and left bundle branch block) because it is known that these individuals have a high incidence of progression to heart block.

In our laboratory the HV interval is measured from the onset of the first rapid His bundle electrogram deflection to the onset of surface electrocardiogram (ECG) QRS activity. A minimum of three orthogonal surface ECG lead recordings are required to determine the HV interval accurately. We make a practice of ignoring ventricular activation in the His bundle recording lead. Although this ventricular activity is often early and may precede detectable QRS activity in the surface leads, it is also quite variable in its morphology and highly dependent on catheter position. We consider the surface electrocardiogram (ECG) a more stable and reliable indication of the onset of ventricular electrical activity, especially when recordings are made over a long period of time, or serially, or when interventions, such as antiarrhythmic drug administration, are being assessed. The normal limits for HV interval in our laboratory are 35-55 milliseconds.

In the normal conduction system it is also unusual to demonstrate block in the His-Purkinje system during rapid atrial pacing because AV nodal Wenckebach block usually occurs earlier and protects the His-Purkinje system from very rapid rates of depolarization. In patients with moderately severe His-Purkinje system disease, such as those with prolonged HV intervals, it is unusual to demonstrate infranodal block during atrial pacing. On the other hand, patients with severe His-Purkinje system disease commonly exhibit additional HV delay and conduction block in the His-Purkinje system during rapid atrial pacing (Figure 2-6).

When the conduction system is normal, it is unusual to be able to determine the His-Purkinje system effective refractory period (see Table 2-2). This is because atrial or His bundle refractoriness is usually encountered before impulses can be induced by atrial depolarization to enter the His-Purkinje system early enough to encounter refractoriness. The relative refractory period of the His-Purkinje system is frequently determinable because right bundle branch block aberration (evidence for relative refractoriness and resultant slowed conduction in the right bundle portion of the His-Purkinje system) is often encountered with closely coupled atrial extrastimuli.

When His-Purkinje system refractory periods cannot be determined by atrial extrastimulation, it may be possible to detect the His bundle potential during retrograde His bundle depolarization induced by ventricular pacing. When this is possible, His-Purkinje system refractory periods during retrograde conduction, which correlate reasonably well with His-Purkinje system refractory periods during antegrade conduction, can usually be determined because the ability to enter the His-Purkinje system is not limited by atrial muscle or AV nodal refractoriness or AV nodal conduction delay. As for the AV node, normal values for His-Purkinje refractory periods related to different adult age brackets do not exist. His-Purkinje functional and effective refractory periods are generally similar to those of the AV node.

Pharmacologic interventions are usually not of great value in assessing the His-Purkinje system. His-Purkinje system conduction and refractoriness are little, if at all, affected by sympathetic stimulation or vagal stimulation or blockade. However, in some patients improvement in AV nodal conduction as a result of isoproterenol or atropine administration may permit documentation of abnormalities in antegrade His-Purkinje system conduction (see also Chapter 6).

Special study techniques *Arrhythmia induction* Techniques for arrhythmia induction are discussed in greater detail in Chapters 9 and 10. For some time it was believed that reentrant arrhythmias alone could be induced by premature electrical stimulation of the appropriate cardiac chamber and that inducibility could serve as reasonably strong evidence of a reentry mechanism. More recent observations in isolated tissue have indicated that nonreentrant tachyarrhythmias (see Chapter 2) can be induced by pacing techniques (Wit and Cranefield, 1976).

Arrhythmias that are typically inducible in the catheterization laboratory include: AV nodal (or junctional) reentrant supraventricular tachycardia, reentrant supraventricular tachycardias utilizing an accessory pathway, atrial flutter (and other atrial tachycardias), atrial fibrillation, SA nodal reentry, ventricular tachycardia, and ventricular fibrillation. Each of these arrhythmias is induced either by delivery of single or multiple extrastimuli at critical intervals, by rapid pacing, or by both. As will be discussed in this chapter and in Chapters 8 and 9, arrhythmia induction is used for several diagnostic purposes and for the selection of antiarrhythmic agents with which to treat the arrhythmia. Pharmacologic interventions may often be valuable in enhancing the inducibility of arrhythmias and in assessing the reentrant pathways involved in maintaining the arrhythmias.

Activation sequence mapping The sequence of electrical activation of cardiac tissues, determined in the electrophysiologic laboratory or in the operating room, is critical in the evaluation of a variety of arrhythmias. The timing and sequence of electrical activation can be determined easily by placing the electrodes in a variety of cardiac locations under fluoroscopic guidance or by direct visualization during surgery (see Chapter 11). The atrial activation sequence can be determined in the catheter laboratory by placing catheters in the coronary sinus, which records left atrial activity at the AV junction, and by placing catheters transvenously in a variety of locations in the right atrium. Atrial activation sequence mapping is used to determine the mechanisms of supraventricular tachycardias, both reentrant and automatic, and to approximate the location of AV bypass fibers.

Endocardial ventricular mapping is performed preoperatively (see Chapter 10) and intraoperatively in patients undergoing surgery for recurrent ventricular tachycardia. In some patients identification of the site of earliest activity during sustained ventricular tachycardia can lead the surgeon to the tissue responsible for ventricular tachycardia. Surgical ablation of that tissue may then eradicate the rhythm disturbance.

The Wolff-Parkinson-White syndrome Special study techniques are used to investigate the Wolff-Parkinson-White syndrome because different sorts of information are sought. The following is a summary of the information usually acquired in studies of patients with the Wolff-Parkinson-White syndrome:

1. Baseline intervals.
2. Extent of preexcitation during incremental right atrial and coronary sinus pacing.
3. Antegrade and retrograde conduction intervals during incremental atrial and ventricular pacing and during premature atrial and ventricular stimulation.
4. Antegrade and retrograde Kent bundle and AV nodal refractory periods.
5. Shortest and average RR interval between preexcited beats during spontaneous or induced atrial fibrillation.
6. Induction of circus movement tachycardia utilizing the bypass fiber by atrial or ventricular pacing.
7. Termination of supraventricular tachycardia by right atrial, coronary sinus, or ventricular pacing programs.
8. Atrial activation sequence mapping (right atrium and coronary sinus) during circus movement tachycardia and during rapid ventricular pacing.
9. Observation of the cycle length of supraventricular tachycardia with a narrow QRS complex and during development of functional right or left bundle branch block.
10. Introduction of ventricular stimuli during supraventricular tachycardia programmed to reach the His bundle immediately after its depolarization to demonstrate advancement of atrial depolarization via the accessory pathway.
11. Assessment of the effect of antiarrhythmic drugs on tachycardia induction, tachycardia cycle length, accessory pathway refractory periods, and ventricular rate during atrial fibrillation.

Detailed explanation of each point would be too lengthy, but a few comments should be made. Supraventricular tachycardia is nearly always inducible by either right atrial, coronary sinus, or ventricular extrastimulation in patients with the Wolff-Parkinson-White syndrome.

Supraventricular tachycardia induction is a crucial step in an accurate diagnosis because it permits examination of the retrograde atrial activation sequence, which not only provides evidence for the presence of an AV bypass fiber but also helps approximate the atrial input site of the bypass fiber. Concealed bypasses (AV bypass fibers that function only in a retrograde manner, from ventricle to atrium, and thus cause no ventricular preexcitation during sinus rhythm or atrial pacing) can be discovered with induction of supraventricular tachycardia or, in a few cases, ventricular pacing (see also Chapter 9).

Determination of the antegrade effective refractory period of the Kent bundle is useful in assessing drug effects and has some value in predicting the maximum rate during atrial fibrillation. However, it is much more valuable to induce atrial fibrillation in patients with Kent bypass fibers to directly assess the maximum rates achieved by the ventricle as a result of transmission across the accessory pathway. Those patients with excessively rapid ventricular response rates are at risk of collapse and even death from spontaneous atrial fibrillation.

The cycle length or rate of supraventricular tachycardia during the development of functional right and left bundle branch block should be established whenever possible because the sidedness of the bypass fiber can be determined by appropriate observations. For example, if a patient with a left free-wall accessory pathway develops left bundle branch block during supraventricular tachycardia, we expect the tachycardia cycle length to increase because left bundle branch block will delay the arrival of circuiting impulses to the left ventricular myocardium and, therefore, to the Kent bypass fiber. The result is a delay in atrial activation and lengthening of the tachycardia cycle length.

INDICATIONS FOR INTRACARDIAC ELECTROPHYSIOLOGIC STUDY

The following is a list of the indications for intracardiac electrophysiologic study at Stanford University Medical Center:

- Arrhythmia assessment
  - Ventricular tachycardia vs. supraventricular tachycardia with aberration
  - Arrhythmia induction for diagnosis
  - Arrhythmia induction for drug selection
  - Activation sequence mapping
  - Tachycardia termination
- Cardiac conduction system disease

Sinus node dysfunction

Syncope of uncertain etiology

Each of these indications will be discussed briefly.

Arrhythmia Assessment

Ventricular tachycardia vs. supraventricular tachycardia with aberration In most instances the surface ECG will provide the necessary clues to distinguish between ventricular tachycardia and supraventricular tachycardia with QRS aberrancy (see Chapter 10). However, in some cases the distinction simply cannot be made by ECG and in others appropriate ECGs are never successfully obtained. Even though we have found that when the distinction cannot be made on 12-lead ECG the rhythm disturbance is nearly always ventricular tachycardia, intracardiac electrophysiologic study is required to make a definitive determination. During electrophysiologic study the tachyarrhythmia must be successfully induced or already present for a differential diagnosis to be possible. Stable His bundle electrogram recording is also required to make the differential diagnosis. If dissociation exists between His bundle electrograms and ventricular electrograms, the diagnosis of ventricular tachycardia is secure. In most instances, however, this will not be possible. The most common finding is disappearance of the His bundle electrogram (within the local ventricular electrogram) at the onset of ventricular tachycardia. AV dissociation is usually also present, but it need not be. In some instances the His electrogram will be visible in front of the local ventricular electrogram during every beat of ventricular tachycardia. This may occur both with and without a 1:1 AV relationship. Ventricular tachycardia can be confidently diagnosed in this circumstance if the HV interval is significantly shorter than that recorded during sinus rhythm. Shortening of the HV interval is usually a result of retrograde capture of the His bundle during a tachycardia developing near or utilizing the specialized conduction system.

Supraventricular tachycardia can be diagnosed with confidence when HV association is present with an HV interval equal to or greater than that recorded during spontaneous sinus rhythm. Observation of the onset of supraventricular tachycardia is often useful because bundle branch block aberration may not develop until after the first few beats. One to one AV conduction is usually present during supraventricular tachycardia, but atrial participation in a reentry circuit localized in the AV node is not required; thus, AV dissociation may be present during true supraventricular tachycardia. Figure 2-7 shows an example of atrial fibrillation with QRS aberrancy and rate regularization, which simulated paroxysmal ventricular tachycardia. His electrogram recordings identified the rhythm as supraventricular rather than ventricular tachycardia.

Arrhythmia induction for diagnosis Some patients with recurrent tachyarrhythmias defy all attempts to record their arrhythmias. Their histories often include diagnoses of tachycardia by a bystander palpating the pulse. In such instances it is reasonable to attempt arrhythmia induction with both atrial and ventricular extrastimulation to document the nature of the arrhythmia and, at the same time, if indicated, to assess antiarrhythmic drug efficacy. Approximately 5% of the arrhythmia inductions performed in our laboratory (or 20 cases per year) are performed primarily for diagnostic purposes.

Arrhythmia induction for drug selection This technique has already been mentioned and will be discussed in greater detail in Chapters 9 and 10 on supraventricular tachycardia and ventricular tachycardia. In 80%-90% of patients with recurrent supraventricular or ventricular tachycardia the rhythm abnormality can be reproduced by extrastimulation in the electrophysiology laboratory. During the latter half of the 1970s researchers discovered that drugs which provided prophylaxis against previously inducible tachyarrhythmias were likely to be effective during chronic therapy (Wu, et al., 1977; Horowitz, et al., 1978; Mason and Winkle, 1978; Mason and Winkle, 1980). Arrhythmia induction has now become an established method for selecting antiarrhythmic drugs in patients with persistent and medically refractory tachyarrhythmias.

Activation sequence mapping Activation sequence mapping has become an important indication for intracardiac electrophysiologic study. We consider it an absolute requirement in the preoperative assessment of patients with the Wolff-Parkinson-White syndrome who are about to undergo surgical ablation of the bypass fiber. It may also be valuable in the preoperative assessment of patients with recurrent ventricular tachycardia. However, in the latter case we feel that accurate localization of putative tachycardia foci is problematic in many patients due to the inaccuracy of fluoroscopic assessment of catheter position and because of the technical difficulty of achieving accurate positioning of electrode catheters within the left ventricular chamber and ignorance regarding tachycardia mechanisms. The use of activation sequence mapping in the operating room is discussed in detail in Chapter 11.

Tachycardia termination Many sustained supraventricular and ventricular tachyarrhythmias can be terminated either by appropriately timed single extrastimuli delivered to the proper chamber or by rapid pacing. Essentially, all AV nodal reentrant supraventricular tachycardias and all those circus movement tachycardias utilizing an accessory pathway can be terminated by atrial or ventricular pacing. In these cases single extrastimuli are often enough to terminate the tachycardia; however, when this is not the case, rapid pacing will invariably extinguish the arrhythmia. It is also possible to pace-terminate some patients with true atrial flutter by using rapid atrial stimulation in excess of the flutter rate. In some cases of atrial flutter a single properly programmed extrastimulus will also terminate the arrhythmia. Failure to capture the atrium because of insufficient current delivery may be responsible in those instances in which the flutter cannot be terminated. In other cases failure to achieve a critically rapid pacing rate or a sufficient duration of rapid pacing may account for the inability to terminate the flutter. When rapid atrial pacing is employed, flutter termination is frequently a consequence of induction of atrial fibrillation; the induced atrial fibrillation is often short-lived.

In 70% of patients inducible ventricular tachycardia can be terminated using ventricular pacing. Termination methods may include single extrastimuli (delivered either by programmed delay or by slow ventricular pacing, sometimes termed "underdrive"), multiple programmed extrastimuli, or rapid ventricular pacing. However, not all episodes of ventricular tachycardia in this 70% of patients can be successfully terminated. If aggressive pacing is attempted to terminate ventricular tachycardia, failure is often complicated by an acceleration of ventricular tachycardia, requiring direct current cardioversion.

We feel that terminating tachyarrhythmias by pacing is often a very satisfactory method of therapy for short-term arrhythmia control and, in rare cases, for the control of chronic arrhythmia by the use of special permanent pacemaker systems (see Chapters 7, 9, and 10).

Figure 2-7 These recordings were obtained in a patient with atrial fibrillation who had frequent episodes of a rapid ventricular rate with wide QRS complexes and relative rate regularization. A differential diagnosis between ventricular tachycardia and rate-related QRS aberration was required. Six surface ECG leads are recorded simultaneously with high right atrial (HRA), right ventricular (RV), and His bundle (HIS) electrograms. The arterial pressure is displayed at the bottom of the recording. The time lines mark 500-millisecond intervals. The high right atrial electrogram shows atrial fibrillation throughout the recording. Intervals between QRS complexes are labeled in milliseconds above the right ventricular electrogram. On the left side of the tracing a variable ventricular response rate is shown with narrow QRS complexes. After an interbeat delay of 510 milliseconds, an early ventricular depolarization 290 milliseconds later is associated with a wide QRS complex. This and the subsequent five beats simulate a run of ventricular tachycardia. However, it can be seen in the His bundle recording that His electrograms with a constant HV interval of 60 milliseconds precede each QRS complex both before and during the period of ventricular aberration. Thus, the arrhythmia diagnosis is atrial fibrillation with sustained QRS aberration rather than ventricular tachycardia. Note that this figure illustrates the Ashman phenomenon: an early cycle following a long cycle is associated with QRS aberration.

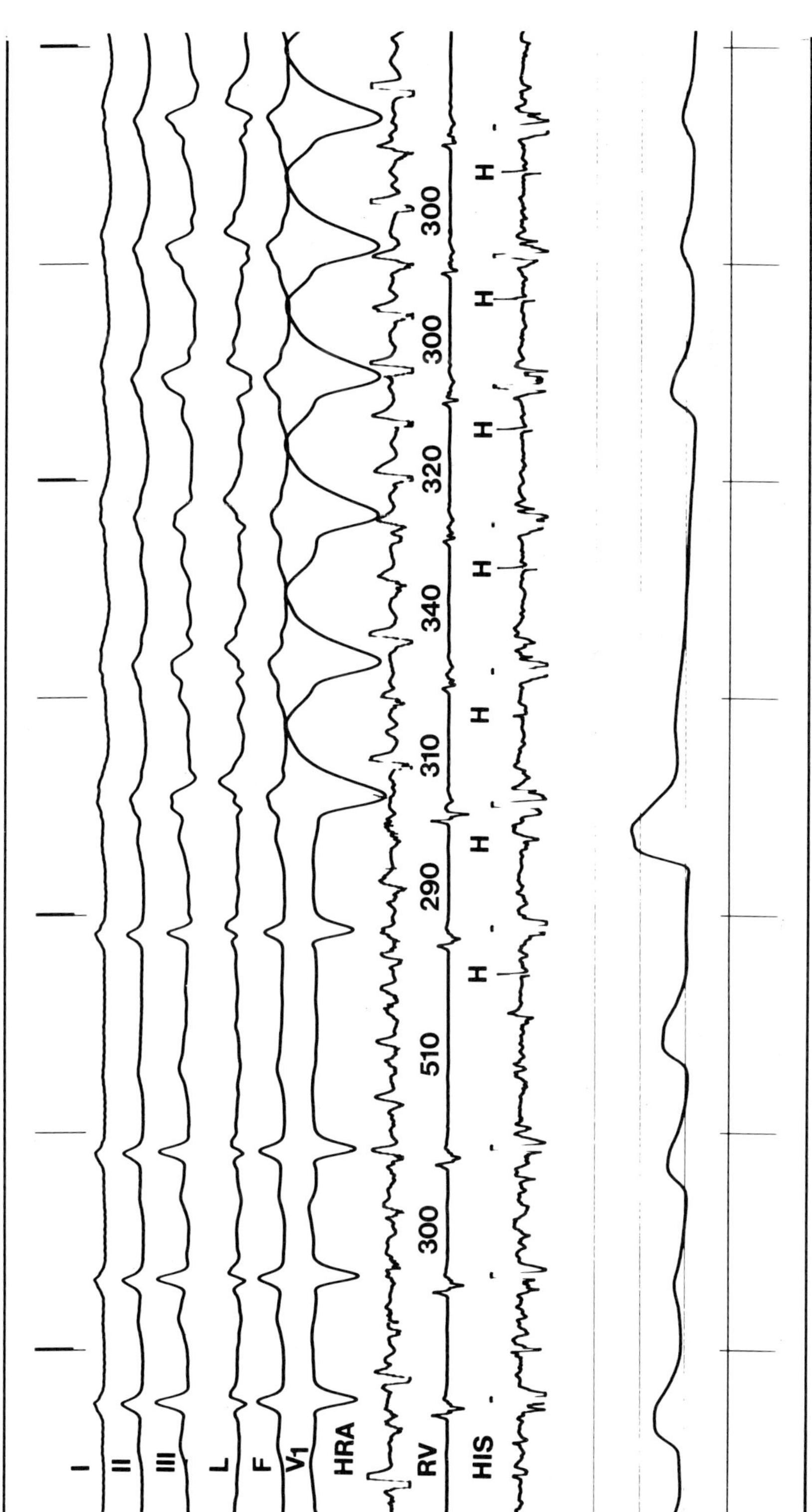
I
II
III
L
F
V_1
HRA
RV
HIS
300
510
290
310
340
320
300
300
H
H
H
H
H
H
H

Cardiac Conduction System Disease

Electrophysiologic study is indicated in various settings to document the site and the extent of conduction block in the cardiac conduction system (see Chapter 6). Successful recording of the His bundle electrogram permits division of AV conduction into supra-Hisian (atrial and AV nodal) and infra-Hisian (His-Purkinje system and ventricular) segments. Thus, His bundle electrocardiography can be used to determine both the site of conduction disease and the extent of disease within that site.

Determination of the site of block may have clinical value in certain circumstances. It is generally true that infranodal conduction block carries a greater risk of eventual complete heart block with inadequate escape rhythms. For example, localization of 2:1 block to the supra-Hisian or the infra-Hisian region can make the difference between a recommendation for or against permanent pacemaker placement in some patients. Figure 2-8 shows an example of 2:1 block in the His-Purkinje system (infra-Hisian).

Although it has now become clear that HV interval prolongation does confer a higher risk of progression to complete heart block in patients with bifascicular block and organic heart disease (Dhingra, et al., 1979), the value of HV interval determination in individual patients with bifascicular block (to determine whether pacemaker implantation is required) is questionable.

On the other hand, a prolonged HV interval seems to be a good predictor of a high likelihood of progression to heart block in patients who develop bifascicular block in the setting of acute myocardial infarction (Lie, et al., 1974). Measurement of the HV interval in patients who develop bifascicular block in the first 1 to 2 days after onset of myocardial infarction can help determine whether temporary prophylactic pacemaker insertion is required. However, because electrode catheter insertion is necessary to determine the HV interval (noninvasive HV interval determination continues to be an experimental technique at this time), electrophysiologic study cannot be used to spare the patient the minimal risk and discomfort of catheter placement. However, the length of the HV interval can help the clinician determine the appropriate time for catheter removal. If the HV interval is normal, it would be reasonable to remove the catheter immediately or to leave it in for only 1 day. If the HV interval is prolonged, removal of the catheter after several days would be reasonable.

Sinus Node Dysfunction

During the early and mid-1970s there was great interest in the use of electrophysiologic investigations to detect sinus node dysfunction. This interest followed on the heels of popularization of the term sick sinus

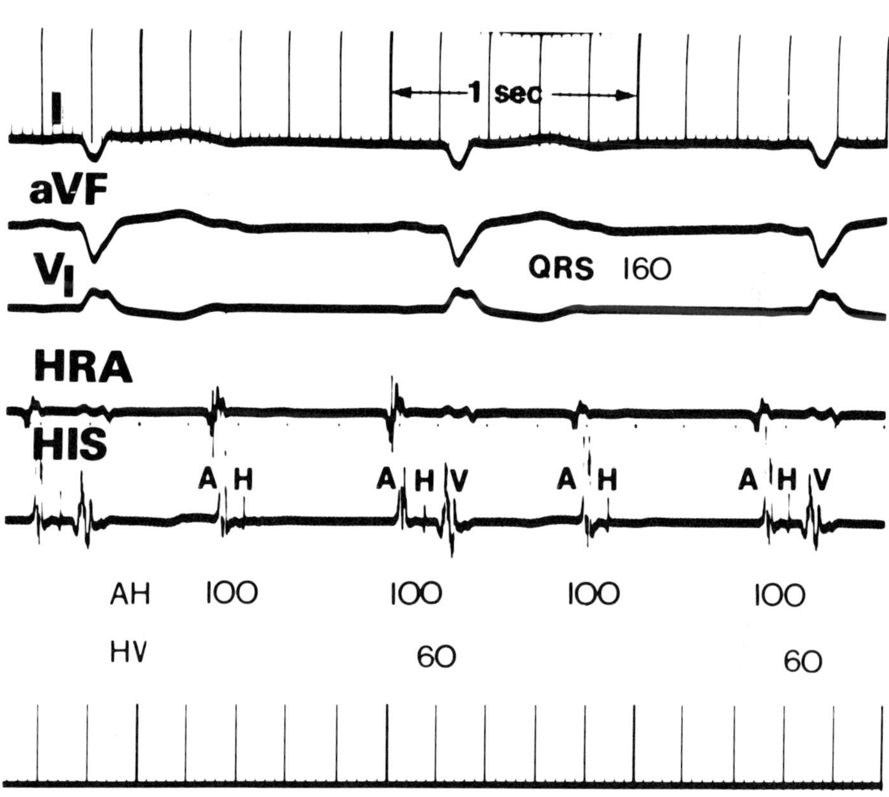

Figure 2-8 Intracardiac recording during 2:1 infranodal block. Three surface leads (I, aVF, V_1) are displayed with high right atrial (HRA) and His bundle (HIS) electrograms. The AH interval is constant (100 milliseconds). The HV interval is 60 milliseconds during conducted beats. Every other supraventricular beat is blocked in the His-Purkinje system, resulting in His bundle deflections without succeeding ventricular depolarizations. Note the presence of right bundle branch block and extreme right axis deviation in the conducted QRS complexes.

syndrome, an alliterative moniker for sinus node dysfunction that is often used interchangeably with the term brady-tachy syndrome. Atrial pacing to determine the sinus node recovery time, as previously described, became a popular method for diagnosing the sick sinus syndrome or brady-tachy syndrome. However, it is now clear that abnormalities of the sinus node recovery time are frequently absent in patients with significant sinus node dysfunction. On the other hand, an abnormal sinus node recovery time is a specific finding that indicates either true sinus node disease or high cardiac vagal tone.

The most effective method for diagnosing sinus node dysfunction is ambulatory monitoring (see Chapter 4). While ambulatory monitoring may document abnormalities, clinical judgment is still required to make a final decision regarding the need for pacemaker placement. Generally speaking, electrophysiologic study will not provide help in making this decision (see also Chapter 6).

Syncope of Uncertain Etiology

Syncope is a common complaint with many possible etiologies. In most patients syncope is not sufficiently recurrent or severe to require extensive evaluation. However, in a small number of patients all attempts to uncover an etiology for recurrent syncope, including extensive neurologic evaluation, fail. In such patients electrophysiologic study may disclose an arrhythmic or conduction disorder that can be potentially responsible for the syncope. However, the incidence of yield from electrophysiologic study of diagnostically helpful information in patients with syncope of unknown etiology is quite small, except, perhaps, in patients with documented structural heart disease (DiMarco, et al., 1981).

In evaluating these patients we thoroughly evaluate sinus node function, including the use of pharmacologic interventions. If sinus node function and AV transmission appear to be intact, we attempt arrhythmia induction, first with atrial pacing and then with ventricular pacing. If all these studies are negative, a small possibility persists that tachyarrhythmias, conduction disease, or sinus node disease are, in fact, responsible for recurrent syncope but are simply not detectable by available methods.

The indications for electrophysiologic study put forward in this chapter are those followed at Stanford University Medical Center. Other clinicians recognize additional indications, and the current list will undoubtedly change in coming years.

REFERENCES

Alanis, J.; Gonzales, H.; and Lopez, E. 1958. Electrical activity of the bundle of His. *J. Physiol.* 142:127.

Bashour, T.; Hemb, R.; and Wickramesekaran, R. 1973. An unusual effect of atropine on overdrive suppression. *Circulation* 48:911.

Dhingra, R. C.; Wyndham, C.; Bauernfeind, R., et al. 1979. Significance of chronic bifascicular block without apparent organic heart disease. *Circulation* 60:33.

DiMarco, J. P.; Garan, H.; Harthorne, W., et al. 1981. Intracardiac electrophysiologic techniques in recurrent syncope of unknown cause. *Ann. Int. Med.* 95:542.

George, C. F.; Conolly, M. E.; Briant, F., et al. 1972. Intravenously administered isoproterenol sulfate dose response curves in man. *Arch. Intern. Med.* 30:361.

Horowitz, L. N.; Josephson, M. E.; Farshidi, A., et al. 1978. Recurrent sustained ventricular tachycardia. 3. Role of the electrophysiologic study in selection of antiarrhythmic regimens. *Circulation* 58:986.

Kossman, C. E.; Berger, A. R.; Rader, B., et al. 1950. Intracardiac and intravascular potentials resulting from electrical activity of the normal human heart. *Circulation* 2:10.

Lasser, R. P.; Haft, J. I.; and Friedberg, C. K. 1968. Relationship of right bundle branch block and marked left axis deviation to complete heart block and syncope. *Circulation* 37:429.

Lie, K. I.; Wellens, H. J. J.; Schuilenburg, R. M., et al. 1974. Factors influencing prognosis of bundle branch block complicating acute anteroseptal infarction: the value of His bundle recordings. *Circulation* 50:935.

Mason, J. W. 1980. Overdrive suppression in the transplanted heart: effect of the autonomic nervous system on human sinus node recovery. *Circulation* 62:688.

Mason, J. W.; and Winkle, R. A. 1978. Electrode catheter arrhythmia induction in the selection and assessment of antiarrhythmic drug therapy for recurrent ventricular tachycardia. *Circulation* 58:971.

Mason, J. W.; and Winkle, R. A. 1980. Accuracy of the ventricular tachycardia induction study for predicting long-term efficacy and inefficacy of antiarrhythmic drugs. *N. Engl. J. Med.* 303:1073.

Scherlag, B. J.; Helfant, R. H.; and Damato, A. N. 1968. Catheterization technique for His bundle stimulation and recording in the intact dog. *J. Appl. Physiol.* 25:425.

Scherlag, B. J.; Low, S. H.; Helfant, R. A., et al. 1969. Catheter technique for recording His bundle activity in man. *Circulation* 39:13.

Wit, A. L.; and Cranefield, P. F. 1976. Triggered activity in cardiac muscle fibers of the simian mitral valve. *Circ. Res.* 38:85.

Wu, D.; Amat-y-Leon, F.; Simpson, R. J., Jr., et al. 1977. Electrophysiologic studies with multiple drugs in patients with atrioventricular reentrant tachycardia utilizing an extranodal pathway. *Circulation* 56:727.

3 Antiarrhythmic Therapy

Roger A. Winkle, M.D.

Associate Professor of Medicine
Stanford University School of Medicine
Stanford, California

PRINCIPLES OF PHARMACOKINETICS

Pharmacokinetics is the study of drug disposition (Greenblatt and Koch-Weser, 1975). The disposition of any drug in the body is the net result of absorption, metabolism in the liver and other organs, removal by the kidneys and other sources, transfer across membranes, and distribution to various tissues. Mathematical models are useful for predicting drug concentrations in the body following intravenous and oral antiarrhythmic drug administration. Although these models may become mathematically complex, one often need only understand the principles involved to utilize antiarrhythmic drugs more safely and effectively.

The rationale for predicting or measuring an antiarrhythmic drug concentration is that the drug concentration frequently correlates better with pharmacologic response and toxicity than does the actual drug dose. Although drug concentration may correlate with drug effect, the ultimate goal of drug therapy is not the achievement of a "therapeutic" drug plasma concentration but rather the production of a desired drug action. Technological advances such as continuous ECG monitoring and intracardiac electrophysiologic studies now permit measurement of a drug's pharmacologic action in each patient being treated. Although it is not the final end point of therapy, knowledge of a drug's plasma concentration is of immense value in patient management. Many instances of apparent drug failure can be explained on the basis that drug plasma concentrations were inadequate, and many instances of drug toxicity can be explained on the basis of failure to account for disease-related alterations in drug disposition. The existence of a high drug plasma concentration indicates that the likelihood of observing a toxic reaction from increasing the dose further may be considerable.

This section of this chapter presents simplified pharmacokinetic principles that apply to antiarrhythmic drugs. Tables summarizing the pharmacokinetics of a large number of commonly used antiarrhythmic drugs are presented later in the chapter.

One Compartment Model

The one compartment model makes several assumptions about drug distribution in the body. It assumes that drug distribution is instantaneous (or at least rapid compared to drug elimination) into a single homogeneous compartment with a constant volume. It also assumes that drug elimination by excretion and metabolism follows first order kinetics. Drugs removed by a first order process have a constant fraction of the drug remaining in the body at any time removed per unit of time. Although a constant fraction of the drug remaining in the body is removed per unit time, increasingly smaller fractions of the initial concentration or initial dose are removed. First order decay of drug concentration follows an exponential curve when drug concentration is plotted linearly as a function of time (Figure 3-1). First order decay can be linearized by plotting the logarithm of drug concentration as a function of time. The concept of drug half-life evolves directly from such a plot and is the amount of time required for the removal of one-half of the drug present in the body at any given time. Approximately 87.5% of the drug dose is removed in three half-lives.

Another important concept of pharmacokinetics is the apparent volume of distribution (V_d). This is the volume through which the drug is assumed to be uniformly distributed. Equation 1 relates the amount of drug in the body (A_b) and the drug concentration (C) in the body fluid being sampled (usually blood or plasma) to the volume of distribution, as follows:

$$A_b = C \cdot V_d \tag{1}$$

The volume of distribution is constant for a given drug and patient. Although drug doses are given in measured amounts, the amount of drug that remains in a patient at any given time cannot easily be directly measured. Instead, drug concentration in blood, plasma, or other bodily fluids is measured. The only time the exact amount of drug in the body is known is immediately after an intravenous bolus is given. At this time the drug distribution (which is assumed to be instantaneous) has occurred and no elimination has yet taken place. The volume of distribution is estimated from equation 1 after an intravenous bolus by extrapolating drug concentration data to zero time. It must be recognized that the volume of distribution is only a proportionality constant and does not have any specific physiologic significance in terms of an actual space or volume. It does not necessarily represent plasma, extracellular fluid, blood, or total body water volumes.

Drug clearance is another important pharmacokinetic concept. Clearance has the dimensions of volume per unit of time and is defined as the volume of blood or plasma from which a drug is totally and irreversibly removed in a given time period. Because most drugs are

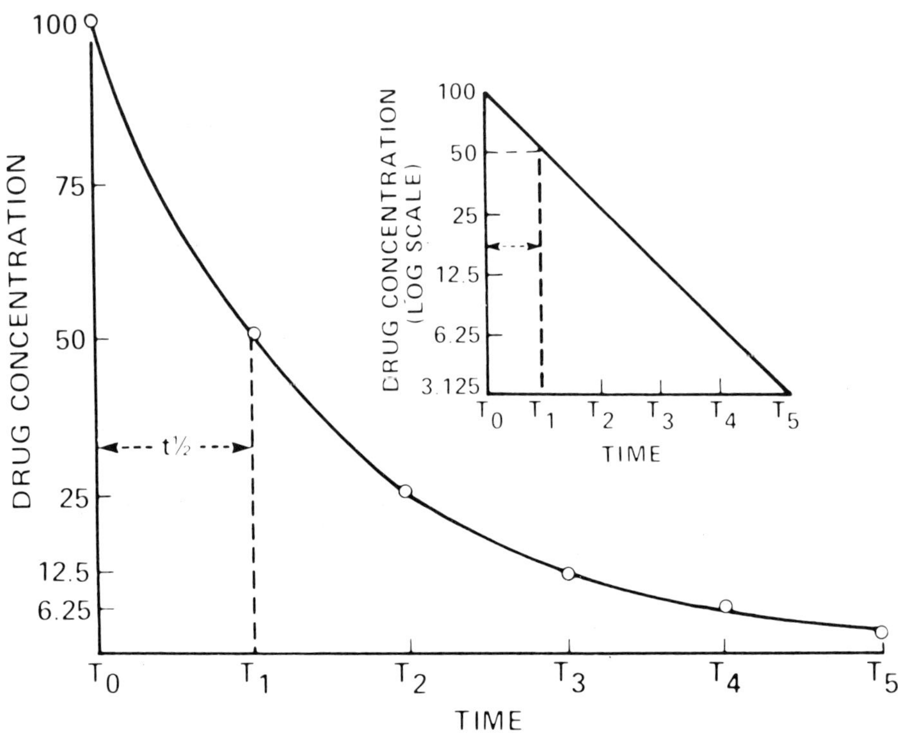

Figure 3-1 Drug concentration versus time for a one compartment model. The inset shows the same curve plotted as the logarithm of drug concentration versus time. Note that plotting the data in this manner linearizes the drug concentration time curve. Time T_1 represents the drug's half-life because concentration falls by 50% from time T_0 to time T_1. (*Source:* Harrison, D. C.; Meffin, P. J.; and Winkle, R. A. 1977. Clinical pharmacokinetics of antiarrhythmic drugs. *Prog. Cardiovas. Dis.* 20:217-242. Used by permission.)

eliminated by renal excretion and hepatic metabolism, the maximum values of clearance possible relate to the blood flow to these organs. This is approximately 1.5 L/min for hepatic blood flow and 1.2 L/min for renal blood flow. Some drugs are removed or metabolized by other organs, and the clearance from various mechanisms is additive. In practice it is difficult to measure directly the clearance from organs other than the kidneys. Therefore, one usually measures total body clearance (which is the sum of all metabolic and excretory processes) and renal clearance. The difference between these two is the nonrenal clearance, which is often very close to the hepatic clearance. For drugs that follow linear pharmacokinetics the total body clearance can be determined following an intravenous dose. The relationship between total body clearance ($C\ell_T$), drug dose (D), and total area under the concentration time curve from 0 to infinite time (AUC_0^∞) is given in equation 2, as follows:

(2) $$C\ell_T = \frac{D}{AUC_0^\infty}$$

Clearance measured by this technique is independent of the mathematical model describing drug distribution and applies equally well for drugs described by one, two, or more compartment models. Clearance cannot usually be calculated following oral drug doses because the fraction of the drug dose that reaches the systemic circulation (systemic availability or bioavailability) is not usually available.

Most clinicians consider that drug half-life ($T_{1/2}$) is the most important determinant of drug disposition. It should be emphasized, however, that half-life is only one portion of the data necessary to assess drug disposition. In fact, drug half-life is directly dependent on the volume of distribution and inversely proportional to clearance:

(3) $$T_{1/2} = \frac{V_d\ 0.693}{C\ell_T}$$

Measurement of the drug half-life may not be an accurate reflection of important changes in drug disposition. An excellent example of this is seen with lidocaine (Thompson, et al., 1973). For patients with congestive heart failure a reduction in lidocaine clearance occurs. However, there is also a proportionately similar change in the drug volume of distribution. Thus, the half-life is not changed significantly by congestive heart failure. On the other hand, because the infusion rate of the drug to achieve any given steady state drug concentration is directly proportional to the clearance, marked reductions in lidocaine infusion rates are necessary in congestive heart failure.

Two Compartment Model

For many drugs distribution is not rapid compared with elimination, and considerable time may elapse before drug concentration in all the tissues shows a constant relationship to that in the blood or plasma. At all times there are a number of distribution processes taking place in individual parts of the body, and to describe them all in detail would require extremely cumbersome mathematical models. Fortunately, for most drugs the change in drug plasma concentration with time can be averaged into fast and slow processes (Figure 3-2). Such a model assumes that the drug is administered into and eliminated from a central compartment

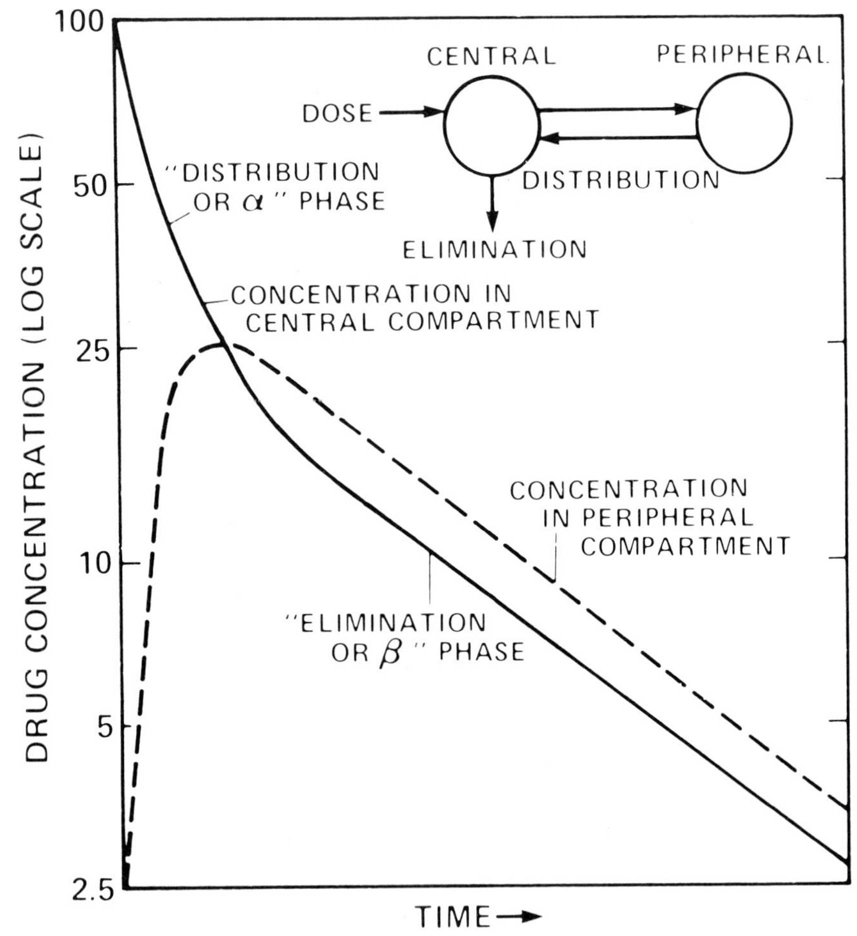

Figure 3-2 A two compartment model. In this model the drug dose is administered into the central compartment and there is reversible distribution between this rapidly equilibrating central compartment and a less rapidly equilibrating peripheral compartment. The drug concentrations are also shown in both the central and peripheral compartments at various times following an intravenous bolus into the central compartment. Drug concentrations in the central compartment (which includes blood) falls rapidly during the initial distribution, or alpha, phase and more slowly during the later elimination, or beta, phase. Note that at later times drug concentrations in both the central and peripheral compartments decline in parallel. This is the so-called period of pseudoequilibrium. During pseudoequilibrium drug concentration in the plasma may correlate directly with pharmacologic effect, even though the drug's site of action may be located in the peripheral compartment. (*Source:* Harrison, D. C.; Meffin, P. J.; and Winkle, R. A. 1977. Clinical pharmacokinetics of antiarrhythmic drugs. *Prog. Cardiovas. Dis.* 20:217-242. Used by permission.)

that consists of plasma and rapidly perfused tissues, such as the central nervous system and the myocardium. After an intravenous bolus all of the drug is initially in this central compartment, in which it rapidly equilibrates. Distribution takes place from this compartment into a more slowly equilibrating peripheral compartment at a rate that is a function of the amount of drug in the central compartment. As the drug is eliminated from the central compartment (again at a rate that is proportional to the amount of drug in the central compartment), a transfer of the drug from the peripheral compartment back to the central compartment occurs.

Frequently, most of the distributive processes are faster than drug elimination, and the term distributive (or alpha) phase is used to describe the plasma concentrations shortly after drug administration. The term elimination (or beta) phase describes drug plasma concentrations that occur later on. Although this descriptive terminology does not truly reflect physiologic events, it does help in understanding the compartmental models as they are used for delineating and predicting drug plasma concentrations. In the post-distributive, or beta, phase the rate of drug loss from the central and peripheral compartments is the same, and a dynamic equilibrium is established in which the drug concentrations in the two compartments decline in parallel. Prior to distributional equilibrium the relationship between the drug concentration in the plasma and in the more slowly equilibrating peripheral compartment is constantly changing. After dynamic equilibrium the drug concentration in the plasma may correlate directly with pharmacologic effect, even though the drug's site of action is located in the peripheral compartment. Plasma concentrations obtained shortly after drug administration may correlate poorly with pharmacologic response if the site of action is in the peripheral compartment.

In a two compartment model two half-lives must be considered. These are $T_{1/2}$ alpha, or the distribution phase half-life, and $T_{1/2}$ beta, or the elimination phase half-life (Figure 3-2). It should be recognized that these are composite mathematical terms that are dependent on the transfer coefficients between compartments and true drug elimination from the central compartment. The half-lives assume considerable clinical importance because $T_{1/2}$ alpha determines the rate at which drug plasma concentrations will fall soon after an intravenous bolus (to potentially subtherapeutic concentrations), and $T_{1/2}$ beta describes the rate at which a steady state is approached during continuous drug administration and the rate at which drug levels fall when chronic drug administration ceases.

In a two compartment model drug distribution is not instantaneous as it is in the single compartment model but is instead time-dependent. A number of volume of distribution terms have come into common use to relate the amount of drug present in the body or in a given compartment to blood or plasma concentrations at various times following drug administration. Immediately after intravenous bolus administration it is assumed that all the drug is in a central compartment and no elimination or distribution has taken place. The volume of the central compartment (V_c) is defined as the dose divided by the sum of the extrapolated concentrations at zero time. The volume of the central compartment is an important factor in determining drug concentrations immediately after an intravenous bolus. The smaller the volume of the central compartment the higher the drug concentration in the blood for a given dose of an antiarrhythmic drug. The volume through which the drug is ultimately distributed during long-term infusions or after multiple chronic oral dosing is also an important factor and is known as the volume of distribution at steady state (Vd_{ss}).

Physiologic Models of Drug Disposition

The physiologic determinants of drug clearance are blood flow to the organ of elimination, the inherent ability of the organ to clear the drug from the blood, and the binding of the drug to plasma proteins and organ cellular components. Hepatic clearance is described by the relationship in equation 4, where $C\ell_H$ is the hepatic clearance, f_b is the fraction of the drug unbound in blood, $C\ell_{INT}$ is the intrinsic clearance (a function of enzyme activity), and Q is the hepatic blood flow:

$$(4) \qquad C\ell_H = Q\left(\frac{f_b \cdot C\ell_{INT}}{Q + f_b \cdot C\ell_{INT}}\right)$$

The parenthetical term in this equation is known as the extraction ratio (E), which can vary between 0 and 1. If all the drug were removed during a single pass through the liver, the extraction ratio would be 1 and the hepatic clearance would be equal to the hepatic blood flow (Q). Drugs with a low clearance are generally insensitive to changes in hepatic blood flow. Clearance is instead affected by changes in the extraction ratio (f_b and $C\ell_{INT}$). Interpatient differences in the extraction ratio or changes in the same patient over time primarily reflect the metabolic activity of liver enzymes, which may differ as a function of genetic makeup, exposure to environmental factors, such as drugs, and disease states. Drugs that are mainly eliminated by the liver and have high total body clearances generally have clearances that are sensitive to changes in hepatic blood flow. When such high clearance drugs are given orally, considerable interpatient variability may exist in drug plasma concentrations because all of the drug must pass through the liver via the portal circulation. Drug metabolism resulting from this initial pass through the liver is known as the first pass effect. The systemic availability of the drug (F) can be estimated in this instance by the following relationship:

(5) $$F = 1 - \frac{C\ell_H}{Q} = 1 - E$$

When clearance approaches hepatic blood flow, small changes in clearance will give rise to large changes in systemic availability.

Systemic Availability

When a drug is administered orally, one should be concerned with the amount of the drug that reaches the system circulation to be available for perfusing the sites of drug action. Many factors may prevent the drug from reaching the systemic circulation, including failure of the drug to be released from its dose form because of solubility problems, local inactivation or metabolism within the gastrointestinal tract or mucosal cells, or a gastrointestinal transit time that is short compared to the time needed for drug dissolution and absorption. In addition, drugs may not be well absorbed by the gastrointestinal mucosa or may be metabolized in the liver during the first pass through. Drugs with a high hepatic clearance have a significant fraction of the total absorbed dose removed during the first pass through the liver. Systemic availability or bioavailability (F) is estimated by comparing the area under the plasma or blood concentration time curve after an oral dose with that obtained after an intravenous dose, as follows:

(6) $$F = \frac{AUC_0^\infty\ (\text{oral})}{AUC_0^\infty\ (\text{IV})} \cdot \frac{D\ (\text{IV})}{D\ (\text{oral})}$$

It is assumed after intravenous dosing that systemic availability is 100%. It should be recognized that determining systemic availability in this way does not enable one to identify the site or mechanism between the oral dose (i.e., the tablet) and the systemic circulation that is responsible for failure of a portion of the drug to reach the systemic blood.

Intravenous Infusion

After a constant intravenous infusion is begun the drug concentration gradually increases to a plateau or steady-state level (Figure 3-3A). The rate at which steady-state drug concentrations are attained is determined by the half-life of the drug. During one half-life infusions reach 50% of steady-state concentration, and in three to four half-lives approximately 90% of steady state is reached. The rate of drug administration does not influence the rate at which steady state is achieved. The latter is controlled strictly by the drug half-life. Rate does, however, determine the actual value of steady-state drug concentration. For drugs with linear

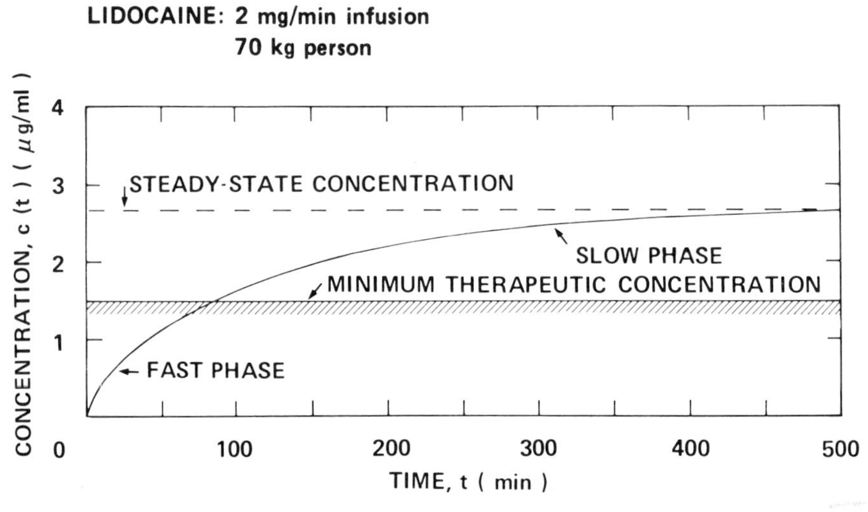

Figure 3-3A Lidocaine plasma concentration following initiation of a 2 mg/min infusion in a patient weighing 70 kg. Note that without a loading dose nearly 100 minutes are required to achieve a minimum therapeutic concentration. Steady state is not achieved until several hours have elapsed.

pharmacokinetics the steady-state drug plasma concentration (C_{SS}) is directly proportional to the infusion rate. In this situation a doubling of the infusion rate will result in a plasma steady-state concentration that is twice what would have resulted from the lower dose. At steady state the rate of drug administration (R) is equal to the rate of drug elimination (i.e., clearance), as follows:

(7) $$\text{Infusion Rate} = \text{rate of elimination}$$
$$= C_{ss} \cdot C\ell_T$$

This equation is useful in determining the infusion rate that is required to reach any given steady-state drug concentration when the clearance is known.

Multiple Oral Doses

After instituting chronic oral therapy the attainment of steady-state drug concentrations is determined by the drug half-life, just as it is in the intravenous infusion situation. At steady state the average dose rate ($\bar{R}$) (amount/time) is equal to the drug elimination rate. By employing the concept of the average drug concentration ($\overline{C}$) during a dosing interval, one can write an equation that is analogous to equation 7, as follows:

$$F \cdot \overline{R} = \overline{C} \cdot C\ell_T \tag{8}$$

This situation is analogous to a constant intravenous infusion because the time required to approach the mean plateau concentration is determined by the drug half-life, and the average drug plasma concentration at steady state is determined by the dosing rate.

Loading Doses and Drug Plasma Concentration Fluctuations During Chronic Oral Dosing

For drugs with long half-lives or in clinical situations in which it is necessary to achieve a therapeutic drug concentration very rapidly, administering the drug at a constant rate, either intravenously or by multiple oral dosing, will not achieve the required drug concentrations rapidly enough (Figure 3-3A). Therefore, a large initial, or loading, dose, which rapidly produces effective drug plasma concentrations, must be given (Figure 3-3B). The appropriate size of the loading dose can be

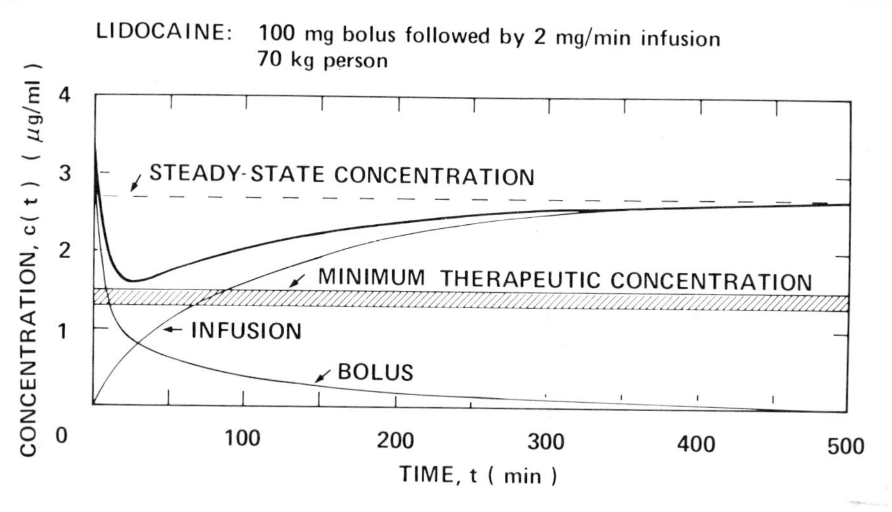

Figure 3-3B The net effect of giving an initial 100 mg bolus followed by a 2 mg/min infusion is shown. The effect of the bolus and infusion are additive. Note that shortly after initiating therapy drug concentration falls to a nadir that is near or sometimes below the minimum therapeutic concentration.

determined using equation 1 if the volume of distribution of the drug is known. For drugs whose distribution is rapid compared to elimination and that have a fairly narrow toxic to therapeutic ratio a rapid decline to subtherapeutic drug plasma concentrations may occur after a loading dose is given. Even if a constant intravenous infusion is started at the time the drug loading dose is given, a period of time during which drug concentrations are subtherapeutic may still exist. In such situations additional small extra doses of drug may be necessary to maintain therapeutic drug plasma concentrations continuously. This is especially important following the intravenous administration of lidocaine (Figure 3-3C).

In patients receiving chronic oral doses drug plasma concentrations fluctuate over one dose interval between some peak and minimal value. For general purposes the mean drug concentration over the dosing interval may be important. However, in individual patients the actual values of the peak and trough drug concentration may be important. Drugs with a short half-life will show a greater difference between peak and trough levels for a given dosing interval. A degree of acceptable

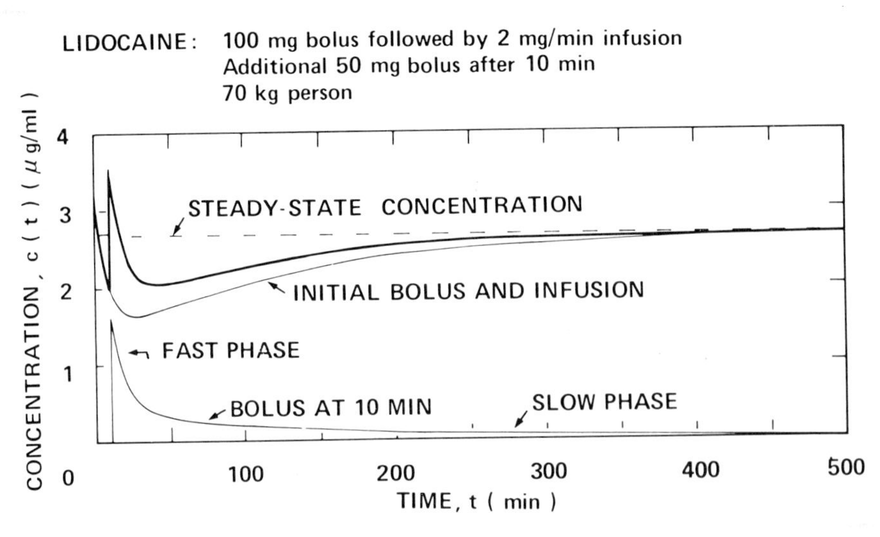

Figure 3-3C The marked fall in lidocaine concentration following initiation of a single bolus and infusion may be avoided by giving one or more additional boli during the initial loading phase. This figure shows the effect of giving an additional 50 mg bolus 10 minutes after the initial 100 mg bolus. Because lidocaine follows linear pharmacokinetics, the effect of this second bolus may be added to the effects of the initial bolus and maintenance infusion shown in Figure 3-3B.

fluctuation over a dosing interval is defined by the toxic to therapeutic ratio of a drug. A drug with a very wide toxic to therapeutic ratio may be administered only infrequently, even if it has a short half-life. In this situation a very large dose of a drug may be given, resulting in very high drug plasma concentrations. Further drug administration will not be necessary for several half-lives or longer because it may take that long for subtherapeutic drug concentrations to occur. On the other hand, a drug with a narrow toxic to therapeutic ratio must be given at more frequent dosing intervals (even if the drug half-life is long) to avoid the wide swings in drug concentration that occur with longer dosing intervals.

When monitoring drug plasma concentration, it is important to recognize that the most stable and reproducible drug plasma concentration during multiple oral dosing is the trough level. This is because peak drug concentration will be affected by the timing of blood specimens and by factors such as the amount of food in the patient's stomach at the time the drug is taken.

Nonlinear Pharmacokinetics

Thus far, only the situation of linear pharmacokinetics in which drug concentrations are proportional to the amount of drug administered has been discussed. A doubling of the dose will result in a doubling of the plasma concentration. In this setting the concentration of drug is below the maximal capacity of the drug elimination systems. In some situations drug concentration can exceed the capacity of the elimination systems so that they become saturated, and a constant amount of drug is removed in a given time. This is termed zero order kinetics. Often, situations between first and zero order kinetics occur in which less drug is removed than would be expected from a first order process, but the elimination system is not completely saturated. For such systems a greater than anticipated increase in drug plasma concentrations occurs for a given increase in dose. The half-life of the drug is not constant but rather increases as the drug plasma concentration increases. This lengthens the time that is required to reach a steady-state concentration as the dose increases. For a pure zero order kinetics situation a constant amount, as opposed to a constant fraction, of the dose is removed in a given time, and if the dosing rate exceeds the rate of removal, the drug concentration will increase indefinitely and never reach a steady state.

Drug Metabolites

Many drugs are converted to one or more metabolites, which are subsequently eliminated from the body. Remarkably little is known about the pharmacologic activity and, more importantly, the clinical significance of antiarrhythmic drug metabolites. In recent years there has been increasing interest in the study of drug metabolites. When considering the clinical importance of drug metabolites, one must assess the metabolite's pharmacologic activity, the relative potency of the active metabolite to the parent compound, and whether the metabolite accumulates sufficiently in the plasma to produce significant effects. Metabolites may have pharmacologic activity that is similar to the parent drug (with the same or different potency) or they may produce effects and side-effects that are different from those of the parent compounds. An active metabolite may contribute to the desired effect of the parent drug, compete with binding sites and diminish the effectiveness of the parent drug, or produce side-effects that limit the usefulness of the parent drug. As a general principle, most drugs with active metabolites do not accumulate them following bolus or short-term intravenous administration (Figure 3-4). Drug metabolites usually achieve importance only following oral drug administration or extremely long intravenous infusions. In most instances the relative potency of active drug metabolites to the parent compound have been determined only in animal models.

Protein Binding

Plasma protein binding of antiarrhythmic drugs may play an important role in modulating therapeutic effects. It is free drug, rather than that bound to plasma proteins, that is in equilibrium with drug receptor sites, and for most drugs the free concentration is a constant fraction of the total concentration with only a moderate interpatient variability. For highly bound (greater than 80%) drugs a small change in the percent protein binding can make a large difference in the free drug concentration. For example, a decrease in the percent protein binding from 80% to 60% would double the free drug fraction from 20% to 40% (Figure 3-5). This would result in a doubling of drug effect. Most drug assays measure total drug concentration, including both bound and unbound drug. If protein binding remains constant, the total concentration will be a direct reflection of the amount of free drug. If, however, there are changes in protein binding as a result of disease states, measurement of total drug concentration may give a misleading estimate of the amount of active (free) drug.

For some drugs protein binding is not constant over the range of plasma concentrations that are utilized clinically. Such changes have been reported for disopyramide (Meffin, et al., 1979) and lidocaine (Tucker, et al., 1970). In this situation protein binding sites presumably become saturated as the drug plasma concentration increases, and the percent of drug that is free or unbound increases disproportionately. Thus, a doubling of the drug dose and/or plasma concentration will result in a greater than doubling of the active free drug.

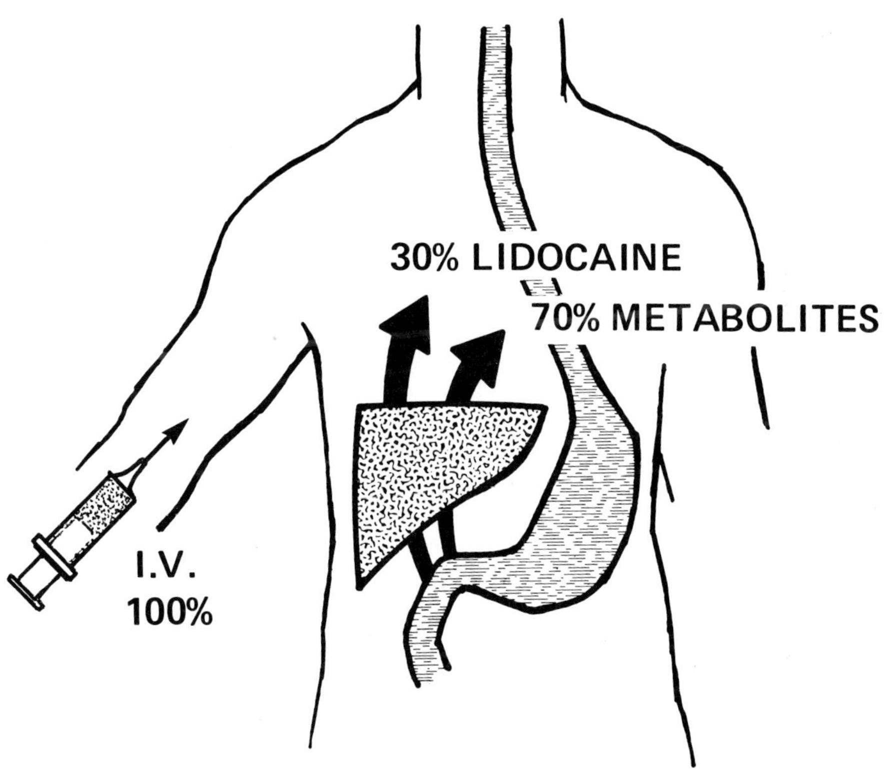

Figure 3-4 The difference between intravenous and oral lidocaine administration. When lidocaine is given directly intravenously, 100% of the drug immediately reaches the systemic circulation. When lidocaine is given orally, all of the drug passes through the liver via the portal circulation. Because of lidocaine's high first pass effect, only 30% of the oral dose of lidocaine reaches the systemic circulation unchanged, and the remainder appears as lidocaine metabolites.

Age

The age of a patient can influence the disposition of some drugs. However, little information is available regarding which antiarrhythmic drugs exhibit such changes or the clinical implications of such changes.

Renal Disease

Renal disease can affect drug disposition in several ways. The most obvious is that renal disease decreases the amount of drug that is

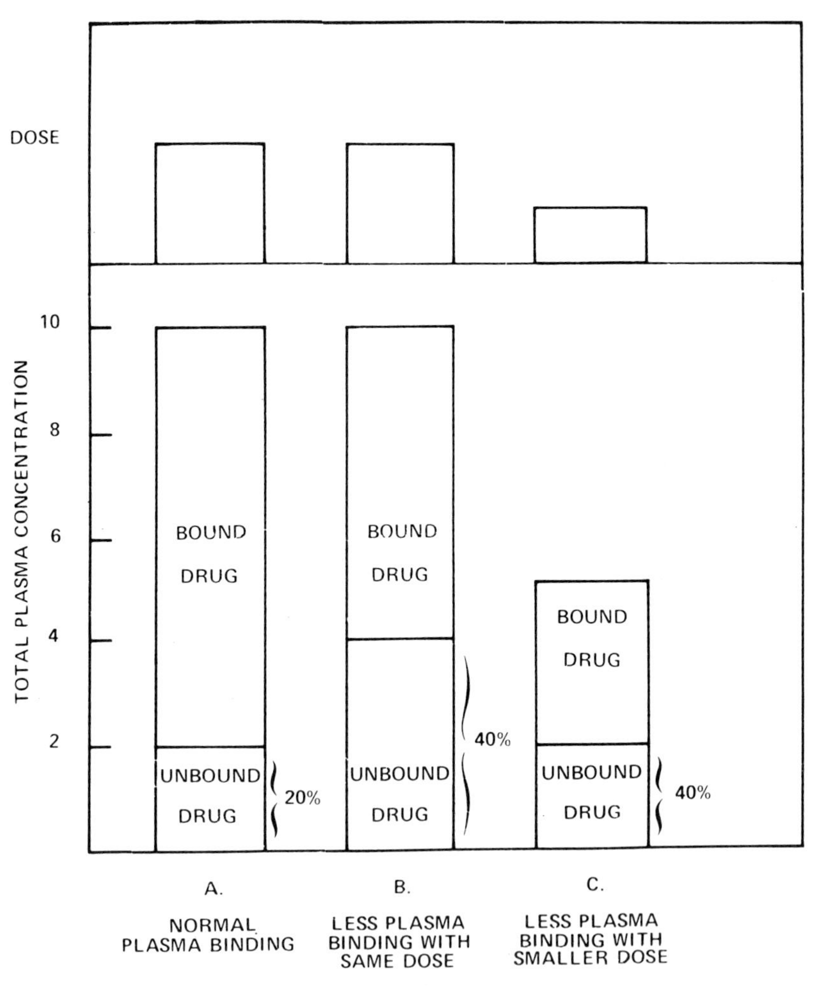

Figure 3-5 Effect of plasma protein binding on the effective plasma concentration of a hypothetical drug. In A 20% of the drug is in the unbound, and hence active, form. In B the same drug dose is given, but the plasma binding decreases and 40% of the drug is unbound. This effectively doubles the concentration of the active drug without changing the measured drug level. C shows how an appropriate reduction in dose allows the same amount of unbound drug as in situation A with only half the measured plasma level. (*Source:* Winkle, R. A.; Glantz, S. A.; and Harrison, D. C. 1975. Pharmacologic therapy of ventricular arrhythmias. *Am. J. Cardiol.* 36:629-650.)

eliminated unchanged in the urine. Drugs that are excreted primarily by the kidneys are most susceptible to such changes, and large reductions in dose may be required in patients with renal disease. It may be possible to develop nomograms indicating the appropriate reduction in dose based on creatinine clearance. In some instances renal disease may alter plasma protein binding of drugs and thus may influence pharmacokinetics. Renal failure can create problems even for some drugs that are metabolized primarily by the liver. Such drugs may have active metabolites that are eliminated by the kidneys and that can accumulate in patients with renal failure, thus accentuating the desired clinical effect or producing unwanted toxicity. In addition, inactive metabolites may accumulate, which can interfere with drug assays or compete with the active compound for binding sites.

Liver Disease

The effects of liver disease on drug disposition are complicated. In most instances there is no need to alter the dose significantly after single oral or intravenous doses because of intrinsic hepatic disease. It is most advisable during long infusions or multiple oral dosing to adjust the dose based on the drug plasma concentration. Because liver disease may affect drug protein binding, it may also be necessary to measure the fraction of the drug that is free.

Congestive Heart Failure

Congestive heart failure can have a profound effect on drug disposition. Heart failure can result in a marked alteration of regional blood flows and can produce changes in drug half-life, clearance, and volume of distribution. Drugs with high hepatic clearances that are blood-flow sensitive, such as lidocaine, may show the greatest changes in drug disposition during congestive heart failure. However, because renal blood flow may be diminished, heart failure may also influence the accumulation of drugs that are excreted by the kidneys.

Therapeutic Range

As discussed at the beginning of this section, one of the bases for the clinical application of pharmacokinetics is the premise that drug effect more closely relates to drug plasma concentration than to the dose administered. However, the therapeutic and toxic ranges of drug plasma concentrations represent no more than a statistical attempt to provide guidelines for drug administration (Figure 3-6). The end point of therapy should be a desired clinical response and not a drug plasma concentration.

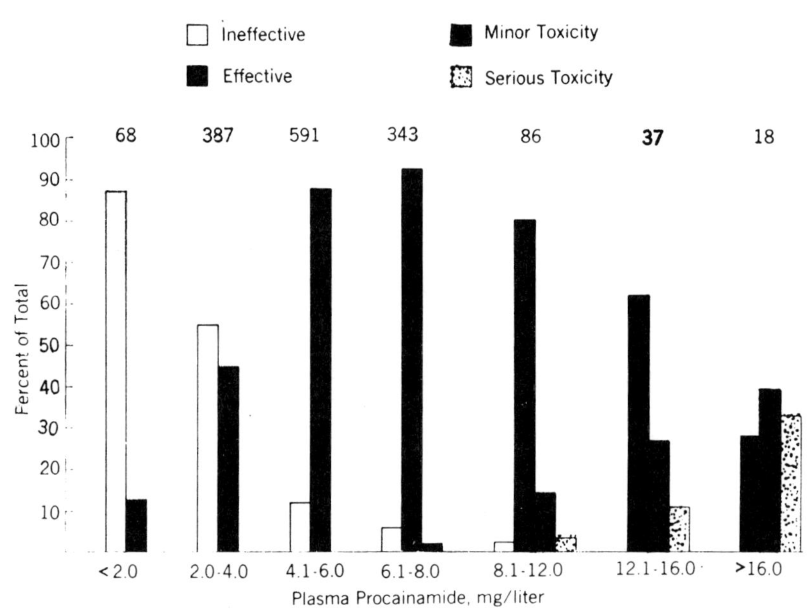

Figure 3-6 This figure shows the data on which the therapeutic concentration of procainamide is based. As can be seen, most patients are ineffectively treated at plasma concentrations below 4 mg/L. At concentrations above 8-12 mg/L the incidence of toxicity increases considerably. It should be noted, however, that some patients respond at concentrations below 4 mg/L, while others tolerate concentrations above 16 mg/L without toxicity. (*Source:* Koch-Weser, J.; and Klein, S. W. 1971. Procainamide dosage schedules, plasma concentrations, and clinical effects. *J.A.M.A.* 215:1454-1460. Copyright 1971, Americal Medical Association.)

Some individual patients may have an adequate clinical response at drug concentrations below those that are considered to be therapeutic, while some patients may experience a desired effect only at drug concentrations that are above what is considered to be in the therapeutic range. Likewise, unwanted side-effects may occur well within the drug's therapeutic range in some patients and may not be present in other patients despite drug plasma concentrations that are higher than the accepted upper limit of normal. The quoted therapeutic ranges represent only those plasma concentrations at which a therapeutic effect often occurs without significant toxicity. Whenever possible, the clinical end point should be monitored in conjunction with drug plasma concentration measurements. The ultimate end point may be either subjective, such as a change in the patient's symptoms, or objective, such as the reduction or elimination of asymptomatic arrhythmias.

CELLULAR BASIS OF ANTIARRHYTHMIC DRUG ACTION

Despite considerable knowledge about the cellular action of antiarrhythmic drugs, large gaps remain in our understanding of how these compounds affect arrhythmias in individual patients. The antiarrhythmic drugs have been divided into several classes based on their characteristic effects on the intracardiac action potential. The most widely utilized classification scheme is a modification of that initially proposed by Singh and Vaughan-Williams (1971). In this classification system the type I, or membrane-active, agents are those that affect the fast sodium channel. This class contains the largest number of antiarrhythmic drugs (see Table 3-1). Other than depressing the upstroke phase 0 of the action potential and slowing conduction in Purkinje fibers, many of the class I drugs have little in common. Some of the type I agents lengthen the action potential duration and refractoriness, whereas others shorten them. For most of these drugs, however, the net effect is to increase the ratio of effective refractory period to action potential duration. The type I agents may also exhibit significant differences in their noncardiac actions. Some, such as quinidine, procainamide, and phenytoin, are potent peripheral vasodilators, and others, such as tocainide, increase systemic vascular resistance. These peripheral drug actions can modulate a drug's direct cardiac effects via baroreceptor activation. Some of the type I agents, such as quinidine, disopyramide, and procainamide, have anticholinergic (vagolytic) effects. Clinical experience has shown that patients can have an excellent response to one type I antiarrhythmic agent and no response to another.

In this classification scheme the beta blocking drugs are considered as a separate class (class II) of antiarrhythmic drugs. Most beta blocking drugs exert their antiarrhythmic actions predominantly via beta blockade, although some, such as propranolol, do have class I membrane activity at higher plasma concentrations (Woosley, et al., 1979). Beta blocking drugs can also influence slow channel-dependent late after-depolarizations because the magnitude of these afterpotentials may be enhanced by catecholamines. The class III antiarrhythmic drugs are those that prolong the action potential duration with little or no effect on the fast or slow channels. Amiodarone and bretylium are the two most widely encountered examples of class III antiarrhythmic agents, although a recent study suggests that amiodarone may indeed have some sodium channel blocking properties (Mason, et al., 1982). Class IV antiarrhythmic drugs are those that block the slow calcium channels. Verapamil is the most widely utilized antiarrhythmic drug in this class, although diltiazem may have similar antiarrhythmic properties. Although nifedipine is a slow channel calcium blocker, it has no effect on the slow channels of the SA or AV nodes and is not considered an antiarrhythmic agent.

Table 3-1 Classification of antiarrhythmic drugs

Category	Action
Type I	Depress fast sodium channels
	A. Quinidine Procainamide Disopyramide Propafenone
	B. Lidocaine Mexiletine Tocainide Phenytoin
	C. Encainide Aprindine Lorcainide Flecainide
Type II	Beta blocking agents
	Acebutolol Alprenolol Atenolol Metoprolol Nadolol Oxprenolol Pindolol Practolol Propranolol Sotalol Timolol
Type III	Prolong refractory period, little effect on conduction
	Amiodarone Bretylium ? N-acetylprocainamide
Type IV	Calcium channel blockers
	Diltiazem Verapamil

The exact mechanism by which a drug's cellular electrophysiologic properties translate into termination or prevention of cardiac arrhythmias is poorly understood. For reentrant arrhythmias, slowing of conduction velocity can convert areas of unidirectional block to areas of bidirectional block and thus prohibit initiation of the arrhythmia. Likewise, acceleration of conduction can eliminate unidirectional block completely. For an already established reentrant arrhythmia critical changes in conduction velocity and/or tissue refractoriness will terminate the arrhythmias.

Calcium channel blockers can theoretically eliminate arrhythmias caused by early and late after-depolarizations. Almost all antiarrhythmic drugs are capable of depressing spontaneous automaticity in one or more types of cardiac tissue, and these properties may also contribute to their antiarrhythmic effects. The antiarrhythmic drugs are presumed to have a greater effect on areas of abnormal electrophysiology as opposed to areas with normal electrophysiology.

CHOICE OF ANTIARRHYTHMIC DRUGS FOR SPECIFIC ARRHYTHMIAS

The large number of antiarrhythmic drugs (Winkle, et al., 1975; Harrison, et al., 1977; Anderson, et al., 1978a) and other treatment modalities that are now available to the clinician can cause confusion as to the therapy of choice for treating a specific arrhythmia. Although there are always certain dangers in trying to establish a "cookbook" approach to the treatment of cardiac arrhythmias, Table 3-2 summarizes the most effective treatments for commonly encountered arrhythmias. It should be emphasized that in many instances the clinical setting will determine the most appropriate treatment modality. For instance, a critically ill patient who is not tolerating a sustained tachyarrhythmia should be treated promptly with cardioversion when this is an option, whereas in more stable clinical situations initial attempts at pharmacologic conversion may be permitted. The specific doses and side-effects of these drugs are given in the next section of this chapter, and the specific arrhythmias are discussed in Chapters 8, 9, and 10. The therapy of arrhythmias caused by digitalis intoxication is covered in detail in Chapter 12.

PHARMACOLOGY, CLINICAL USES, AND SIDE-EFFECTS OF THE ANTIARRHYTHMIC DRUGS

During the 1970s many new compounds were introduced for the pharmacologic termination or prevention of cardiac arrhythmias. The increase in knowledge of the clinical pharmacology and basic and clinical electrophysiology permits the more rational use of these compounds. No single compound represents a "miracle drug" that can control arrhythmias in all patients without side-effects. Detailed knowledge of each drug (available to the physician) and a thorough understanding of the patient and the arrhythmia being treated will optimize the chance of drug success and minimize the chance of side-effects. The following section will provide information about the pharmacology, clinical uses, and side-effects of a number of traditional and investigational antiarrhythmic drugs. Table 3-3 summarizes these data.

Table 3-2 Therapy of commonly encountered (nondigitalis intoxication-induced) arrhythmias

Arrhythmia	Immediate or prompt termination	Chronic prophylaxis
Intra-AV nodal reentry supraventricular tachycardia (SVT)*	Vagal maneuvers IV verapamil IV edrophonium IV digitalis IV propranolol IV procainamide Pacemaker Cardioversion	Digitalis Beta blocking drug Verapamil Quinidine Procainamide Disopyramide‡ Amiodarone
AV reciprocating using AV node and bypass*	Vagal maneuvers IV verapamil IV edrophonium IV propranolol IV procainamide Pacemaker Cardioversion	**First choice** Quinidine Lorcainide Amiodarone **Second choice** Procainamide Disopyramide‡ Verapamil† Digoxin†
Atrial fibrillation and flutter	Cardioversion Oral quinidine loading Pacemaker (flutter only) For rate control Digoxin† Verapamil† Beta blocking drug	**First choice** Quinidine Amiodarone **Second choice** Procainamide Verapamil Disopyramide‡
Ventricular ectopic beats or nonsustained ventricular salvos	IV lidocaine IV procainamide	**First choice** Quinidine Lorcainide Flecainide Encainide Propafenone **Second choice** Procainamide Mexiletine Tocainide Disopyramide‡ Beta blocking drugs‡
Sustained ventricular tachycardia	IV lidocaine Cardioversion IV procainamide	**First choice** Quinidine Lorcainide Amiodarone

Arrhythmia	Immediate or prompt termination	Chronic prophylaxis
		Second choice Procainamide Mexiletine Tocainide Verapamil Beta blocking drugs‡ **Toxic but effective** Encainide Aprindine Disopyramide‡
Polymorphic ventricular tachycardia caused by QT prolongation	Overdrive pacemaker Isoproterenol infusion	Withdraw drugs
Ventricular fibrillation	Cardioversion Cardioversion plus IV lidocaine Cardioversion plus IV bretylium	Treatment same as for sustained ventricular tachycardia

*Frequently the mechanism is not known at the time of acute therapy (commonly called PSVT).

†If antegrade preexcitation (i.e., Wolff-Parkinson-White syndrome) is present, electrophysiologic study is required prior to use.

‡If ventricular function permits.

CLASS I AND III DRUGS

Amiodarone

Pharmacology Amiodarone was first introduced as an antianginal agent, but it has since been found to be an effective antiarrhythmic drug. Although it has a slight intrinsic myocardial depressant effect, its vasodilating properties reduce afterload and increase coronary blood flow, and it is well tolerated in most patients with left ventricular dysfunction. The primary electrophysiologic effect of amiodarone is a prolongation of atrial and ventricular muscle action potential duration with a minor effect on the rate of phase 4 diastolic depolarization (Singh and Vaughan-Williams, 1970). In humans it prolongs the refractory periods of the atrium, AV node, and ventricle and causes some AH and HV interval prolongation (Wellens, et al., 1976). Amiodarone also prolongs the refractoriness of accessory pathways in preexcitation syndromes with a

Table 3-3 Pharmacokinetic properties, dose, and important side-effects of antiarrhythmic drugs

	Amiodarone	Aprindine	Bretylium
Administration	Oral	Oral	Oral, parenteral
Therapeutic plasma range (μg/mL)	0.2-5.0	1-2	0.070-0.46
Systemic availability	—	>90%	0.22 (0.11-0.32)
Plasma clearance (mL/min/kg)	—	2.6	18 (oral) 4.4 (IV)
Volume of distribution (L/kg)	—	V_c 1.7 Vd_{ss} 3.7	Vd_{ss} 3.4
Half-life*	13-60 days	$t_{1/2\alpha}$ 1.7 h $t_{1/2\beta}$ 30 h	13.5 h
Percentage of dose excreted unchanged in urine	<1%	<1%	>80%
Plasma protein binding	—	85%-95%	1%
Commonly used dose	200-800 mg/day	Loading: 200-400 mg Maintenance: 100-200 mg/day, 1-2 doses	IV: 5 mg/kg, slow injection bolus Maintenance: 1-4 mg/min Oral: 200-600 mg q8h
Side-effects	Corneal deposits, altered thyroid function, liver dysfunction, CNS (cerebellar), pulmonary fibrosis	CNS (tremor), conduction block, agranulocytosis	Hypotension, nausea and vomiting, parotid pain
Known active metabolites	desethylamiodarone (? active)	desethylaprindine	—

Diltiazem	Disopyramide	Encainide	Flecainide
Oral, parenteral	Oral, parenteral	Oral, parenteral	Oral, parenteral
—	3-6 (total drug)	Uncertain because of active metabolites	0.3-1.3
—	0.83	0.42 (0.07-0.82)	95
16	3.4†	13	—
$V_{d_{ss}}$ 4.0	V_c 0.13† $V_{d_{ss}}$ 1.3	—	—
2-8 h	$t_{½\alpha}$ 2 min $t_{½\beta}$ 4.5 h	1.5-3.0 h (metabolites longer)	18.8 h
<5%	52%	Low	—
70%-86%	35%-95% over therapeutic range (concentration-dependent)	—	—
IV: 15-25 mg Oral: 60-90 mg q6h	150-300 mg q6h	Oral: 25-50 mg q6-8h IV: 1 mg/kg over 15 minutes	Oral: 100-300 mg q12h
Pedal edema	Cardiac depression, anticholinergic, malignant arrhythmias	Cardiac (malignant arrhythmias, excessive QRS widening), CNS (dizziness, visual disturbances)	CNS (blurred vision, lightheadedness, (ataxia), elevated alkaline phosphatase, malignant arrhythmias
desacetyl-diltiazem	mono-N-dealkylated disopyramide	0-demethyl-encainide; 3-methoxy-0-demethylencainide	

Table 3-3 (Continued)

	Lidocaine	Lorcainide	Mexiletine
Administration	Parenteral	Oral, parenteral	Oral
Therapeutic plasma range (μg/mL)	2-6	0.050-0.200 (lorcainide) 0.080-0.400 (norlorcainide)	0.5-2.0
Systemic availability	Low	Low (single dose) High (multiple doses)	High
Plasma clearance (mL/min/kg)	10	23	$\cong$ 5
Volume of distribution (L/kg)	V_c 0.5 $V_{d_{ss}}$ 1.3	—	$V_{d_{ss}} \cong 5$
Half-life*	$t_{1/2\alpha}$ 8 min $t_{1/2\beta}$ 108 min	7-10 h ($\cong$ 24 h norlorcainide)	10-20 h
Percentage of dose excreted unchanged in urine	<5%	3%	10%
Plasma protein binding	40%-80%	73%-85%	70%
Commonly used dose	Loading: 1-2 mg/kg slow injection Maintenance: 20-40 μg/kg/min	Oral: 100-200 mg q12h IV: 1 mg/kg over 15 minutes	Loading: 400-600 mg Maintenance: 150-300 mg orally q6-8h
Side-effects	CNS	CNS (sleep disturbances, tremor) hyponatremia	CNS (tremor), cardiovascular (IV)
Known active metabolites	monoethyl-glycinexylidide; glycinexylidide	norlorcainide	—

N-acetyl-procainamide	Phenytoin	Procainamide	Propafenone
Oral	Oral, parenteral	Oral, parenteral	Oral, parenteral
—	10-18	4-10	0.06-1.0
0.85	0.98	0.75-0.90	Nonlinear
3	≅ 0.3 at linear kinetics	11.8	—
V_c 0.7 $V_{d_{ss}}$ 1.5	$V_{d_{ss}}$ 0.5-0.8	V_c 0.1 $V_{d_{ss}}$ 2.2	—
6-11 h	Dose-dependent (8-60 h; average 22 h)	$t_{½α}$ 5 min $t_{½β}$ 2.5-4.7 h	3-6 h
85%	<5%	50%-60%	—
11%	88%-96%	15%	—
Oral: 1000-2500 mg q8h	Oral: 200-400 mg/day in 1-2 doses IV: 10-12 mg/kg slowly, over 40-60 minutes	Oral: 250-1000 mg q4h IV: loading 10-12 mg/kg over 40-60 minutes	Oral: 150-300 mg q6-8h IV: 1-2 mg/kg over 10 minutes
Nausea, visual disturbances	CNS, cardio-vascular	Hypotension, immunologic	Funny taste, dry mouth, gastrointestinal CNS, hepatitis
—	—	N-acetyl-procainamide	—

Table 3-3 (Continued)

	Quinidine	Tocainide	Verapamil
Administration	Oral, parenteral	Oral, parenteral	Oral, parenteral
Therapeutic plasma range (μg/mL)	2-5	4-10	—
Systemic availability	0.8 (0.4-0.9)	1.0	0.22-0.35
Plasma clearance (mL/min/kg)	4.7 (1.5-7.0)	2.2	8-20
Volume of distribution (L/kg)	V_c 0.9 Vd_{ss} 3.0	V_c 1.0 Vd_{ss} 1.6	Vd_{ss} 3-6
Half-life*	6.3 (3-16) h	13.5 h	4-8 h
Percentage of dose excreted unchanged in urine	20%	40% (20%-70%)	<1%
Plasma protein binding	60%-90%	50%	90%
Commonly used dose	Oral: 200-600 mg q6-8h IV: slowly 6-10 mg/kg over 20-45 minutes	Oral: 400-600 mg q8h	Oral: 80-160 mg q8h IV: 10-20 mg, slow injection
Side-effects	Cardiac, gastro-intestinal, hematologic, fever	CNS (tremor), nausea	Cardiac depression, hypotension, constipation
Known active metabolites	3-hydroxyquinidine	—	norverapamil

*Elimination half-life ($t_{1/2\beta}$) unless stated otherwise.

†Calculated from concentration of unbound (free drug).

Abbreviations: V_c = volume of the central compartment; Vd_{ss} = volume of distribution at steady state; $t_{1/2\beta}$ = slow or elimination half-life; $t_{1/2\alpha}$ = fast or distribution half-life; IV = intravenous; CNS = central nervous system.

Table compiled with data from: Anderson, et al., 1978; Anderson, et al., 1980; Anderson, et al., 1981a; Anderson, et al., 1981b; Keefe, et al., 1982; Winkle, et al., 1981c; Harris, et al., 1981; Haffajee, et al., 1981; Kates, 1982; Duff, et al., 1981; Kates, et al., 1981.

greater effect on AV than on VA conduction. On the surface ECG amiodarone causes a slowing of the sinus rate, PR interval prolongation, and ventricular repolarization abnormalities, including T and U wave changes and prolonged QT intervals. Amiodarone is used predominantly in its oral form as a once daily dose of 200-800 mg. The lower doses are often effective in the control of supraventricular arrhythmias, and the higher doses are required to treat malignant ventricular arrhythmias. Following single oral doses of 800 mg peak plasma concentrations of amiodarone of 2.8-7.7 μg/mL have been reported (Haffajee, et al., 1981). These levels fall rapidly, and during chronic oral maintenance therapy steady state is not achieved for several weeks or longer. This explains the clinical observation that following the institution of chronic oral maintenance therapy antiarrhythmic effect may not be seen for several weeks (Rosenbaum, et al., 1974). At the time of arrhythmia control, plasma concentrations of amiodarone are 0.2-5.2 μg/mL and those of its metabolite desethylamiodarone are 0.3-4.7 μg/mL (Harris, et al., 1981). The relative contribution of each of these plasma concentrations to the antiarrhythmic activity is unknown. When the drug is discontinued, antiarrhythmic effect may persist for 1 month or longer. Following drug withdrawal the half-life of amiodarone has been measured from 13 to 60 days, and the drug can be detected in the plasma for over 1 year.

Therapeutic uses Amiodarone has a broad range of clinical uses (Rosenbaum, et al., 1974; Rosenbaum, et al., 1976). It is effective in the treatment of all paroxysmal supraventricular arrhythmias, including atrial fibrillation, atrial flutter, and reentrant supraventricular tachycardias. Amiodarone is especially useful in the prevention of reciprocating tachycardia associated with the preexcitation syndromes and can prevent a rapid ventricular response to atrial fibrillation and flutter in these conditions. It can suppress ventricular ectopic activity and prevent sustained and life-threatening ventricular tachycardia and fibrillation. Patients with the latter condition may not experience recurrences of sustained ventricular tachycardia or fibrillation while taking amiodarone, even though these arrhythmias remain inducible during electrophysiologic drug testing.

Side-effects Amiodarone is an iodinated compound and may interfere with thyroid metabolism, causing hypo- or hyperthyroidism (Pritchard, et al., 1975). Thyroid function tests should be performed during long-term amiodarone administration, although only a few patients will develop clinically important abnormalities. Corneal microdeposits occur in all patients receiving amiodarone; however, they interfere with vision in only a few patients and are completely reversible upon cessation of therapy. Amiodarone may elevate serum digoxin levels and may potentiate the action of oral anticoagulants. Photosensitivity dermatitis occurs in a high percentage of fair-skinned patients who are treated in sunny climates. Infrequently, a bluish or gray discoloration of the skin may also occur, and some patients develop petechiae, especially on the forearms. Patients may occasionally develop gastrointestinal side-effects such as nausea, vomiting, and constipation. When nausea is related to large drug doses, it may be minimized by giving the drug in divided doses. Cerebellar signs and symptoms may occur after many months of receiving high doses but usually respond to a dose reduction. Liver function abnormalities and more severe hepatic dysfunction may occur, as well as occasional cases of interstitial pulmonary infiltrates. These pulmonary infiltrates may be life-threatening (Sobel and Rakita, 1982) and may occur in up to 10% of patients treated with higher doses of amiodarone. The drug should be used with caution in patients who have serious conduction delays or pronounced sinus node dysfunction. In rate cases amiodarone will worsen ventricular arrhythmias. This can be an especially difficult side-effect to deal with because of the long persistence of the drug's effects.

Aprindine

Pharmacology Aprindine is a membrane active agent whose predominant electrophysiologic effect is to slow the upstroke velocity of phase 0 of the action potential in isolated atrial, ventricular, and Purkinje fibers (Verdonck, et al., 1974; Elharrar, et al., 1975). Aprindine shortens the action potential duration (APD) and the effective refractory period (ERP) in isolated Purkinje fibers but increases the ratio of the ERP to APD (Steinberg and Greenspan, 1976). In man a prolongation of the PR interval occurs, which is caused by prolongation of both AH and HV intervals, and an increase in the QRS duration of 10%-20% happens in therapeutic doses (Schlepper and Neuss, 1974; Zipes, et al., 1977). Aprindine lengthens the effective refractory period of the atria, AV node, and ventricle. The drug is also successful in blocking conduction in accessory pathways in the Wolff-Parkinson-White syndrome and has its greatest effect on AV as opposed to VA conduction (Zipes, et al., 1977). The drug has a modest hemodynamic depressant effect but only rarely aggravates congestive heart failure. Intravenous doses of up to 200 mg may be administered at a rate not exceeding 20 mg/min. Measurements of arterial pressure and ECG recordings should be performed frequently during intravenous infusion. Oral aprindine therapy is usually given as a loading dose of 200-400 mg followed by maintenance doses of 100-200 mg/day given in two divided doses. The drug is well absorbed after oral administration except in the first few hours following a myocardial infarction. Less than 1% of the dose is excreted unchanged in the urine. Aprindine has complex pharmacokinetics following multiple oral dosing and has a long half-life of 24-30 hours. The drug is 85%-95% bound to plasma proteins (Fasola and Carmichael, 1974).

Therapeutic uses Aprindine has a broad spectrum of antiarrhythmic activity. It is effective against a variety of paroxysmal supraventricular arrhythmias, including atrial fibrillation, atrial flutter, reentry within the AV node, and reciprocating tachycardia in the Wolff-Parkinson-White syndrome (Zipes, et al., 1977). Aprindine can successfully block AV conduction via accessory pathways and is useful in the treatment of atrial fibrillation and flutter in patients with the Wolff-Parkinson-White syndrome. The drug is effective against ventricular ectopic activity and recurrent sustained ventricular tachycardia and fibrillation (Fasola and Carmichael, 1974).

Side-effects Aprindine has a narrow therapeutic to toxic ratio. The usual therapeutic plasma concentration is 1-2 μg/mL, and troublesome neurologic side-effects such as dizziness, tremor, and, on rare occasions, seizures can occur at levels in or just above this range. Careful titration of the dose may minimize these side-effects. Underlying conduction system disease and severe left ventricular dysfunction may be exacerbated by aprindine. Gastrointestinal side-effects are infrequent, but there have been a few cases of cholestatic jaundice reported. The occurrence of agranulocytosis has limited the widespread distribution of this drug, and hematologic function should be monitored frequently during therapy. In most instances this potentially fatal side-effect can be reversed by discontinuing the drug.

Bretylium

Pharmacology Bretylium was introduced as an antihypertensive agent and was subsequently found to have antiarrhythmic activity. The drug causes an initial release of norepinephrine from adrenergic nerve endings, which causes a sympathomimetic action. This results in a rise in heart rate, arterial pressure, and myocardial contractility. The drug subsequently blocks norepinephrine release, causing a fall in blood pressure that is especially prominent when the patient assumes an upright posture. The initial electrophysiologic effects of the drug mimic catecholamine administration; however, it subsequently lengthens the action potential duration and effective refractory period of His-Purkinje fibers (Wit, et al., 1970; Bigger and Jaffe, 1971). Bretylium has little effect on atrial muscle (Papp and Vaughan-Williams, 1969), but has potent antifibrillatory action in ventricular muscle (Bacaner, 1966). Bretylium is frequently administered intravenously in nonemergency situations in a dose of 5-10 mg/kg given slowly and as a rapid bolus in the presence of recurring or sustained ventricular fibrillation. Following successful intravenous administration, a maintenance dose of 1-2 mg/min may be given by constant infusion. The drug is absorbed erratically after oral administration, and the usual oral dose is 200-600 mg every 6-8 hours. Bretylium is excreted largely unchanged in the urine. The half-life is approximately 10-13.5 hours (Romhilt, et al., 1972; Anderson, et al., 1980a; Anderson, et al., 1981).

Therapeutic uses Bretylium plays only a very minimal role in the treatment of supraventricular arrhythmias. Its primary use is for managing refractory ventricular tachycardia and fibrillation. On rare occasions it may chemically defibrillate the ventricles (Sanna and Arcidiacono, 1973), but it is most often used to successfully defibrillate previously resistant ventricular fibrillation (Holder, et al., 1977). Bretylium is generally a second-line agent in this situation to be used after lidocaine has failed. It is also valuable in maintaining sinus rhythm when successful defibrillation occurs but ventricular tachycardia or fibrillation promptly recurs. Bretylium should not be given to patients with hemodynamically well-tolerated ventricular tachycardia unless cardioversion and other drugs have failed, because the drug may fail to convert the arrhythmia and the patient may be left with a hypotensive ventricular tachycardia. In this situation the hypotension is caused by bretylium's peripheral action and not the arrhythmia.

Side-effects The most frequent side-effect of bretylium is hypotension caused by its adrenergic neuronal effects. This is usually postural, but severe hypotension may occur even in the supine state. Excessive hypotension may be treated by cautious volume expansion or by the use of norepinephrine. However, catecholamine hypersensitivity may develop, and pressor agents should be administered initially in lower than usual doses. Nausea and vomiting may occur and are often related to excessive hypotension. Postural hypotension resulting from bretylium often limits the long-term oral use of the drug, although tolerance is said to develop after long periods of treatment. Preliminary studies suggest that concomitant administration of tricyclic antidepressants can minimize the hypotensive effects of bretylium without antagonizing its antiarrhythmic effects (Reele, et al., 1978). Limited data are available about the effects of long-term oral use of the drug, but pain and tenderness of the parotid glands may occur. Aggravation of ventricular arrhythmias shortly after administration of bretylium caused by catecholamine release from adrenergic nerve endings is a theoretical, although poorly documented, adverse effect.

Disopyramide

Pharmacology Disopyramide is a membrane-active agent whose direct effect is to slow conduction in the atrium, AV node, His-Purkinje system, and ventricular muscle and to prolong the refractory period of the atrium, AV node, and ventricle (Dreifus, et al., 1973; Kus and Sasyniuk, 1975; Danilo, et al., 1977). The drug also suppresses phase 4 diastolic depolarization in most cardiac tissues. Its direct effects on the sinus node and AV node are often opposed by its vagolytic effects, and the net effect on the sinus node automaticity and AV nodal conduction may be minimal. Disopyramide may prolong the HV interval and QRS duration and can precipitate conduction disturbances in patients with preexisting disease. It may cause modest prolongation of the PR and QRS intervals at higher doses and routinely prolongs the QT interval. The drug slows conduction in accessory pathways in the Wolff-Parkinson-White syndrome (Spurrell, et al., 1975). Disopyramide may be used orally or intravenously and is nearly completely absorbed following oral administration. The usual oral dose is 100-150 mg every 6 hours, and the therapeutic concentration is 3-6 μg/mL. The fraction of the drug that binds to plasma proteins is a function of plasma concentration, and the percent of free (and presumably active) drug increases at higher plasma concentrations (Meffin, et al., 1979). Disopyramide has serious myocardial depressant effects (see the section on toxicity), and for this reason we only use it in selected cases.

Therapeutic uses Disopyramide is effective in the treatment of a broad spectrum of arrhythmias, including atrial fibrillation and flutter, AV nodal reentrant supraventricular tachycardia and reciprocating tachycardia, and atrial fibrillation or flutter that occurs in association with the Wolff-Parkinson-White syndrome. Disopyramide effectively suppresses ventricular ectopic activity (Vismara, et al., 1974) and is used in treating recurrent ventricular tachycardia and fibrillation (Vismara, et al., 1977).

Side-effects The most frequent side-effects of disopyramide are caused by its anticholinergic actions. Dry mouth is almost universal in patients receiving adequate doses. Although bothersome, this side-effect rarely limits long-term therapy. Constipation, blurred vision, and urinary hesitancy can also occur. The latter problem limits the use of the drug in elderly males, especially those who have prostatic symptoms. Acute and chronic urinary obstruction, urinary tract infection, and obstructive uropathy can also occur. Disopyramide can aggravate conduction disturbances and can precipitate serious, life-threatening ventricular arrhythmias. These are generally associated with QT prolongation and a torsade de pointe ECG morphology similar to that seen in quinidine syncope. The most serious side-effect of the drug is myocardial depression. In critically ill patients with preexisting depression of myocardial function disopyramide can precipitate cardiogenic shock (Story, et al., 1979). If the cardiogenic shock is not recognized as caused by the drug, it may be attributed to the patient's underlying heart disease and may result in death. Cardiogenic shock usually resolves promptly with appropriate supportive therapy and discontinuation of the drug. Many patients with a history of left ventricular dysfunction will develop worsening of heart failure during chronic oral therapy (Podrid, et al., 1980).

Encainide

Pharmacology Encainide is a membrane-active antiarrhythmic drug whose predominant effect is on cardiac conduction. It significantly decreases the rate of rise of the upstroke (phase 0) of the action potential and minimally shortens the action potential duration in isolated His-Purkinje fibers (Gibson, et al., 1978). Immediately following intravenous doses in humans it has little effect on atrial, AV nodal, or ventricular refractory periods but causes a 20%-40% prolongation of the HV interval and intraventricular conduction as measured by the QRS duration (Sami, et al., 1979). Changes reflected on the surface ECG during long-term therapy include prolongation of the PR interval and widening of the QRS complex up to 40%-50% in some patients. Little prolongation of the overall QT interval occurs other than that accounted for by prolongation of the QRS complex. Studies on encainide done an hour or so after intravenous dosing or during oral therapy have shown prolongation of refractoriness of the atrium, AV node, and ventricle, presumably caused by the accumulation of active metabolites. The drug exhibits marked interpatient variation in bioavailability and has a half-life that averages less than 3 hours (Winkle, et al., 1981c). Encainide has several metabolites with half-lives that are longer than the parent compound, and these metabolites contribute to the drug's antiarrhythmic action (Winkle, et al., 1981d) (Figure 3-7). These metabolites may not reach steady state until after 5-7 days of encainide therapy. The usual intravenous dose of encainide is 1 mg/kg, and oral maintenance doses range from 100 to 240 mg/day given in three or four divided doses. Single intravenous doses of the drug result in a modest decrease in cardiac output, but the drug can be safely given to most patients with left ventricular dysfunction without clinical deterioration.

Therapeutic uses Encainide is one of the most effective agents for suppressing chronic ventricular ectopic activity and frequently results in complete or nearly complete suppression of this arrhythmia (Roden, et al., 1980a; Winkle, et al., 1981). It is also valuable in treating recurrent sustained ventricular tachycardia (Mason and Peters, 1981). Although encainide is effective for treating selected patients with supraventricular arrhythmias, little systematic study of its value in treating these arrhythmias has been conducted.

Side-effects Although encainide routinely prolongs the PR interval and QRS duration by up to 25%-50%, second- or third-degree heart block is uncommon. Neurologic side-effects include blurred vision, paresthesias, and dizziness. The most serious side-effect of encainide is the production of life-threatening ventricular tachyarrhythmias. These arrhythmias are uncommon in patients without a history of previous sustained ventricular

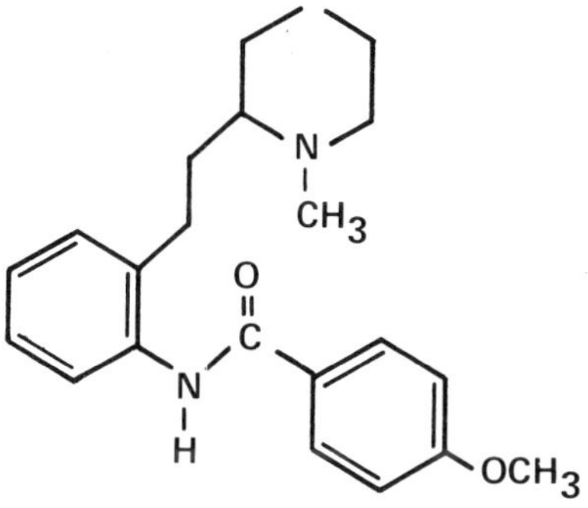

ENCAINIDE

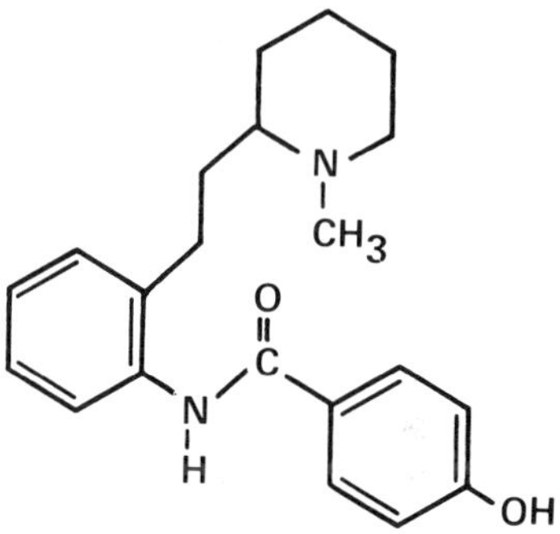

O-DEMETHYLENCAINIDE (ODE)

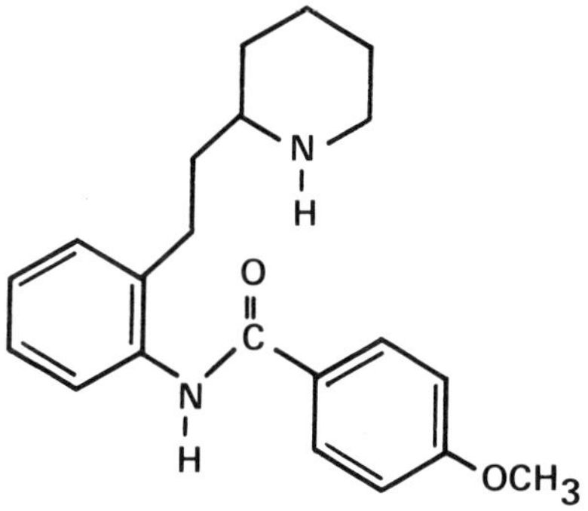

N-DEMETHYLENCAINIDE (NDE)

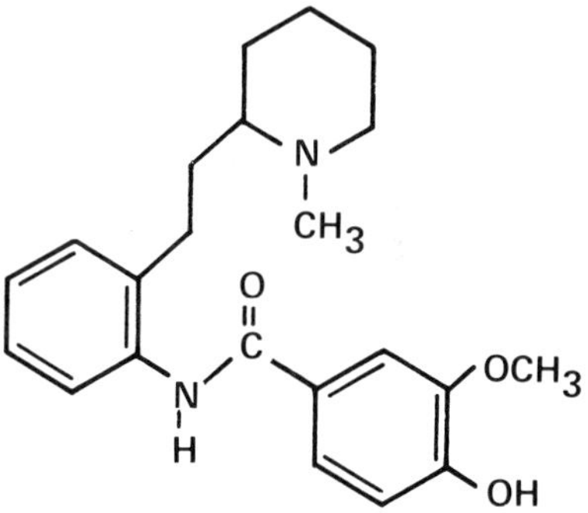

3-METHOXY-ODE (MODE)

Figure 3-7 Encainide and three of its known metabolites. ODE and MODE are present in approximately 90% of patients who are receiving encainide at plasma concentrations that are approximately five times those of unchanged encainide. NDE is produced in only a minority of patients receiving encainide.

tachycardia or fibrillation. In this latter group, however, ventricular arrhythmias occur in up to 12% of patients (Winkle, et al., 1981b). They may occur 1-2 hours after a single, large intravenous or oral dose and/or 20-40 hours after institution of chronic oral maintenance therapy or after a dose increase. These arrhythmias are not necessarily preceded by QT prolongation, are frequently sustained, may require cardiopulmonary resuscitation, and can be difficult to treat. All patients with a history of sustained ventricular tachycardia or fibrillation should receive encainide only in a hospital setting where monitoring and full resuscitative capabilities are available. Patients should not have a dose increase more frequently than every 72 hours and should not be discharged from the hospital until they have been on their final dose of encainide for at least 72 hours.

Flecainide

Pharmacology Flecainide acetate is a new fluorinated antiarrhythmic compound that has been recently introduced for clinical trials. In an animal model it prolongs the effective refractory period of the atrium slightly, prolongs the refractory period of the AV node, and lengthens the AH and HV conduction times (Hodess, et al., 1979). In humans therapeutic concentrations of the drug result in an average 37% prolongation of the PR interval, 26% prolongation of the QRS interval, and a 14% prolongation of the QT interval (Duff, et al., 1981). Although the hemodynamic actions have not been directly studied, no apparent changes have been noted on two-dimensional echocardiography during oral therapy. The half-life of flecainide averages 18.8-20.3 hours in patients with ventricular ectopic beats (Anderson, et al., 1981b; Duff, et al., 1981). Suppression of ventricular ectopic beats occurs at plasma concentrations that range from approximately 300 to 1300 ng/mL. Most patients can receive twice daily dosing with a usual total daily dose of 200-600 mg. The toxic and therapeutic ranges appear to overlap.

Therapeutic uses The only clinical trials of flecainide to date have evaluated its efficacy for the suppression of chronic ventricular ectopic beats (Hodges, et al., 1982). The drug is highly effective in the suppression of ventricular ectopic beats in most patients, showing a greater than 90% reduction and suppression of repetitive forms. No studies of its safety and/or efficacy in patients with more serious ventricular arrhythmias have been reported.

Side-effects Frequently occurring side-effects of flecainide include blurred vision and dizziness or light-headedness. A few patients have noted an unusual taste, flushing, tinnitus, sleepiness, parethesias, and headaches. During long-term therapy some patients have exhibited a slightly elevated alkaline phosphatase (Duff, et al., 1981). Because the drug is a fluorinated compound, it has been speculated that the elevated alkaline phosphatase results from some alteration in bone metabolism. In Duff's study several patients experienced a paradoxical increase in the frequency of ventricular ectopic beats during therapy with flecainide, and ventricular tachycardia has appeared for the first time in one patient who had previously only shown ventricular ectopic beats. Recently it has been suspected of inducing malignant arrhythmias in some patients.

Lidocaine

Pharmacology Lidocaine is a local anesthetic antiarrhythmic drug that slows phase 0 upstroke velocity and shortens the action potential duration in isolated healthy His-Purkinje fibers (Singh and Vaughan-Williams, 1971); its electrophysiologic actions may differ in diseased tissues. It has little effect on atrial tissue. In humans the drug shortens ventricular refractoriness minimally (Josephson, et al., 1972) and has little effect on cardiac conduction. In usual doses lidocaine has no significant hemodynamic effects, and it may be administered to patients with severe left ventricular dysfunction. Following a single pass through the liver lidocaine undergoes a 70% degradation (Stenson, et al., 1971) to a number of pharmacologically active metabolites, and it is not usually given orally because these metabolites may cause central nervous system toxicity (Figure 3-4). The drug is administered intravenously as a loading bolus followed by a maintenance infusion. The usual loading dose is 100-175 mg administered as a slow infusion over 5-10 minutes or as multiple small boli. The usual rate of the maintenance infusion is 1-4 mg/min. The dose of lidocaine that is chosen should take into account the patient's body weight. In patients with heart failure the volume of distribution is diminished, and the inital loading bolus should be somewhat smaller (Thompson, et al., 1973). Because the rate of removal of lidocaine depends on hepatic blood flow, reduced maintenance infusion rates should be given to patients with congestive heart failure or cardiogenic shock. Lidocaine may show some tendency to accumulate with infusion lasting longer than 24 hours (LeLorier, et al., 1977). The usual therapeutic plasma concentration is 1-6 μg/mL; toxicity occasionally occurs in this range but more frequently develops at higher plasma concentrations. The recent ability of laboratories to rapidly measure lidocaine concentration may increase the clinical usefulness of this drug.

Therapeutic uses Lidocaine's major use is in the treatment of serious ventricular arrhythmias that occur in the hospitalized patient. The drug suppresses ventricular ectopic activity effectively in a variety of clinical settings and can control recurrent sustained ventricular tachycardia in a small number of patients. Routine administration of lidocaine to patients with acute myocardial infarction can diminish the occurrence of primary ventricular fibrillation (Lie, et al., 1974). This is the largest single clinical indication for lidocaine therapy. The drug has little or no effect on supraventricular arrhythmias but may be valuable in blocking conduction through accessory pathways in the Wolff-Parkinson-White syndrome in the presence of atrial fibrillation or flutter (Rosen, et al., 1972), although its use in this situation is still controversial.

Side effects The most frequently encountered side-effects of lidocaine are caused by its central nervous system action, and include drowsiness, parasthesias, slurred speech, dizziness, tinnitus, disorientation, psychosis, focal tremor, grand mal seizures, and respiratory arrest. These potentially serious side-effects occur most frequently when large intravenous boli are given too rapidly; however, they occasionally occur during long-term maintenance infusion. These side-effects are usually preventable by careful clinical monitoring of the patient and ready access to lidocaine plasma concentration measurements. There are occasional reports of sinus arrest caused by lidocaine (Cheng and Wadhwa, 1973), and heart block may be precipitated in patients with preexisting infranodal disease (Gupta, et al., 1974).

Lorcainide

Pharmacology Lorcainide is a type I antiarrhythmic agent whose predominant cellular effect is to slow the rate of rise of phase 0 of the action potential. Following intravenous doses it has little effect on atrial and ventricular refractoriness and causes significant prolongation of the HV interval and QRS duration. The drug blocks conduction through accessory pathways effectively in patients with the Wolff-Parkinson-White syndrome (Baer, et al., 1978). The pharmacokinetics of lorcainide are not fully understood, but early reports suggest that it has saturable presystemic elimination; therefore, the bioavailability is low after the first few doses but increases to nearly 100% following multiple oral doses (Jahnchen, et al., 1979; Meinertz, et al., 1979). Lorcainide has a metabolite, norlorcainide, that accumulates during chronic oral administration to plasma concentrations greater than those of the parent compound (Keefe, et al., 1982). This metabolite may contribute to lorcainide's antiarrhythmic actions, because an increase in its antiarrhythmic activity over several days to weeks following the institution of oral therapy has been noted. The half-life of lorcainide is approximately 9 hours, and the half-life of norlorcainide is considerably longer. Following the initiation of chronic oral therapy with lorcainide the plasma concentration of lorcainide does not reach steady state until after 4-5 days, while that of norlorcainide does not achieve steady state until 7-10 days have passed. Thus, dose adjustments should be made only after the conclusion of approximately 1 week of therapy. The usual dose of lorcainide is 1.5-2 mg/kg intravenously over 15-20 minutes or 200-400 mg/day orally in two divided doses. The plasma concentrations of lorcainide and norlorcainide associated with ventricular premature beat suppression are approximately 50-200 and 80-400 ng/mL, respectively (Keefe, et al., 1982). Lorcainide has a modest myocardial depressant effect and can worsen congestive heart failure, especially at higher doses.

Therapeutic uses Lorcainide has been evaluated primarily as an agent for treating ventricular arrhythmias (Kesteloot and Stroobandt, 1977; Cocco and Strozzi, 1978; Klotz, et al., 1979). It suppresses ventricular ectopic beats effectively (Keefe, et al., 1982) and can treat and prevent sustained ventricular tachycardia. The drug is successful in treating supraventricular arrhythmias associated with the Wolff-Parkinson-White syndrome, including reciprocating tachycardia and rapid conduction through the accessory pathway in atrial fibrillation and flutter. Lorcainide may be effective against a variety of atrial arrhythmias but has received little clinical evaluation in this area.

Side-effects Lorcainide has significant neurologic side-effects, including dizziness, tremor, and blurred vision following intravenous infusion. During chronic oral therapy patients frequently complain of slight tremor and severe sleep disturbances, including frequent awakenings and vivid dreams. The tremor often first appears after 1-2 weeks of therapy and may reflect a slow accumulation of norlorcainide. This side-effect often requires a slight dose decrease. The sleep disturbances begin after 1-2 days of treatment and frequently subside after several weeks of therapy. The sleep disturbance is often very severe and frightening to the patient. It can be prevented in most patients with prophylactic nighttime benzodiazepine hypnotics during the early weeks of therapy. Lorcainide should be used with caution in patients with preexisting conduction disturbances. In a small number of patients the drug may precipitate or aggravate sustained ventricular tachyarrhythmias. Hyponatremia may occur in a small number of patients treated with lorcainide.

Mexiletine

Pharmacology Mexiletine causes depression of the phase 0 upstroke velocity and a minimal shortening of action potential duration in isolated Purkinje fibers (Yamaguchi, et al., in press). Intravenous doses have only a minimal depressant effect on the sinus node in normal people but may depress sinus node function in patients with preexisting disease. In some patients mexiletine causes a modest prolongation of His-Purkinje conduction time, and there is no consistent effect on atrial ventricular refractoriness or AV nodal conduction and refractoriness (Roos, et al., 1976). There are conflicting reports of the drug's effect on accessory bypass tracts in the Wolff-Parkinson-White syndrome. Intravenous doses of mexiletine are associated with a modest depression of myocardial function, which is most severe in patients with preexisting abnormalities. Intravenous therapy requires several loading infusions during the early distribution phase because of the drug's high apparent volume of distribution. Mexiletine is well absorbed after oral administration with nearly complete systemic bioavailability. Oral therapy may be started with a loading dose of 400-600 mg followed by 150-300 mg every 6-8 hours (Talbot, et al., 1973). The half-life in study volunteers is approximately 10 hours but may be longer in patients (Clark, et al., 1973). Mexiletine undergoes considerable metabolism with approximately 8% excreted unchanged in the urine. However, little is known about the pharmacologic activity of the metabolites of mexiletine. Therapeutic plasma concentration is 0.5-2 μg/mL and toxicity may be seen at plasma concentrations only slightly above this range.

Therapeutic uses Mexiletine has undergone its most extensive clinical trials for the treatment of ventricular arrhythmias. It is effective for patients with acute or chronic ventricular ectopic activity (Talbot, et al., 1976) and sustained or recurrent ventricular tachycardia. Mexiletine may be effective even when lidocaine fails to control the ventricular arrhythmia (Campbell, et al., 1973). The drug has not been widely evaluated in the management of supraventricular arrhythmias, but one would not expect mexiletine to have a major effect on these rhythm disturbances.

Side-effects Mexiletine therapy has been associated with side-effects in a high percentage of the patients treated in the early post-myocardial infarction phase (Campbell, et al., 1973). In this setting the drug may cause unacceptable bradycardia and hypotension, worsening of intrinsic conduction system disease, asystole, and neurologic side-effects such as tremor, dizziness, nausea, vomiting, blurred vision, paresthesias, ataxia, confusion, and drowsiness. Chronic oral dosing is associated with mild or less frequent toxicity, usually first occurring as tremor (Talbot, et al., 1976). Mexiletine's side-effects are generally dose-related and may be minimized by careful dose titration. Toxicity occurs at plasma concentrations only slightly above the therapeutic concentration range, and considerable individual susceptibility to toxicity exists. Serious myocardial depression may be precipitated in patients who have preexisting abnormalities of left ventricular function. The drug is contraindicated in patients with serious left ventricular dysfunction, bradyarrhythmias, and abnormalities of His-Purkinje conduction. Because the incidence of serious side-effects is considerably greater in the early stages of myocardial infarction, mexiletine is unlikely to replace lidocaine in this setting.

Phenytoin (Formerly Diphenylhydantoin)

Pharmacology Phenytoin is a widely used anticonvulsant that also has electrophysiologic effects that permit its use as an antiarrhythmic in selected situations. Following intravenous doses the drug causes significant systemic arteriolar vasodilatation and may have myocardial depressant effects at higher doses. The usual intravenous dose of phenytoin is up to

1 g administered at a rate not exceeding 50 mg/min and preferably at 25 mg/min. An excessive fall in arterial pressure may require a temporary discontinuation of the infusion. The drug is extensively metabolized by the liver and less than 5% appears unchanged in the urine (Kutt, et al., 1964). At doses and plasma concentrations of phenytoin that are below the usual therapeutic range the drug exhibits linear pharmacokinetics. However, in the therapeutic range of 10-18 μg/mL (Bigger, et al., 1968) the drug follows nonlinear kinetics, and small increases or decreases in dose may result in large changes in plasma concentration (Gerber and Wagner, 1972). The half-life of phenytoin increases with increasing dose and plasma concentration because of the nonlinear kinetics, and in the therapeutic plasma concentration range it averages 22 hours (Arnold and Gerber, 1970). The usual daily maintenance dose of 300-500 mg may be administered once daily. The wide range of interpatient variability in plasma concentration for a given dose requires that the dose be adjusted by measuring plasma concentrations. A variety of drugs alter the metabolic pathway of phenytoin and may increase or inhibit drug metabolism, resulting in clinically significant changes in plasma concentration (Winkle, et al., 1975). Plasma concentration should be rechecked any time other medications change. Phenytoin may also affect the metabolism of other drugs. One clinically important drug-drug interaction is the phenytoin-induced lowering of plasma quinidine concentration, often to subtherapeutic levels, when phenytoin is added to quinidine therapy (Data, et al., 1976). Phenytoin is normally 93% bound to plasma proteins (Lunde, et al., 1970) but liver disease and uremia may increase the free-drug fraction, and effective therapeutic levels and toxicity may occur in some patients with these conditions despite low total plasma drug concentrations.

Therapeutic uses Phenytoin's primary clinical use is in the treatment of digitalis-induced arrhythmias. In this situation it is effective for treating atrial tachycardia with or without block and is successful against a variety of ventricular arrhythmias. Phenytoin has the advantage of not exacerbating the AV block that is frequently associated with digitalis intoxication. For serious ventricular arrhythmias caused by digitalis toxicity lidocaine may still be the agent of choice, but phenytoin should be the second drug used if lidocaine fails to control life-threatening ventricular arrhythmias. In other settings phenytoin's role as an antiarrhythmic drug is less certain, but it may be effective in selected patients with serious ventricular arrhythmias and may play a role in the treatment of patients with the long QT interval syndrome.

Side-effects Many of the central nervous system side-effects of phenytoin are related to plasma concentration. Nystagmus frequently occurs at plasma concentrations above 20 μg/mL, ataxia at 30 μg/mL, and lethargy at 40 μg/mL (Kutt, et al., 1964). Side-effects during long-term therapy may include nausea, vertigo, rash, gingival hyperplasia, pseudolymphoma, folate-responsive megaloblastic anemia, peripheral neuropathy, hyperglycemia, and paradoxical seizures. In rare instances phenytoin may accelerate AV conduction and increase the ventricular response in atrial fibrillation and flutter (Grissom, et al., 1967). The intravenous administration of phenytoin at rates above 50 mg/min may precipitate respiratory arrest, hypotension, ventricular arrhythmias, asystole, heart block, ventricular fibrillation, and death. Significant hypotension may occur even at lower infusion rates. Hypotension usually responds to a temporary discontinuation of the intravenous infusion but may occasionally require fluid administration and the use of pressors. In many instances the infusion may be resumed after the arterial pressure has risen.

Procainamide

Pharmacology Procainamide causes a slowing of the upstroke velocity of phase 0 of the action potential and prolongation of action potential duration in isolated His-Purkinje fibers. In humans it results in a prolongation of atrial and ventricular refractory periods and modest prolongation of the HV interval and QRS duration at higher plasma concentrations. The action of procainamide on the AV node has not been fully described, but it probably results from a combination of direct depressant effects that are opposed by vagolytic effects in such a way that the overall effect is minimal in most patients. The drug routinely prolongs the QT interval to a modest extent and may prolong the QRS and PR intervals at higher doses. Procainamide prolongs the refractoriness of accessory pathways in the Wolff-Parkinson-White syndrome. At the usual therapeutic doses procainamide has little myocardial depressant effect (Miller, et al., 1973) but may exacerbate ventricular dysfunction at higher doses. Following intravenous infusion it routinely results in a modest fall in arterial pressure because of its peripheral vasodilating properties. The usual intravenous dose is up to 1 g administered at a rate not to exceed 50 mg/min and preferably not faster than 25 mg/min. If intravenous procainamide is successful, maintenance infusions may be continued at 1-4 mg/min with the infusion rate adjusted in accordance with plasma concentrations. Some reduction in dose may be required in patients with serious congestive heart failure. The average half-life of procainamide is approximately 3-4 hours (Koch-Weser and Klein, 1971), thus necessitating oral maintenance doses of 250-1000 mg every 4 hours. Recently, several sustained release procainamide preparations have been approved for general use. These promise to diminish the required frequency of dosing to every 6-8 hours. However, in our limited clinical experience to date these preparations have resulted in erratic procainamide levels in some patients, including one patient who experienced severe electrical toxicity and died when the amount of drug in his system suddenly "jumped" to toxic levels, which suggested erratic bolus absorption of the sustained release drug. Because of the large interpatient variation, plasma concentrations and clinical response should be used to select the proper dose. The usual range of effective plasma concentration is 4-10 μg/mL (Figure 3-6) but many patients with serious ventricular arrhythmias may respond only at higher concentrations. One should keep in mind, however, the increased risk of toxicity when using these higher plasma concentrations. Systemic bioavailability after oral dosing is 75%, but absorption may be erratic in the first few hours after a myocardial infarction (Koch-Weser, 1971). Procainamide is only 15% bound to plasma proteins, and 40% is excreted unchanged in the urine (Mark, et al., 1951; Koch-Weser, 1971). Some dose adjustment may be required in patients with renal disease.

Procainamide is metabolized by the liver to n-acetylprocainamide (NAPA) (Dreyfuss, et al., 1972). The rate of acetylation to NAPA shows a bimodal distribution with patients being either slow or fast acetylators (Karlsson and Molin, 1975; Reidenberg, et al., 1976). The plasma concentration of NAPA during chronic long-term oral therapy is similar to that of procainamide. The pharmacologic activity of NAPA has been extensively investigated, and the drug has different electrophysiologic and pharmacokinetic properties from its parent compound. N-acetylprocainamide has little or no effect on resting His-Purkinje conduction at clinically achieved concentrations (Jaillon and Winkle, 1979; Jaillon, et al., 1981) (Figure 3-8) and should not be considered as a substitute for procainamide, despite its longer half-life of 10 hours (Atkinson, et al., 1977; Winkle, et al., 1981a) and lack of the complication of systemic lupus erythematosus during long-term therapy (Lertora, et al., 1979). Patients who respond to procainamide do not necessarily respond to NAPA (Roden, et al., 1980b), and the routine monitoring of NAPA concentrations has little place in the management of patients receiving procainamide. N-acetylprocainamide is almost entirely excreted by the kidneys and may accumulate to toxic concentrations in patients with impaired renal function.

Therapeutic uses Procainamide is effective against a broad spectrum of arrhythmias, including atrial fibrillation and flutter. In AV nodal reentrant supraventricular tachycardia procainamide is often effective because it blocks conduction in the retrograde fast pathway (Wu, et al., 1978). Because it blocks both antegrade and retrograde conduction in the accessory pathways in the Wolff-Parkinson-White syndrome, it may be effective for long-term prophylaxis against reciprocating tachycardias in this condition and can be used to block rapid conduction to the ventricles during atrial fibrillation and flutter (Sellers, et al., 1977). Procainamide is effective against all types of ventricular arrhythmias. In the early post-myocardial infarction setting it is often the drug of second choice when lidocaine fails to control ventricular irritability. It may also be

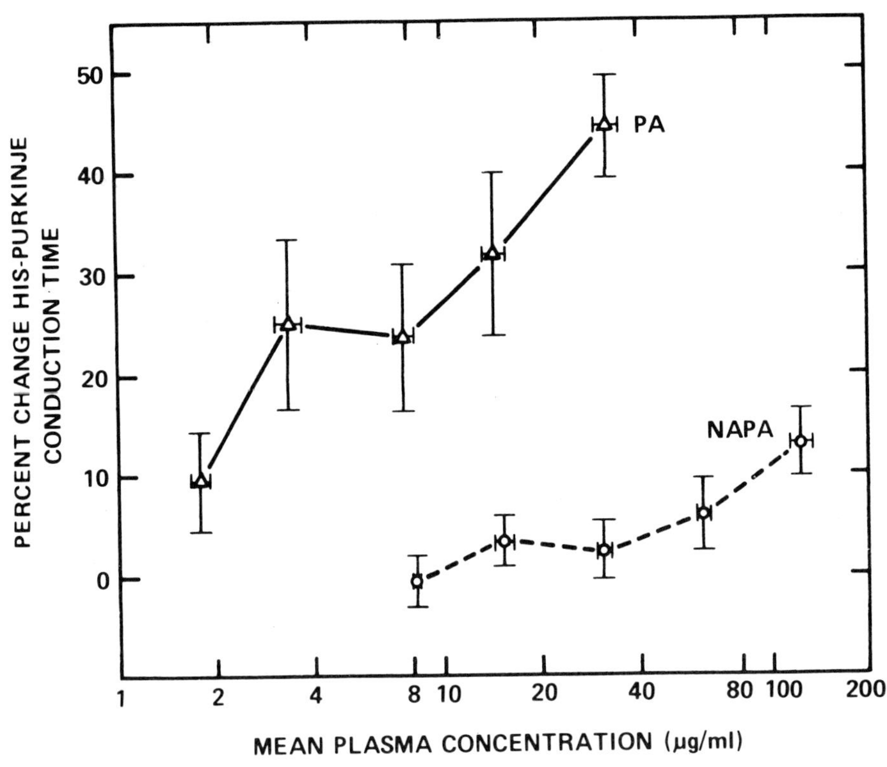

Figure 3-8 This figure shows the effects of procainamide (PA) and n-acetylprocainamide (NAPA) on the His-Purkinje conduction time (HV interval) in the dog. Procainamide causes a significant concentration-dependent increase of the HV interval, whereas NAPA prolongs the HV interval only at concentrations of 80-100 μg/mL. (*Source:* Jaillon, P.; and Winkle, R. A. 1979. Electrophysiologic comparative study of procainamide and n-acetylprocainamide in anesthetized dogs: concentration-response relationships. *Circulation* 60:1385-1394. By permission of the American Heart Association, Inc.)

used for long-term prophylaxis against recurrent sustained ventricular tachycardia, although higher than usual doses and plasma concentrations may be required in many patients. In most situations where long-term antiarrhythmic therapy is desirable procainamide is not the drug of choice because of its potential for long-term side-effects.

Side-effects Rapid intravenous infusion of procainamide may lead to severe myocardial depression, conduction disturbances, ventricular arrhythmias, and death. These side-effects are unusual with infusions of 25 mg/min, although hypotension frequently occurs. Intravenous infusion of procainamide requires continuous ECG monitoring and frequent monitoring of arterial pressure. Hypotension usually resolves promptly when the infusion is discontinued but may require the use of fluids and pressors. In many instances the infusion may be restarted when arterial pressure begins to rise. Long-term therapy with procainamide is associated with development of antinuclear antibodies and a clinical drug-induced lupus syndrome in many patients (Blomgren, et al., 1972). These patients may only complain of a flulike syndrome, or they may exhibit the more characteristic symptoms of fever, arthritis, arthralgia, pleurisy, and pericarditis. Patients with these side-effects rarely have renal or central nervous system involvement. Rash, fever, and agranulocytosis may occur even after a single dose. Because of its potential for conduction system disturbances, procainamide should be used cautiously in patients with preexisting conduction abnormalities.

Propafenone

Pharmacology Propafenone is a type I antiarrhythmic agent that causes a concentration-dependent decrease in the rate of rise of the phase 0 upstroke of the action potential in isolated papillary muscles of guinea pigs (Kohlhardt and Seifert, 1980). In addition to sodium channel blocking properties, propafenone has beta blocking properties in isolated tissue preparations and a weak and probably clinically insignificant calcium channel blocking effect (Ledda, et al., 1981). In humans propafenone causes a concentration-dependent prolongation of the PR and QRS intervals (Keller, et al., 1978; Connolly, et al., 1982). Intracardiac electrophysiologic studies in humans show a prolongation of the AH and HV intervals, as well as prolongation of the atrial and ventricular effective refractory periods. The drug also prolongs the antegrade and retrograde refractory periods of bypass fibers in patients with the Wolff-Parkinson-White syndrome (Waleffe, et al., 1981). The average reported elimination half-life has ranged from 3 hours (Seipel and Breithardt, 1980) to 6 hours (Connolly, et al., 1982). The drug exhibits nonlinear bioavailability with a tenfold increase in mean steady-state plasma concentration observed for a threefold increase in daily dose from 300 to 900 mg. The drug has a wide interpatient range of mean steady-state plasma concentrations for a given dose. In one study, although the mean therapeutic plasma concentration was 588 ng/mL, effective concentrations varied in individual patients from 64 to 1044 ng/mL (Connolly, et al., 1982). Pairs and runs are suppressed at plasma concentrations below those required for suppression of ventricular ectopic beats. The usual intravenous dose is 1-2 mg given over 10-15 minutes, and the range of oral doses is from 450 to 900 mg/day divided into three or four doses. The wide range of interpatient variability in half-life, plasma concentration for a given dose, and therapeutic plasma concentration require careful individualization of therapy with propafenone.

Therapeutic uses Propafenone has been most widely evaluated for the therapy of ventricular arrhythmias. It provides nearly complete suppression of ventricular ectopic beats in a high percentage of patients (Connolly, et al., 1982). The drug is also useful in some patients with recurrent sustained ventricular tachycardia and is reported to be effective for preventing paroxysmal atrial fibrillation and flutter. Propafenone terminates reentrant arrhythmias utilizing the AV node or reciprocating tachycardias using the AV node and an accessory bypass fiber when administered intravenously. Long-term oral therapy in a small number of patients has prevented recurrences of these reentrant supraventricular tachycardias.

Side-effects Intravenous propafenone has been reported to cause excessive bradycardia in patients with preexisting sinus node abnormalities and AV block in patients with abnormalities of AV conduction (Seipel and Breithardt, 1980). Many patients complain of either a funny taste or a dry mouth. These side-effects are generally well tolerated. Occasional patients report nausea, constipation, dizziness, disorientation, diaphoresis, or visual disturbances. Propafenone therapy is associated with a cholastatic hepatitis, although the exact incidence of its occurrence is unknown at this time. Connolly and colleagues (1982) reported worsening of ventricular arrhythmias in two of 13 patients who were receiving the drug for chronic ventricular ectopic beats. The drug may occasionally worsen left ventricular dysfunction.

Quinidine

Pharmacology Quinidine's effect on isolated Purkinje fibers is to slow the rate of rise of phase 0 upstroke and prolong action potential duration. Electrophysiologic effects in humans include prolongation of atrial and ventricular refractory periods and a direct depressant effect on the sinus node and AV node, which are countered by the drug's vagolytic properties (Mason, et al., 1977) in such a way that no net change in the sinus rate or AV nodal conduction occurs. The drug prolongs the PR and QRS intervals slightly in higher doses. QT interval prolongation occurs regularly and is dose-dependent. Excessive QT interval prolongation may necessitate limiting the dose in some patients. Quinidine's hemodynamic actions include both arteriolar and venous vasodilating properties. Although in high doses it is a direct myocardial depressant, in most patients with left ventricular dysfunction its vasodilating properties usually overcome its direct depressant effects. In patients who are dependent on high filling pressures to maintain cardiac output quinidine can cause a precipitous fall in cardiac output, which does, however, usually respond to the administration of fluid. Although quinidine has not traditionally been given intravenously, it may be given cautiously in the gluconate preparation in doses of 5-10 mg/kg at a rate not to exceed 25-30 mg/min.

Hypotension commonly occurs during this infusion, and arterial pressure must be constantly monitored. Concomitant infusion of normal saline (1-2 L) will usually minimize the hypotension. If an excessive fall in blood pressure occurs, the drug should be discontinued. On occasion the infusion may be resumed when the blood pressure returns toward predrug levels.

Quinidine is metabolized in the liver to several compounds that may have antiarrhythmic action, although their contribution to the clinical actions of quinidine is unknown. Approximately 10% of quinidine is excreted unchanged in the urine (Gerhardt, et al., 1969). Therapeutic plasma concentrations vary depending on the assay used but are generally approximately 2-4 μg/mL. Quinidine is usually well absorbed after oral administration with an average systemic availability of 72% (Ueda, et al., 1977). The drug has a variable half-life, which averages 6-7 hours (Ueda, et al., 1976). The oral dose of quinidine sulfate is 800-2000 mg/day in four divided doses with higher doses required for quinidine gluconate. Clinical response and plasma concentration measurements should be used as guidelines for determining the appropriate quinidine dose. Because many of the quinidine metabolites accumulate in patients with renal failure, assays that specifically measure unchanged quinidine should be used in this setting (Kessler, et al., 1974). Anticonvulsants such as phenobarbital and phenytoin stimulate the hepatic metabolism of quinidine and may result in clinically important declines in drug plasma concentration (Data, et al., 1976). An important drug interaction occurs between quinidine and digoxin, which results in a twofold or greater rise in digoxin plasma concentrations in patients receiving digoxin who are given quinidine, and in some patients digitalis intoxication may be precipitated (Leahey, et al., 1978). When quinidine is started in a patient receiving chronic digoxin, we usually omit the digoxin dose for 1 day, restart the digoxin at one-half its previous level, and monitor digoxin levels and the patient's clinical status carefully.

Therapeutic uses Quinidine has a broad spectrum of antiarrhythmic actions. It is effective against all types of supraventricular arrhythmias and is the drug of choice for paroxysmal atrial fibrillation and flutter. The drug blocks conduction through accessory pathways in the Wolff-Parkinson-White syndrome successfully and may be used to treat both reciprocating tachycardias and rapid ventricular responses to atrial fibrillation and flutter in this condition (Sellers, et al., 1977). Quinidine suppresses chronic ventricular ectopic activity effectively and is successful in treating patients with recurrent sustained ventricular tachycardia and fibrillation.

Side-effects Hypotension is common following the intravenous administration of quinidine, and if infusion rates are too rapid, cardiovascular collapse may occur. During chronic oral therapy gastrointestinal side-effects such as frequent loose stools or diarrhea and nausea and vomiting may limit therapy in up to one-third of patients. A number of idiosyncratic reactions can occur including rash, fever, thrombocytopenia, hepatic toxicity, and hemolytic anemia. The vagolytic actions of quinidine may increase conduction to the ventricles in cases of atrial fibrillation and flutter, and in the case of the latter this may precipitate 1:1 conduction by slowing the flutter rate and improving conduction to the ventricles. The most serious side-effect of quinidine is a drug-induced ventricular tachyarrhythmia (Selzer and Wray, 1964). This rhythm may occur after a single dose, after multiple doses, or after long-term chronic therapy. It is characterized by excessive QT interval prolongation or the development of bizarre QT-U waves. The typical ECG morphology of this rhythm is that of torsade de pointes with the arrhythmia initiated by early cycle premature ventricular beats. The condition is usually self-terminating but may be fatal in a small percentage of patients. When this arrhythmia occurs, it can be treated effectively by withdrawing quinidine, by rapid overdrive pacing of the atrium or ventricles, and/or by infusion of isoproterenol. Quinidine may precipitate heart block in some patients with preexisting abnormalities of His-Purkinje conduction, and in high doses it may aggravate bradyarrhythmias in patients with severe sinus node dysfunction.

Tocainide

Pharmacology Tocainide is structurally similar to glycinexylidide, a naturally occurring lidocaine metabolite (Figure 3-9). Electrophysiologically, the drug is similar to lidocaine (Anderson, et al., 1978b; Moore, et al., 1978). In isolated Purkinje fibers it depresses phase 0 upstroke of the action potential and minimally shortens action potential duration. Following intravenous doses in humans it causes a small but consistent decrease of ventricular refractoriness but no consistent change in sinus node function and AV nodal conduction of His-Purkinje or intraventricular conduction times. The hemodynamic effects (Winkle, et al., 1978a) of intravenous tocainide are a modest increase in systemic and pulmonary vascular resistance and aortic and pulmonary artery pressures. A minimal elevation in left ventricular end-diastolic pressure occurs, which may be a direct or reflex action of the drug. Clinically, the drug is well tolerated in patients who have significant left ventricular dysfunction. Following oral therapy tocainide is almost 100% systemically available, has a half-life of 13 hours, and obeys linear pharmacokinetics (Lalka, et al., 1977). Forty percent of the dose is excreted unchanged in the urine, and the dose may have to be diminished slightly in patients with renal impairment. The intravenous dose is 1 mg/kg/min for 15-20 minutes, and the oral dose is 1200-2400 mg/day in two or three divided doses. The drug has reasonably stable interpatient pharmacokinetics, but a wide range of

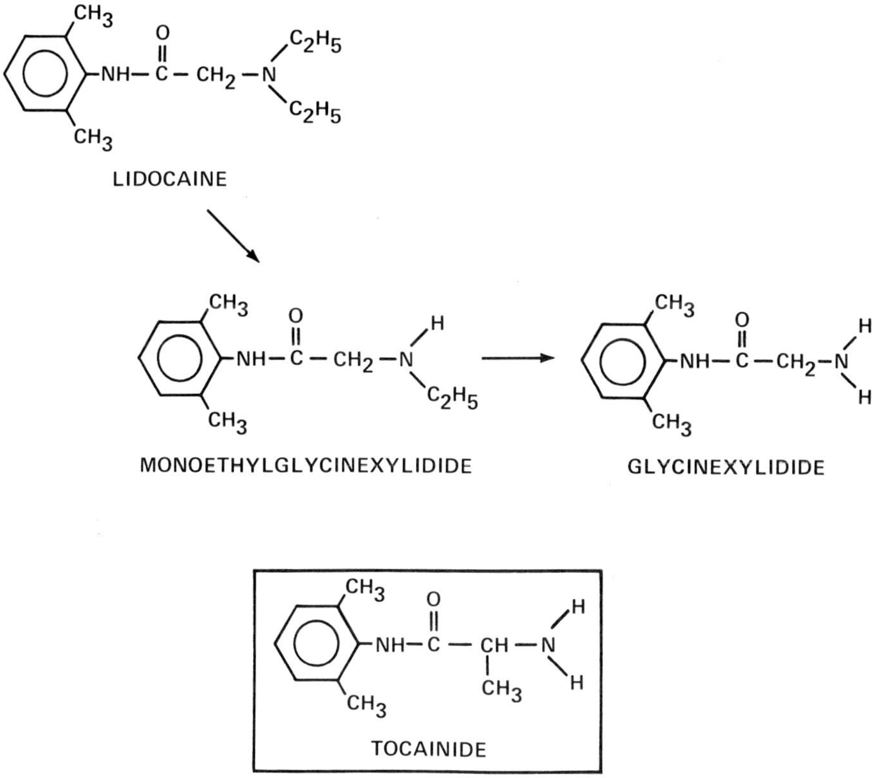

LIDOCAINE

MONOETHYLGLYCINEXYLIDIDE

GLYCINEXYLIDIDE

TOCAINIDE

Figure 3-9 This figure shows the initial steps in the metabolism of lidocaine. The first step in lidocaine metabolism involves the removal of a single ethyl group from the terminal nitrogen to give monoethylglycinexylidide. The next step is to remove the second ethyl group, giving glycinexylidide. After the pharmacologic activity of these metabolites was evaluated lidocaine, which is structurally similar to glycinexylidide, was synthesized.

individual patient sensitivity to its therapeutic actions and side-effects does exist. Most patients experiencing an adequate antiarrhythmic response have plasma concentrations between 6 and 12 μg/mL (Winkle, et al., 1976; Woosley, et al., 1977). Side-effects are common at plasma concentrations above this and may even occur within this range.

Therapeutic uses The only clinical trials of tocainide to date have evaluated its action in the treatment of ventricular arrhythmias (Winkle, et al., 1978c). Tocainide suppresses chronic ventricular ectopic beats and can be effective against recurrent sustained ventricular tachycardia and fibrillation, especially in patients who are responsive to lidocaine. However, a one to one correspondence to lidocaine efficacy does not exist, and some patients whose arrhythmias respond to lidocaine may fail to respond to tocainide. The drug can suppress ventricular ectopic activity occurring in the early phases of an acute myocardial infarction, but there are no data to evaluate its effect on preventing primary ventricular fibrillation in this situation. No studies have been conducted to date assessing the effect of tocainide on supraventricular arrhythmias or evaluating its action on accessory pathways in the Wolff-Parkinson-White syndrome.

Side-effects Following intravenous administration some patients may exhibit bradycardia and hypotension, although the exact incidence of this reaction is uncertain because large numbers of patients have not been treated intravenously. During chronic oral therapy side-effects are common and sensitivity to side-effects is variable. For most patients side-effects occur at plasma concentrations only slightly above those associated with effective arrhythmia control, and careful dose titration is necessary. Side-effects include tremor (especially of the hands) and nausea in a high percentage of patients. Other, less frequent side-effects include fever, rash, arthralgias, immune complex glomerulonephritis, changes in mental status, diplopia, blurred vision, and nightsweats (Winkle, et al., 1980). Central nervous system toxicity may occur at the time of peak plasma concentration, especially when the drug is taken on an empty stomach. This side-effect can be minimized by taking the drug with food. Side-effects are also reduced by administering the drug daily in three divided doses, despite its 13-hour half-life, to minimize the peaks and valleys in drug plasma concentration. Minor toxicity may occur in up to two-thirds of patients receiving long-term tocainide therapy but rarely requires drug discontinuation. More serious side-effects occur in approximately 10% of patients and may necessitate discontinuing the drug.

Beta Blocking Drugs

Pharmacology The beta-adrenergic blocking agents (Table 3-4) play a role in the treatment of certain arrhythmias. Although there may be subtle differences in the mode of antiarrhythmic action, most of these drugs rely predominantly on their beta-adrenergic receptor blocking properties. Beta blockade causes a slowing of the sinus node and other pacemaker discharge rates and a slowing of conduction through and prolongation of refractoriness of the AV node. At high doses some of the beta blocking drugs have a direct membrane depressant effect, but this is not usually clinically important for their antiarrhythmic activity (Coltart, et al., 1971). The beta blockers are divided into the nonspecific beta blockers, which block both the beta-1 receptors (cardiac, renin

Table 3-4 Comparative pharmacology of the beta blocking drugs*

	Cardio-selectivity	ISA	Membrane activity	Relative beta blocking potency	Usual IV dose (mg)	Usual total daily oral dose (mg)	Pharmacodynamic half-life (hours)	CNS penetration	Route of elimination	Clinically important active metabolites
Acebutolol	±	+	+	0.3	30	600-1200	24	0	renal, hepatic	yes
Alprenolol	0	++	+	1	15	400	—	—	hepatic	yes
Atenolol	++	0	0	1	10	50-200	24	0	renal	no
Metoprolol	+	0	±	1	—	100-400	10-12	+	hepatic	no
Nadolol	0	0	0	1.5	—	80-240	39	0	renal	no
Oxprenolol	0	++	+	0.5-1.0	15	160-320	13	+	hepatic	—
Pindolol	0	+++	+	6	1	20-40	8	+	renal, hepatic	—
Practolol	+	++	0	0.3	30	400-1200	—	—	—	—
Propranolol	0	0	++	1	10	80-320	11	+	hepatic	yes
Sotalol	0	0	0	0.3	30	80-480	24	0	renal	—
Timolol	0	0	0	6	—	30-60	15	+	renal, hepatic	—

*Table compiled with data from: Vukovich, et al., 1979; Regardh and Johnsson, 1980; Heel, et al., 1979; Heel, et al., 1980; Jackson, 1980.

Key: ± = possible effect or conflicting data; + = mild; ++ = moderate; +++ = strong; — = not available.

release) and the beta-2 receptors (bronchiole, vasodilatation, tremor), and those that are termed cardioselective and block only the beta-1 receptors. This distinction is most important when treating patients with obstructive pulmonary disease. However, even cardioselective drugs have some beta-2 blocking activity in higher doses and must be used cautiously in patients with pulmonary airway obstruction. The beta blocking drugs depress myocardial function in most patients and can precipitate heart failure in those individuals with serious impairment of ventricular function. Some of the beta blocking drugs also have partial agonist properties, commonly referred to as intrinsic sympathomimetic activity (ISA). Drugs with ISA have less myocardial depressant activity and cause less sinus slowing. A number of the beta blocking drugs possess a duration of action (pharmacodynamic half-life) that is longer than their pharmacologic half-life, possibly because of active metabolites, and several of these need only be administered once a day. The beta blocking drugs also differ with regard to their lipid solubility. Those that are most lipid soluble cross the blood-brain barrier more readily and cause more nonspecific complaints such as fatigue and depression. Beta blocking drugs also differ with regard to their primary route of elimination, a factor that may play a role in drug selection in patients who have renal or hepatic impairment.

Therapeutic uses The beta blocking drugs are sometimes successful in the termination and prevention of supraventricular tachycardias, especially those utilizing the AV node. Because of their effect on conduction and refractoriness in the AV node, these drugs may be useful in slowing the ventricular response to atrial fibrillation and flutter when digitalis alone is ineffective or is contraindicated. The beta blockers are also effective in treating arrhythmias caused by excessive catecholamines (pheochromocytoma) or digitalis intoxication. The depressant effects of these drugs on AV conduction may be additive to those of digitalis, however, and their use in the treatment of digitalis toxicity requires the prophylactic insertion of a temporary pacemaker. Beta blocking drugs may have a special role in treating ventricular tachyarrhythmias associated with the long QT syndrome, where they help to minimize the effects of the autonomic imbalance between the left and right stellate ganglia. Beta blocking drugs also suppress ventricular ectopic beats in some patients (Gradman, et al., 1977; Winkle, et al., 1978b; Woosley, et al., 1979). They are useful in treating palpitations in patients with the mitral valve prolapse syndrome (Winkle, et al., 1977) and are occasionally effective against recurrent sustained ventricular tachycardia and fibrillation, especially when these arrhythmias are precipitated by exercise. Clinical trials have shown that alprenolol (Wilhelmsson, et al., 1974), practolol (Multicentre International Study, 1975), timolol (The Norwegian Multicentre Study Group, 1981), and propranolol are successful in preventing sudden death in patients in the 1-year period following acute myocardial infarction. The mechanism by which sudden death is prevented is unknown. The beta blocking drugs have little effect on antegrade conduction over accessory pathways and are not useful in slowing the ventricular response to atrial fibrillation and flutter in patients with the Wolff-Parkinson-White syndrome (Rosen, et al., 1972). They may play a role in therapy of this syndrome when rapid conduction over a bypass tract occurs only during catecholamine stimulation.

Side-effects Beta blocking drugs are contraindicated in patients with serious left ventricular dysfunction who may be dependent on catecholamine stimulation to maintain cardiac output. Although sinus bradycardia occurs routinely during beta blockade therapy, it rarely limits the use of the drug. An occasional patient with preexisting sinus node dysfunction may experience excessive bradycardia. The use of beta blocking drugs with ISA may be helpful in some patients with sinus node disease. Similarly, AV block may be precipitated in patients with preexisting abnormalities. The nonspecific beta blocking drugs aggravate obstructive pulmonary airway disease, and even the cardioselective drugs must be used cautiously in such patients. Chronic oral therapy is frequently associated with complaints of fatigue and depression, especially with the drugs that readily enter the central nervous system. Beta blocking drugs may occasionally cause impotence, nausea, and diarrhea and may aggravate peripheral vascular insufficiency. These drugs must be used with caution in patients with diabetes because they may mask the sympathetic response to insulin-induced hypoglycemia, and they may also aggravate the tendency toward hypoglycemia. In patients with coronary artery disease and angina sudden withdrawal of beta blocking drugs may precipitate a rebound increase in anginal symptoms or, occasionally, myocardial infarction and death (Diaz, et al., 1974). Thus, beta blocking drugs should not be discontinued abruptly in these patients unless they are in a carefully controlled hospital setting.

CALCIUM ANTAGONISTS

Verapamil

Pharmacology Verapamil is a representative of the class of drugs that are called the calcium antagonists. The electrophysiologic effects of verapamil are primarily mediated through the blocking of the slow channels of membrane ionic currents, which are predominantly dependent on calcium ion flux. Verapamil acts mainly on the cells of the SA and AV nodes (which are predominantly dependent on slow channel responses). In these tissues verapamil slows phase 4 spontaneous diastolic depolarization, reduces the rate of rise of the action potential, and prolongs action potential duration (Zipes and Fischer, 1974). The drug is much less active in tissues of the atria, ventricles, and the specialized His-Purkinje conduction system, all of which are primarily dependent on the fast sodium channels. In experimental situations the drug is active against catecholamine-induced delayed after-depolarizations and rhythms caused by triggered automaticity. Because the drug's effect on calcium currents is not limited to cardiac tissue, but also effects vascular smooth muscle, the drug is a potent coronary and peripheral vasodilator. These actions give it additional clinical usefulness in the treatment of angina pectoris, coronary artery spasm, and other conditions. The peripheral vasodilating actions of verapamil offset some of its direct myocardial depressant effects; therefore, the drug can frequently be given to patients with modest left ventricular dysfunction without their suffering clinical deterioration. The reflex increase in sympathetic tone caused by vasodilatation tends to counteract verapamil's direct depressant effect on the sinus node, and the overall result is usually that little change occurs in sinus rate. The drug's effect on AV nodal tissue is to prolong conduction times and refractoriness by a direct action as opposed to the autonomically mediated effects that occur with digitalis, quinidine, and certain other drugs. Verapamil has no direct effect on or may even shorten refractoriness of the bypass tracts associated with the Wolff-Parkinson-White syndrome (Sung, et al., 1980). The usual intravenous dose of the drug is 10-25 mg administered slowly until the desired clinical result or side-effects occur. After initial loading a maintenance infusion of 0.0025 mg/kg/min may be given as needed. Intravenous administration may be associated with excessive peripheral vasodilatation, resulting in moderate degrees of hypotension in some patients. Verapamil has a high first pass effect following oral administration, and the usual oral dose is 80-160 mg administered every 6-8 hours. Little systematic study has been conducted on verapamil's many metabolites, although some may have pharmacologic activity. One metabolite, norverapamil, is present during long-term oral therapy in plasma concentrations that exceed the parent compound.

Therapeutic uses The major clinical use of verapamil to date has been in the treatment of arrhythmias involving the AV node (Rinkenberger, et al., 1980; Sung, et al., 1980). Following intravenous administration the drug terminates reentrant tachycardias that use the AV node exclusively, or the AV node in conjunction with accessory pathways in approximately 90% of patients. The drug is also effective in treating some patients who have other types of atrial tachycardias. The drug slows the ventricular response uniformly in patients with atrial fibrillation and flutter. Long-term oral verapamil administration can control the ventricular response to atrial fibrillation and flutter in patients who have inadequate rate control resulting from digitalis or beta blockade and can prevent recurrences of paroxysmal supraventricular tachycardias in many patients. On occasion the drug causes spontaneous termination of atrial fibrillation or flutter. Because it has little effect on accessory bypass tracts, it is not useful for slowing the ventricular response to these rhythms in patients with the Wolff-Parkinson-White syndrome. In fact, verapamil may actually accelerate conduction over the bypass by decreasing retrograde concealed penetration by QRS complexes conducted over the AV node (Rinkenberger, et al., 1980) or by shortening the refractory period of the bypass. Verapamil has received only limited evaluation in patients with ventricular arrhythmias, and reports to date are inconsistent. However, it is clear that in some patients verapamil can terminate and/or prevent ventricular arrhythmias successfully.

Side-effects Following intravenous infusion of verapamil a transient and mild fall in arterial pressure frequently occurs, which occasionally may be excessive and require discontinuation of the drug and specific therapy for the hypotension. Verapamil can precipitate marked bradycardia and asystole in patients with preexisting sinus node disease. Because many of the direct effects of the drug are counteracted by reflex increases in sympathetic tone, side-effects may be considerably more common when verapamil is given in conjunction with beta blockade, and the drug must be used with extreme caution or not at all in patients receiving beta blocking drugs. Verapamil can precipitate AV nodal block in high doses in patients with preexisting condition abnormalities. Because of its effect on AV nodal conduction, the drug should not be used to treat digitalis intoxication-induced arrhythmias without prior insertion of a temporary prophylactic ventricular pacemaker. Because verapamil does have some direct myocardial depressant effect, it should be avoided in patients with advanced uncontrolled heart failure unless the heart failure is caused by a rapid supraventricular arrhythmia that might respond to verapamil administration. Long-term therapy is generally very well tolerated with many patients complaining only of mild gastrointestinal intolerance and constipation. Rare cases of vertigo, headaches, and nervousness have been described. The drug interacts with digoxin, causing significant rises in digoxin plasma concentrations that could lead to digitalis intoxication (Klein, et al., 1982). Concomitant use of verapamil with digitalis, while frequently effective, should be done with caution.

Diltiazem

Pharmacology Diltiazem is a calcium antagonist drug with a clinical spectrum of uses similar to those of verapamil. The clinical pharmacology of diltiazem has not been studied as extensively as has verapamil's, and the limited data available have been reviewed recently by Kates (Kates, 1982). Diltiazem is a benzothiazepine derivative. It undergoes deacetylation, and the deacetylated metabolite is then 0-demethylated or N-demethylated. One metabolite, desacetyldiltiazem, is present in plasma concentrations that are 15%-35% of those of the parent compound. This metabolite is reported to have 40%-50% of the activity of diltiazem (Rovei, et al., 1980). Concomitant administration of diazepam may cause a 20%-30% lowering of diltiazem blood levels (Morselli, et al., 1979). The drug is 80%-86% protein bound, and less than 5% is excreted unchanged in the urine. The very limited data that are available suggest a half-life of 2-8 hours. A recent intracardiac electrophysiologic study (Mitchell, et al., 1982) of intravenous diltiazem showed that the drug depresses SA node function slightly and prolongs AV nodal conduction time and AV nodal functional and effective refractory periods. The electrophysiologic effects of diltiazem on the AV and SA node are additive to those of digoxin. The usual intravenous dose of diltiazem is 15-25 mg, and typical oral maintenance doses are 60-90 mg every 6 hours.

Therapeutic uses Although diltiazem has been used extensively in the treatment of coronary artery spasm and angina pectoris, it has received only limited evaluation as an antiarrhythmic agent (Rozanski, et al., 1982). Based on its electrophysiologic profile, one would expect the drug to have an antiarrhythmic spectrum similar to that of verapamil.

Side-effects During long-term oral dosing the most common side-effect of diltiazem is slight pedal edema. Occasional patients complain of paresthesias. Based on the drug's electrophysiologic profile, one might expect the drug to have the potential for aggravating preexisting sinus node disease or causing AV conduction disturbances in patients who have preexisting abnormalities or following drug overdoses.

Nifedipine

Nifedipine is another of the calcium channel blocking agents. It is different from verapamil and diltiazem in that it does not affect the SA or AV nodes to any significant extent. Thus, the drug has no known potential role as an antiarrhythmic agent. This should be kept in mind because in our practice we have seen a number of clinicians using this agent inappropriately to treat arrhythmias. The drug does have potent peripheral vasodilating properties and is useful in the treatment of coronary spasm, angina pectoris, hypertension, and other conditions.

OTHER DRUGS

Atropine

Pharmacology Atropine is a potent anticholinergic agent that increases the rate of spontaneous phase 4 diastolic depolarization of supraventricular pacemakers in the sinus node, atrium, and junctional tissues and shortens the refractoriness of and conduction times through the AV node. The net result is a shortening of the PR interval and an increase in the sinus rate. The drug has few direct hemodynamic effects, but in patients with a fixed stroke volume the increase in cardiac rate may increase cardiac output. The usual dose is 1 mg, which is given as a rapid intravenous bolus. Doses of less than 0.5 mg may on occasion produce a paradoxical slowing of the heart rate and lengthening of AV conduction time. Atropine acts within a few minutes, and its effects persist for several hours. Patients with intrinsic sinus or AV node disease may be less responsive to atropine.

Therapeutic uses Atropine is useful for accelerating sinus bradycardia associated with hypotension, such as may occur following an acute inferior myocardial infarction or during a vasovagal episode. It is also effective in reversing block in the AV node associated with inferior myocardial infarction or digitalis, propranolol, or verapamil therapy. In the setting of complete AV nodal block it is often useful for accelerating the rate of any junctional escape rhythms.

Side-effects Atropine's generalized anticholinergic effects result in a dry mouth, dilated pupils, blurred vision (secondary to inability to accommodate), and urinary retention (especially in elderly males). The drug may precipitate acute attacks of glaucoma and when given chronically may result in constipation. On occasion atropine may cause some central nervous system aberrations. The classical description of atropine overdose is a patient who is "red as a beet, dry as a prune, and crazy as a loon." In some patients AV nodal conduction is enhanced to the extent that infranodal conduction disturbances may be unmasked. Sinus tachycardia resulting from atropine may precipitate angina in patients with coronary artery disease.

Digitalis

A detailed description of digitalis' side-effects is given in Chapter 12. Most clinicians are well versed in the use of digoxin, and a lengthy description of the drug's pharmacology is beyond the scope of this chapter. However, given the widespread role of digoxin in the treatment of cardiac arrhythmias, a few general comments are in order here. There is little need for clinicians to use any cardiac glycoside other than digoxin. Given intravenously, the drug has a rapid onset of effect with peak action in approximately 30 minutes. After oral dosing, the peak effect occurs within several hours. The digitalizing dose is 1.0-1.5 mg, which is usually given as several divided doses over 12-24 hours. The drug is well absorbed and has a half-life of approximately 30 hours. Its marked renal excretion requires a decrease in the maintenance dose in patients with renal impairment; dosing should be based on monitoring of plasma concentration. The usual therapeutic digoxin plasma concentration is 1-2 ng/mL but patients taking the drug for control of ventricular response to atrial fibrillation or flutter may require slightly higher plasma concentrations. The usual maintenance dose is 0.25-0.375 mg/day, although older patients may require less and occasional patients may require more. The cardiac glycosides are frequently effective in terminating reentrant arrhythmias that use the AV node or for slowing the ventricular response to atrial fibrillation or flutter. These effects result from the drug's cholinergic action, which decreases the slope of phase 4 spontaneous diastolic depolarization (especially in abnormal tissues) and slows conduction and prolongs refractoriness of the AV node. Digoxin has recently been replaced by verapamil as the drug of choice in the termination of acute paroxysmal supraventricular tachycardia or the immediate slowing of the ventricular response to atrial fibrillation or flutter. However, there are still many patients (especially those with ventricular dysfunction) in whom the positive inotropic effects of digoxin are preferred to the uncertain or negative inotropic effects of verapamil. In addition to slowing the ventricular response to atrial fibrillation or flutter, digoxin may on occasion terminate these arrhythmias, especially when they are of recent onset. For the long-term chronic suppressive therapy of supraventricular arrhythmias digoxin is one of the least expensive and best tolerated antiarrhythmic drugs. It is effective in preventing recurrences of reentrant arrhythmias involving the AV node, in suppressing certain ectopic atrial tachycardias, and in maintaining a slow ventricular response to atrial fibrillation or flutter. The effects of digoxin are additive to those of beta blocking drugs and verapamil, and the drug may be used in combination with these agents. In our experience digoxin plays little, if any, role in the treatment of ventricular arrhythmias.

A detailed description of digitalis toxicity is given in Chapter 12. It is worth emphasizing, however, that many of the toxic effects of cardiac glycosides are exacerbated by hypokalemia, and patients who are receiving diuretics are at special risk. Digoxin interacts with quinidine, verapamil, and amiodarone, and the addition of any of these drugs to digoxin will cause an increase in the digoxin level and may result in digitalis intoxication. Digoxin or any other cardiac glycoside is contraindicated in the treatment of atrial fibrillation in patients with the Wolff-Parkinson-White syndrome because the drug may enhance conduction over bypass fibers and may result in an increased ventricular response. Digoxin should not be used to treat paroxysmal supraventricular tachycardia in patients with the preexcitation syndrome without prior electrophysiologic study to document its safety because these patients are at risk of developing paroxysmal atrial fibrillation.

Edrophonium

Edrophonium (Tensilon) is a potent cholinergic agent. Its vagotonic effects are frequently effective in evaluating the type of supraventricular tachycardia (Moss and Aledort, 1966; Spitzer, et al., 1967) or for actually terminating supraventricular tachycardias. This is especially true for those reentrant arrhythmias that involve the AV node, such as intranodal reentry or AV reciprocating tachycardias utilizing the AV node antegradely and a bypass tract retrogradely. Edrophonium is generally given as a 5-10 mg rapid intravenous dose. Patients receiving digitalis (Gould, et al., 1971) or those who have had a recent myocardial infarction (Rossen, et al., 1976) should be given smaller initial doses because the effects of edrophonium may be additive to the enhanced vagal tone already present in these settings, and transient complete heart block may occur. Edrophonium is usually well tolerated but may result in abdominal cramping because of its effect on gastrointestinal motility. A continuous infusion of edrophonium may be started in patients with atrial fibrillation or flutter and a rapid ventricular response. The initial infusion rate is 0.5 mg/min, and the rate may be increased gradually up to 2 mg/min as needed to maintain the appropriate degree of AV block (Frieden, et al., 1971).

Magnesium

Although magnesium is not generally considered an antiarrhythmic agent, we have occasionally experienced dramatic control of life-threatening ventricular arrhythmias by the administration of one to two ampules of magnesium sulfate. The drug has been most effective in treating the recurrent ventricular tachycardias and fibrillation that require multiple cardioversions and are resistant to a number of antiarrhythmic drugs, and it is occasionally useful when such arrhythmias are caused by drug toxicity. Several patients have been maintained on a continuous intravenous infusion. Magnesium is a vasodilator and excessive hypotension may occur, especially when the drug is given in conjunction with other vasodilating antiarrhythmic agents. The drug seems to be effective even in patients who are not hypomagnesemic.

Pressors

Some supraventricular tachycardias can be terminated by elevating arterial pressure to increase vagal tone via the baroreceptor reflexes. This is especially helpful in hypotensive patients who have paroxysmal supraventricular tachycardia and in whom carotid sinus massage alone is not effective. Although small rapid intravenous boli of phenylephrine may be given, we prefer to begin a continuous infusion of either phenylephrine (Neo-synephrine) or levarterenol (Levophed) so as to increase arterial pressure gently. These drugs must be used cautiously to avoid excessive increases in arterial pressure.

Vagal Stimulation

A variety of techniques for enhancing vagal tone can be successful in evaluating or terminating supraventricular tachycardias. The simplest of these for the patient to perform is a Valsalva maneuver. Patients may also be taught to use the diving reflex, which consists of holding one's breath and immersing the face in a basin of cold water. Gagging or vomiting may also elevate vagal tone. If the patient is not incapacitated by the arrhythmia, leaning over the side of a bed raises arterial pressure effectively and can enhance cardiac vagal tone. The most useful form of vagal stimulation is carotid sinus massage, which is generally performed by the physician. Before performing this maneuver clinicians should question the patient concerning any possible history of cerebrovascular disease, such as previous strokes or a history of transient ischemic attacks, and the carotid arteries should be auscultated for the presence of bruits. Carotid sinus massage should be started on the right side with the patient in the supine position and the head turned to the left. Carotid sinus massage is usually fairly vigorous and, if effective, probably results in transient carotid artery occlusion. The massage should be maintained for several seconds or longer. If it is not effective on the right side, the left carotid sinus may be massaged. One should never perform simultaneous bilateral carotid massage. Carotid sinus massage should always be performed with the patient connected to a continuous ECG recording machine and with the availability of full resuscitative capabilities. Pressure on the eyeball to enhance vagal tone should not be used because of the danger of retinal detachment or other ocular injuries.

REFERENCES

Anderson, J. L.; Harrison, D. C.; Meffin, P. J., et al. 1978a. Antiarrhythmic drugs: clinical pharmacology and therapeutic uses. *Drugs* 15:271-309.

Anderson, J. L.; Mason, J. W.; Winkle, R. A., et al. 1978b. Clinical electrophysiologic effects of tocainide. *Circulation* 57:685-691.

Anderson, J. L.; Patterson, E.; Wagner, J. G., et al. 1980. Oral and intravenous bretylium disposition. *Clin. Pharmacol. Ther.* 28:468-478.

Anderson, J. L.; Patterson, E.; Wagner, J. G., et al. 1981a. Clinical pharmacokinetics of intravenous and oral bretylium tosylate in survivors of ventricular tachycardia or fibrillation: clinical application of a new assay for bretylium. *J. Cardiovasc. Pharmacol.* 3:485-499.

Anderson, J. L.; Stewart, J. R.; Perry, B. A., et al. 1981b. Oral flecainide acetate for the treatment of ventricular arrhythmias. *N. Engl. J. Med.* 305:473-477.

Arnold, K.; and Gerber, N. 1970. The rate of decline of diphenylhydantoin in human plasma. *Clin. Pharmacol. Ther.* 11:121-134.

Atkinson, A. J.; Lee, W. K.; Quinn, M. L., et al. 1977. Dose ranging trial of N-acetylprocainamide in patients with premature ventricular contractions. *Clin. Pharmacol. Ther.* 21:575-587.

Bacaner, M. B. 1966. Bretylium tosylate for suppression of induced ventricular fibrillation. *Am. J. Cardiol.* 17:528-534.

Baer, F.; Farre, J.; Gorgels, A., et al. 1978. Electrophysiological effects of lorcainide, a new antiarrhythmic drug, in man. *Circulation* 57 and 58 (*Suppl.* II):II-248.

Bigger, J. T., Jr.; and Jaffe, C. C. 1971. The effect of bretylium tosylate on the electrophysiologic properties of ventricular muscle and Purkinje fibers. *Am. J. Cardiol.* 27:82-92.

Bigger, J. T., Jr.; Schmidt, D. H.; and Kutt, H. 1968. Relationship between the plasma level of diphenylhydantoin sodium and its cardiac antiarrhythmic effects. *Circulation* 39:363-374.

Blomgren, S. E.; Condemi, J. J.; and Vaughan, J. H. 1972. Procainamide-induced lupus erythematosus. Clinical and laboratory observations. *Am. J. Med.* 52:338-348.

Campbell, N. P. S.; Kelly, J. G.; Shanks, R. G., et al. 1973. Mexiletine (K8 1173) in the management of ventricular dysrhythmias. *Lancet:* 404-407.

Campbell, R. W. F.; Achuff, S. C.; Pottage, A., et al. 1979. Mexiletine in the prophylaxis of ventricular arrhythmias during acute myocardial infarction. *J. Cardiovasc. Pharmacol.* 1:43-52.

Cheng, T. O.; and Wadhwa, K. 1973. Sinus standstill following intravenous lidocaine administration. *J.A.M.A.* 223:790-792.

Clark, R. A.; Julian, D. G.; Nimmo, J., et al. 1973. Clinical pharmacological studies of K8 1173—a new antiarrhythmic agent. Proceedings of the Pharmacological Society, 3rd-5th January. *Br. J. Pharmacol.* 47: 622P.

Cocco, G.; and Strozzi, C. 1978. Initial clinical experience of lorcainide (Ro 13-1042), a new antiarrhythmic agent. *Eur. J. Clin. Pharmacol.* 14:105-109.

Coltart, D. J.; Gibson, D. G.; and Shand, D. G. 1971. Plasma propranolol levels associated with suppression of ventricular ectopic beats. *Br. Med. J.* 1:490-491.

Connolly, S. J.; Kates, R. E.; Lebsack, C., et al. 1982. Clinical pharmacology of propafenone. *Circulation* 66 (*Suppl.* II):II-68.

Danilo, P.; Hordof, A. J.; and Rosen, M. R. 1977. Effects of disopyramide on electrophysiologic properties of canine cardiac Purkinje fibers. *J. Pharmacol. Exp. Ther.* 201:701-708.

Data, J. L.; Wilkinson, G. R.; and Nies, A. S. 1976. Interaction of quinidine with anticonvulsant drugs. *N. Engl. J. Med.* 294:699-702.

Diaz, R. G.; Somberg, J.; Freeman, E., et al. 1974. Myocardial infarction after propranolol withdrawal. *Am. Heart J.* 88:257-258.

Dreifus, L. S.; Zbigniew, F.; Sexton, D. M., et al. 1973. Electrophysiological and clinical effects of a new antiarrhythmic agent: disopyramide. *Am. J. Cardiol.* 31:129.

Dreyfuss, J.; Bigger, J. T.; Cohen, A. I., et al. 1972. Metabolism of procainamide in rhesus monkey and man. *Clin. Pharmacol. Ther.* 13:366-371.

Duff, H. J.; Roden, D. M.; Maffucci, R. J., et al. 1981. Suppression of resistant ventricular arrhythmias by twice daily dosing with flecainide. *Am. J. Cardiol.* 48:1133-1140.

Elharrar, V.; Foster, P. R.; and Zipes, D. P. 1975. Effects of aprindine HC1 on cardiac tissues. *J. Pharmacol. Exp. Ther.* 195:201-205.

Fasola, A. F.; and Carmichael, R. 1974. The pharmacology and clinical evaluation of aprindine—a new antiarrhythmic agent. *Acta Cardiol. (Brux)* 18 (*Suppl.*):217-333.

Fasola, A. F.; Nobel, R. J.; and Zipes, D. P. 1977. Treatment of recurrent ventricular tachycardia and fibrillation with aprindine. *Am. J. Cardiol.* 39:903-909.

Frieden, J.; Cooper, J. A.; and Grossman, J. I. 1971. Continuous infusion of edrophonium (Tensilon) in treating supraventricular arrhythmias. *Am. J. Cardiol.* 27:294-297.

Gerber, N.; and Wagner, J. C. 1972. Explanation of dose-dependent decline of diphenylhydantoin plasma levels by fitting to the integrated form of the Michaelis-Menten equation. *Res. Commun. Chem. Pathol. Pharmacol.* 3:455-466.

Gerhardt, R. E.; Knouss, R. F.; Thyrum, P. T., et al. 1969. Quinidine excretion in aciduria and alkaluria. *Ann. Intern. Med.* 71:927-933.

Gibson, J. K.; Somani, P.; and Bassett, A. L. 1978. Electrophysiologic effects of encainide (MJ 9067) on canine Purkinje fibers. *Eur. J. Pharmacol.* 52:161-169.

Gould, L.; Zahir, M.; and Gomprecht, R. F. 1971. Cardiac arrest during edrophonium administration. *Am. Heart J.* 81:437-438.

Gradman, A. H.; Winkle, R. A.; Fitzgerald, J. W., et al. 1977. Suppression of premature ventricular contractions by acebutolol. *Circulation* 55:785-791.

Greenblatt, D. J.; and Koch-Weser, J. 1975. Drug therapy: clinical pharmacokinetics (first of two parts). *N. Engl. J. Med.* 293:702-705.

Greenblatt, D. J.; and Koch-Weser, J. 1975. Drug therapy: clinical pharmacokinetics (second of two parts). *N. Engl. J. Med.* 293:964-970.

Grissom, J. H.; Sy, B. G.; Duffy, J. P., et al. 1967. Dangerous consequence from use of phenytoin in atrial flutter. *Br. Med. J.* 4:34.

Gupta, P. K.; Lichstein, E.; and Chadda, K. D. 1974. Lidocaine-induced heart block in patients with bundle branch block. *Am. J. Cardiol.* 33:487-492.

Haffajee, C.; Lesko, L.; Canada, A., et al. 1981. Clinical pharmacokinetics of amiodarone. *Circulation* 64 (*Suppl.* IV):IV-263.

Harris, L.; McKenna, W. J.; Rowland, E., et al. 1981. Plasma amiodarone and desethylamiodarone levels in chronic oral therapy. *Circulation* 64 (*Suppl.* IV):IV-263.

Harrison, D. C.; Meffin, P. J.; and Winkle, R. A. 1977. Clinical pharmacokinetics of antiarrhythmic drugs. *Prog. Cardiovasc. Dis.* 20:217-242.

Heel, R. C.; Brogden, R. N.; Pakes, G. E., et al. 1980. Nadolol: a review of its pharmacological properties and therapeutic efficacy in hypertension and angina pectoris. *Drugs* 20:1-23.

Heel, R. C.; Brogden, R. N.; Speight, T. M., et al. 1979. Atenolol: a review of its pharmacological properties and therapeutic efficacy in angina pectoris and hypertension. *Drugs* 17:425-460.

Hodess, A. B.; Follansbee, W. P.; Spear, J. F., et al. 1979. Electrophysiological effects of a new antiarrhythmic agent, flecainide, on the intact canine heart. *J. Cardiovasc. Pharmacol.* 1:427-439.

Hodges, M.; Haugland, J. M.; Granud, G., et al. 1982. Suppression of ventricular ectopic depolarizations by flecainide acetate, a new antiarrhythmic agent. *Circulation* 65:879-885.

Holder, D. A.; Sniderman, A. D.; Fraser, G., et al. 1977. Experience with bretylium tosylate by a hospital cardiac arrest team. *Circulation* 55:541-544.

Jackson, G. 1980. Comparative efficacy and safety of beta blockers in angina pectoris. *Primary Cardiology Supplement* 1:97-101.

Jahnchen, E.; Bechtold, H.; Kasper, W., et al. 1979. Lorcainide: I. Saturable presystemic elimination. *Clin. Pharmacol. Ther.* 26:187-195.

Jaillon, P.; and Winkle, R. A. 1979. Electrophysiologic comparative study of procainamide and n-acetylprocainamide in anesthetized dogs: concentration-response relationships. *Circulation* 60:1385-1394.

Jaillon, P.; Rubenson, D.; Peters, F., et al. 1981. Electrophysiologic effects of n-acetylprocainamide in man. *Am. J. Cardiol.* 47:1134-1140.

Josephson, M. E.; Caracta, A. R.; Lau, S. H., et al. 1972. Effects of lidocaine on refractory periods in man. *Am. Heart J.* 84:778-786.

Karlsson, E.; and Molin, L. 1975. Polymorphic acetylation of procainamide in healthy subjects. *Acta Med. Scand.* 197:299-302.

Kates, R. E. 1982. Calcium antagonists:pharmacokinetic properties. *Drugs* (in press).

Kates, R. E.; Keefe, D. L. D.; Schwartz, J., et al. 1981. Verapamil disposition kinetics in chronic atrial fibrillation. *Clin. Pharmacol. Ther.* 30:44-51.

Keefe, D. L.; Kates, R. E.; Rodriguez, I., et al. 1982. Pharmacodynamics of the initiation of oral lorcainide therapy. *Circulation* 66 (*Suppl.* II): II-69.

Keller, K.; Meyer-Estorf, G.; Beck, O. A., et al. 1978. Correlation between serum concentration and pharmacological effect on atrioventricular conduction time of the antiarrhythmic drug propafenone. *Eur. J. Clin. Pharmacol.* 13:17-20.

Kessler, K. M.; Lowenthal, D. T.; Warner, H., et al. 1974. Quinidine elimination in patients with congestive heart failure or poor renal function. *N. Engl. J. Med.* 290:706-709.

Kesteloot, H.; and Stroobandt, R. 1977. Clinical experience with lorcainide (R 15 889), a new antiarrhythmic drug. *Arch. Interna Pharmacodynam. Therapie* 230:225-234.

Klein, H. O.; Lang, R.; Weiss, E., et al. 1982. The influence of verapamil on serum digoxin concentration. *Circulation* 65:998-1003.

Klotz, U.; Muller-Seydlitz, P. M.; and Heimburg, P. 1979. Lorcainide infusion in the treatment of ventricular premature beats (VPB). *Eur. J. Clin. Pharmacol.* 16:1-6.

Koch-Weser, J. 1971. Pharmacokinetics of procainamide in man. *Ann. N. Y. Acad. Sci.* 179:370-382.

Koch-Weser, J.; and Klein, S. W. 1971. Procainamide dosage schedules, plasma concentrations, and clinical effects. *J.A.M.A.* 215:1454-1460.

Kohlhardt, M.; and Seifert, C. 1980. Inhibition of $\dot{V}_{max}$ of the action potential by propafenone and its voltage-, time-, and pH-dependence in mammalian ventricular myocardium. *Naunyn-Schmiedeberg's Arch. Pharmacol.* 315:55-62.

Kus, T.; and Sasyniuk, B. L. 1975. Electrophysiological actions of disopyramide phosphate on canine ventricular muscle and Purkinje fibers. *Circ. Res.* 37:844.

Kutt, H.; Winters, W.; Kokenge, R., et al. 1964. Diphenylhydantoin metabolism, blood levels, and toxicity. *Arch. Neurol.* 11:642-648.

Lalka, D.; Meyer, M. B.; Duce, R. D., et al. 1977. Kinetics of the oral antiarrhythmic lidocaine congener, tocainide. *Clin. Pharmacol. Ther.* 19:757-766.

Leahey, E. B., Jr.; Reiffel, J. A.; Drusin, R. E., et al. 1978. Interaction between digoxin and quinidine. *J.A.M.A.* 240:533-534.

Ledda, F.; Mantelli, L.; Manzini, S., et al. 1981. Electrophysiological and antiarrhythmic properties of propafenone in isolated cardiac preparations. *J. Cardiovasc. Pharmacol.* 3:1162-1173.

LeLorier, J.; Grenon, D.; Latour, Y., et al. 1977. Pharmacokinetics of lidocaine after prolonged intravenous infusions in uncomplicated myocardial infarction. *Ann. Intern. Med.* 87:700-702.

Lertora, J. J.; Atkinson, A. J.; Kushner, W., et al. 1979. Long-term antiarrhythmic therapy with n-acetylprocainamide. *Clin. Pharmacol. Ther.* 25:273-282.

Lie, K. I.; Wellens, H. J. J.; Van Capelle, F. J. L., et al. 1974. Lidocaine in the prevention of primary ventricular fibrillation. A double-blind, randomized study of 212 consecutive patients. *N. Engl. J. Med.* 291: 1324-1326.

Lunde, P. M.; Rane, A.; Yaffe, S. J., et al. 1970. Plasma protein binding of diphenylhydantoin in man. Interaction with other drugs and the effect of temperature and plasma dilution. *Clin. Pharmacol. Ther.* 11: 846-855.

Mark, L. C.; Kayden, H. J.; Steele, J. M., et al. 1951. The physiological disposition and cardiac effects of procainamide. *J. Pharmacol. Exp. Ther.* 102:5-15.

Mason, J. W.; and Peters, F. A. 1981. Antiarrhythmic efficacy of encainide in patients with refractory recurrent ventricular tachycardia. *Circulation* 63:670-675.

Mason, J. W.; Winkle, R. A.; Rider, A. K., et al. 1977. The electrophysiologic effects of quinidine in the transplanted human heart. *J. Clin. Invest.* 59:481-489.

Mason, J. W.; Hondeghem, L. M.; Katsung, B. G. 1982. Amiodarone blocks inactivated Na^+ channels. *Circulation* 66 (*Suppl.* II):II-292.

Meffin, P. J.; Robert, E. W.; Winkle, R. A., et al. 1979. Role of concentration-dependent plasma protein binding in disopyramide disposition. *J. Pharmacokin. Biopharmaceut.* 7:29-46.

Meinertz, T.; Kasper, W.; Kersting, F., et al. 1979. Lorcainide. II. Plasma concentration-effect relationship. *Clin. Pharmacol. Ther.* 26:196-204.

Miller, R. R.; Hilliard, G.; Lies, J. E., et al. 1973. Hemodynamic effects of procainamide in patients with acute myocardial infarction and comparison with lidocaine. *Am. J. Med.* 55:161-167.

Mitchell, L. B.; Jutzy, K. R.; Lewis, S. J., et al. 1982. Intracardiac electrophysiologic study of intravenous diltiazem and combined diltiazem-digoxin in patients. *Am. Heart J.* 103:57-66.

Moore, E. N.; Spear, J. F.; Horowitz, L. N., et al. 1978. Electrophysiologic properties of a new antiarrhythmic drug—tocainide. *Am. J. Cardiol.* 41:703-709.

Morselli, P. L.; Rovei, V.; Mitchard, M., et al. 1979. Pharmacokinetics and metabolism of diltiazem in man (observations on healthy volunteers and angina pectoris patients). In *New drug therapy with a calcium antagonist*. R. Bing, editor. Amsterdam-Princeton: Excerpta Medica, pp. 152-168.

Moss, A. J.; and Aledort, L. M. 1966. Use of edrophonium (Tensilon) in the evaluation of supraventricular tachycardias. *Am. J. Cardiol.* 17:58-62.

Multicentre International Study. 1975. Improvement in prognosis of myocardial infarction by long-term beta-adrenoreceptor blockade using practolol. *Br. Med. J.* 3:735-740.

Mungall, D. R.; Robichaux, R. P.; Perry, W., et al. 1980. Effects of quinidine on serum digoxin concentration. A prospective study. *Ann. Intern. Med.* 93:689-693.

The Norwegian Multicenter Study Group. 1981. Timolol-induced reduction in mortality and reinfarction in patients surviving acute myocardial infarction. *N. Engl. J. Med.* 304:801-807.

Papp, J. G.; and Vaughan Williams, E. M. 1969. The effect on intracellular atrial potentials of bretylium in relation to its local anesthetic potency. *Br. J. Pharmacol.* 35:352-360.

Podrid, P. J.; Schoeneberger, A.; and Lown, B. 1980. Congestive heart failure caused by oral disopyramide. *N. Engl. J. Med.* 302:614-617.

Pritchard, D. A.; Singh, B. N.; and Hurley, P. J. 1975. Effects of amiodarone on thyroid function in patients with ischaemic heart disease. *Br. Heart J.* 37:856-860.

Reele, S.; Woosley, R. L.; and Oates, J. A. 1978. Pharmacologic reversal of the hypotensive effect that complicates antiarrhythmic therapy with bretylium (abstract). *Circulation* (*Suppl.* 57) 58:II-247.

Regardh, C. G.; and Johnsson, G. 1980. Clinical pharmacokinetics of metoprolol. *Clin. Pharmacokinet.* 5:557-569.

Reidenberg, M. M.; Drayer, D. E.; Levy, M., et al. 1976. Polymorphic acetylation of procainamide in man. *Clin. Pharmacol. Ther.* 17:722-730.

Rinkenberger, R. L.; Prystowsky, E. N.; Heger, J. J., et al. 1980. Effects of intravenous and chronic oral verapamil administration in patients with supraventricular tachyarrhythmias. *Circulation* 62:996-1010.

Roden, D. M.; Reele, S. B.; Higgins, S. B., et al. 1980a. Total suppression of ventricular arrhythmias by encainide: pharmacokinetic and electrocardiographic characteristics. *N. Engl. J. Med.* 302:877-882.

Roden, D. M.; Reele, S. B.; Higgins, S. B., et al. 1980b. Antiarrhythmic efficacy, pharmacokinetics, and safety of n-acetylprocainamide in human subjects: comparison with procainamide. *Am. J. Cardiol.* 46:463-468.

Romhilt, D. W.; Bloomfield, S. S.; Lipicky, R. J., et al. 1972. Evaluation of bretylium tosylate for the treatment of premature ventricular contractions. *Circulation* 45:800-807.

Roos, J. C.; Paalman, A. C. A.; and Dunning, A. J. 1976. Electrophysiologic effects of mexiletine in man. *Br. Heart J.* 38:1262-1271.

Rosen, K. M.; Barwolf, C.; Ehasani, A., et al. 1972. Effects of lidocaine and propranolol on the normal and anomalous pathways in patients with preexcitation. *Am. J. Cardiol.* 30:601-809.

Rosenbaum, M. B.; Chiale, P. A.; Halpern, M. S., et al. 1976. Clinical efficacy of amiodarone as an antiarrhythmic drug. *Am. J. Cardiol.* 34: 215-223.

Rosenbaum, M. B.; Chiale, P. A.; Rigiba, D., et al. 1974. Control of tachyarrhythmias associated with Wolff-Parkinson-White syndrome by amiodarone hydrochloride. *Am. J. Cardiol.* 34:215-223.

Rossen, R. M.; Krikorian, J.; and Hancock, W. 1976. Ventricular asystole after edrophonium chloride administration. *J.A.M.A.* 235: 1041-1042.

Rovei, V.; Gomeni, R.; Mitchard, M., et al. 1980. Pharmacokinetics and metabolism of diltiazem in man. *Acta Cardiologica* 35:35-45.

Rozanski, J. J.; Zaman, L.; and Castellanos, A. 1982. Electrophysiologic effects of diltiazem hydrochloride on supraventricular tachycardia. *Am. J. Cardiol.* 49:621-628.

Sami, M.; Mason, J. W.; Peters, F., et al. 1979. Clinical electrophysiologic effects of encainide, a newly developed antiarrhythmic agent. *Am. J. Cardiol.* 44:526-532.

Sanna, G.; and Arcidiacono, R. 1973. Chemical ventricular defibrillation of the human heart with bretylium tosylate. *Am. J. Cardiol.* 32:982-987.

Schlepper, M.; and Neuss, H. 1974. Changes in refractory periods in the AV conduction system induced by antiarrhythmic drugs. A study using His bundle recordings. *Acta Cardiol. (Brux)* 18 (*Suppl.*):269-277.

Seipel, L.; and Breithardt, G. 1980. Propafenone—a new antiarrhythmic drug. *Eur. Heart J.* 1:309-313.

Sellers, T. D.; Campbell, R. W. F.; Bashore, T. M., et al. 1977. Effects of procainamide and quinidine sulfate in the Wolff-Parkinson-White syndrome. *Circulation* 55:15-22.

Selzer, A.; and Wray, H. W. 1964. Quinidine syncope: paroxysmal ventricular fibrillation occurring during treatment of chronic atrial arrhythmias. *Circulation* 30:17-26.

Shand, D. G.; and Rangno, R. E. 1972. The disposition of propranolol. I. Elimination during oral absorption in man. *Pharmacology* 7:159-168.

Singh, B. N.; and Vaughan-Williams, E. M. 1970. The effect of amiodarone, a new antianginal drug, on cardiac muscle. *Br. J. Pharmacol.* 39:657-667.

Singh, B. N.; and Vaughan-Williams, E. M. 1971. Effect of altering potassium concentration on the action of lidocaine and diphenylhydantoin on rabbit atrial and ventricular muscle. *Circ. Res.* 29:286-295.

Sobel, S. M.; and Rakita, L. 1982. Pneumonitis and pulmonary fibrosis associated with amiodarone treatment: a possible complication of a new antiarrhythmic drug. *Circulation* 65:819-824.

Spitzer, S.; Mason, D.; Lemmon, W. M., et al. 1967. Use of edrophonium (Tensilon) in the evaluation of supraventricular tachycardia. *Am. J. Med. Sci.* 254:477-482.

Spurrell, R. A. J., Thorburn, C. W.; Camm, J., et al. 1975. Effects of disopyramide on electrophysiological properties of specialized conduction system in man and accessory atrioventricular pathway in Wolff-Parkinson-White syndrome. *Br. Heart J.* 37:861-870.

Steinberg, M. I.; and Greenspan, K. 1976. Intracellular electrophysiological alterations in canine cardiac conducting tissue induced by aprindine and lidocaine. *Cardiovasc. Res.* 10:236-244.

Stenson, R. E.; Constantino, R. T.; and Harrison, D. C. 1971. Interrelationships of hepatic blood flow, cardiac output, and blood levels of lidocaine in man. *Circulation* 43:205-211.

Story, J. R.; Abdulla, A. M.; and Frank, M. J. 1979. Cardiogenic shock and disopyramide phosphate. *J.A.M.A.* 242:654-655.

Sung, R. J.; Elser, B.; and McAllister, R. G., Jr. 1980. Intravenous verapamil for termination of reentrant supraventricular tachycardias. Intracardiac studies correlated with plasma verapamil concentrations. *Ann. Intern. Med.* 93:682-689.

Talbot, R. G.; Nimmo, J.; Julian, D. G., et al. 1973. Treatment of ventricular arrhythmias with mexiletine (K8 1173). *Lancet* 2:399-407.

Talbot, R. G.; Julian, D. G.; and Prescott, L. F. 1976. Long-term treatment of ventricular arrhythmias with oral mexiletine. *Am. Heart J.* 91:58-65.

Thompson, P. D.; Melmon, K. L.; Richardson, J. A., et al. 1973. Lidocaine pharmacokinetics in advanced heart failure, liver disease, and renal failure in humans. *Ann. Intern. Med.* 78:499-508.

Tucker, G. T.; Boyes, R. N.; Bridenbaugh, P. O., et al. 1970. Binding of anilide-type local anesthetics in human plasma. I. Relationships between binding, physiochemical properties, and anesthetic activity. *Anesthesiology* 33:287-303.

Ueda, C. T.; Hirschfeld, D. S.; Scheinman, M. M., et al. 1976. Disposition kinetics of quinidine. *Clin. Pharmacol. Ther.* 19:30-36.

Ueda, C. T.; Williamson, B. J.; and Dzindzio, B. S. 1977. Absolute quinidine bioavailability. *Clin. Pharmacol. Ther.* 20:260-265.

Verdonck, F.; Vereecke, J.; and Vlengels, A. 1974. Electrophysiological effects of aprindine on isolated heart preparations. *Eur. J. Pharmacol.* 16:338-347.

Vismara, L. A.; Mason, D. T.; and Amsterdam, E. A. 1974. Disopyramide phosphate: clinical efficacy of a new oral antiarrhythmic drug. *Clin. Pharmacol. Ther.* 16:330-335.

Vismara, L. A.; Vera, Z.; Miller, R. R., et al. 1977. Efficacy of disopyramide phosphate in the treatment of refractory ventricular tachycardia. *Am. J. Cardiol.* 39:1027-1034.

Vukovich, R. A.; Foley, J. E.; Brown, B., et al. 1979. Effect of β-blockers on exercise double product (systolic blood pressure × heart rate). *Br. J. Clin. Pharmacol.* 7 (*Suppl.* 2):167S-172S.

Waleffe, A.; Mary-Rabine, L.; de Rijbel, R., et al. 1981. Electrophysiological effects of propafenone studied with programmed electrical stimulation of the heart in patients with recurrent paroxysmal supraventricular tachycardia. *Eur. Heart J.* 2:345-352.

Walle, T.; and Gaffney, T. E. 1972. Propranolol metabolism in man and dog: mass spectrometric identification of six new metabolites. *J. Pharmacol. Exp. Ther.* 182:83-92.

Wellens, H. J. J.; Lie, K. I.; and Bar, F. W. 1976. Effect of amiodarone in the Wolff-Parkinson-White syndrome. *Am. J. Cardiol.* 38:189-194.

Wilhelmsson, C.; Wilhemsen, L.; Veden, J. A., et al. 1974. Reduction of sudden deaths after myocardial infarction by treatment with alprenolol. Preliminary results. *Lancet* 2:890-1160.

Winkle, R. A.; Glantz, S. A.; and Harrison, D. C. 1975. Pharmacologic therapy of ventricular arrhythmias. *Am. J. Cardiol.* 36:629-650.

Winkle, R. A.; Meffin, P. J.; Fitzgerald, J. W., et al. 1976. Clinical efficacy and pharmacokinetics of a new orally effective antiarrhythmic, tocainide. *Circulation* 54:884-889.

Winkle, R. A.; Lopes, M. G.; Goodman, D. J., et al. 1977. Propranolol for patients with mitral valve prolapse. *Am. Heart J.* 93:422-427.

Winkle, R. A.; Anderson, J. L.; Peters, F., et al. 1978a. The hemodynamic effects of intravenous tocainide in patients with heart disease. *Circulation* 57:788-792.

Winkle, R. A.; Gradman, A. H.; Fitzgerald, J. W., et al. 1978b. Antiarrhythmic drug effect assessed from ventricular arrhythmia reduction in the ambulatory electrocardiogram and treadmill test: comparison of propranolol, procainamide, and quinidine. *Am. J. Cardiol.* 42:473-480.

Winkle, R. A.; Meffin, P. J.; and Harrison, D. C. 1978c. Long-term tocainide therapy for ventricular arrhythmias. *Circulation* 57:1008-1016.

Winkle, R. A.; Mason, J. W.; and Harrison, D. C. 1980. Tocainide for drug-resistant ventricular arrhythmias: efficacy, side effects, and lidocaine responsiveness for predicting tocainide success. *Am. Heart J.* 100:1031-1036.

Winkle, R. A.; Jaillon, P.; Kates, R. E., et al. 1981a. Clinical pharmacology and antiarrhythmic efficacy of n-acetylprocainamide. *Am. J. Cardiol.* 47:123-130.

Winkle, R. A.; Mason, J. W.; Griffin, J. C., et al. 1981b. Malignant ventricular tachyarrhythmias associated with the use of encainide. *Am. Heart J.* 102:857-864.

Winkle, R. A.; Peters, F.; Kates, R. E., et al. 1981c. The clinical pharmacology and antiarrhythmic efficacy of encainide in patients with chronic ventricular arrhythmias. *Circulation* 64:290-296.

Winkle, R. A.; Peters, F.; Kates, R. E., et al. 1981d. The contribution of encainide metabolites to long-term antiarrhythmic efficacy. *Circulation* 64 (*Suppl.* IV):IV-264.

Wit, A. L., Steiner, C.; and Damato, A. N. 1970. Electrophysiologic effects of bretylium tosylate on single fibers of the canine specialized conducting system and ventricle. *J. Pharmacol. Exp. Ther.* 173:344-356.

Woosley, R. L.; McDevitt, D. G.; Nies, A. S., et al. 1977. Suppression of ventricular ectopic depolarizations by tocainide. *Circulation* 56:980-984.

Woosley, R. L.; Kornhauser, D.; Smith, R., et al. 1979. Suppression of chronic ventricular arrhythmias with propranolol. *Circulation* 60:819-827.

Wu, D.; Denes, P.; Bauernfeind, R., et al. 1978. Effects of procainamide on atrioventricular nodal reentrant paroxysmal tachycardia. *Circulation* 57:1171-1179.

Yamaguchi, I.; Singh, B. N.; and Mandel, W. J. In press. Electrophysiological actions of mexiletine on isolated rabbit atria and canine ventricular muscle and Purkinje fibers. *Cardiovasc. Res.*

Zipes, D. P.; and Fischer, J. C. 1974. Effects of agents which inhibit the slow channel on sinus node automaticity and atrioventricular conduction in the dog. *Circ. Res.* 34:184-192.

Zipes, D. P.; Gavin, W. E.; and Foster, P. R. 1977. Aprindine for treatment of supraventricular tachycardias with particular application to Wolff-Parkinson-White syndrome. *Am. J. Cardiol.* 40:586-595.

4 Ambulatory Electrocardiography

Roger A. Winkle, M.D.

Associate Professor of Medicine
Stanford University School of Medicine
Stanford, California

EQUIPMENT

During the past 10 years there has been a marked increase in the number of manufacturers of ambulatory ECG equipment and in the types of recording playback devices that are available. This equipment is expensive, and most clinicians will be limited to using the type of equipment that is available in their local area. A detailed review of each manufacturers' specifications is beyond the scope of this chapter. However, understanding the general types of recording and playback devices available is important so that the physician can employ the type of recording system that is most likely to assist with any given clinical problem.

Recording Devices

Continuous recorders This type of ambulatory ECG recorder is currently the most widely used. Battery-operated recorders are available in either AM or FM recording modes. Both types are suitable for the diagnosis of arrhythmias. These devices permit the recording of two channels of ECG data, have timing channels to compensate for recording and playback speed changes and tape stretch, and have patient-activated event markers for correlating ECG data with patient symptoms and activities. The recorders are connected to the patient with short leads that are affixed to the skin with gel-type patch electrodes. Their small size allows the patient a wide range of activity during the recording session. The most important advantage of continuous recording is that all ECG data are available for later detailed analysis. This permits the diagnosis of both asymptomatic and symptomatic arrhythmic events. The major disadvantage of continuous recorders is the relatively limited duration (usually 24 hours) of recording; therefore, they are not ideally suited for evaluating patient symptoms that occur only infrequently.

Intermittent recorders These battery-operated recording devices are attached to the patient in a manner similar to the continuous recorders. They differ from the continuous systems in that they record the ECG signal only intermittently. Depending on the manufacturer, these recorders may sample ECGs at preselected intervals, such as 30 seconds every 15 minutes, or may record the ECG or advance a counter only when predefined events occur, such as ventricular ectopic beats or tachy- or bradyarrhythmias. In this latter type of system the physician is dependent on the machine to detect the events to be recorded because no permanent record is made of all ECG data, and there is no way of subsequently knowing what the recorder failed to detect. These devices may also be activated by the patient when symptoms occur and typically can be worn for several days with the major limitation on time duration being skin irritation at the site of the electrode. Because symptomatic arrhythmias may be of very transient duration and determining the onset of an arrhythmia is often crucial in making a proper diagnosis, intermittently recording patient-activated devices should have a brief delay loop to be maximally useful. These systems are most valuable for use with patients whose symptoms occur once every few days.

Transtelephonic ECG monitoring These small devices (Hasin, et al., 1976; Grodman, et al., 1979; Juson, et al., 1979) are carried by the patient for protracted periods of time (often weeks or months) but do not remain in contact with the patient's skin continuously. When an ECG recording is to be made, the patient places two electrodes in contact with the skin (often by holding the electrodes on the chest or under the axillae), dials a telephone number, and holds the recording device near the telephone mouthpiece (Figure 4-1A). At the hospital or in the physician's office a recording device is automatically activated and makes a brief ECG rhythm strip (Figure 4-1B). This device is most valuable in patients with infrequent and sustained symptomatic arrhythmias (Figure 4-2). Because the patient may not be near a telephone when an arrhythmia occurs, many of these devices have the ability to store brief strips which may be subsequently transmitted. The device may also be used to make routine intermittent ECG recordings in patients with cardiac pacemakers. The base recording station may be placed in a coronary care unit where trained nursing personnel are available to provide instantaneous observation of transmitted ECGs and give immediate feedback to the patient and his or her physician. An alternative arrangement is to leave the receiving recorder unmanned and review all previously transmitted strips at a later time.

Playback Devices

The ECG playback or scanner unit is most important in the analysis of the continuous type of ambulatory ECG recording because large amounts of prerecorded ECG data must be edited and infrequent or isolated arrhythmic events identified. There are two main types of playback units. One type prints all ECG data rapidly in a miniaturized format on light-sensitive paper. For example, 1 hour of ECG data may be presented per page for a rapid arrhythmia screen with the areas of interest expanded

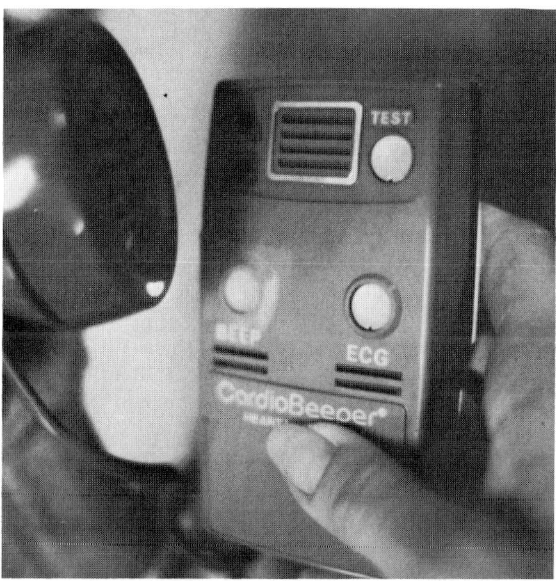

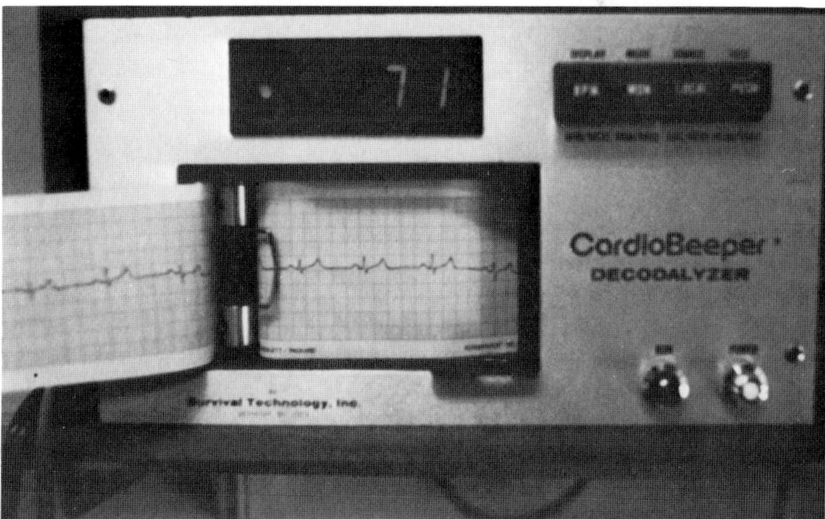

Figure 4-1 Transtelephonic ECG monitoring. Figure 4-1A shows a patient holding the transtelephonic transmitting device near the mouthpiece of a telephone. The transmitter is connected to the patient by means of two short cables with dry electrodes that are placed in each axilla to transmit a lead I ECG. The signal goes over the telephone lines to the base receiving station, which is shown in Figure 4-1B. The base station demodulates the signal and produces a standard ECG rhythm strip.

BASELINE TRANSTELEPHONIC ECG

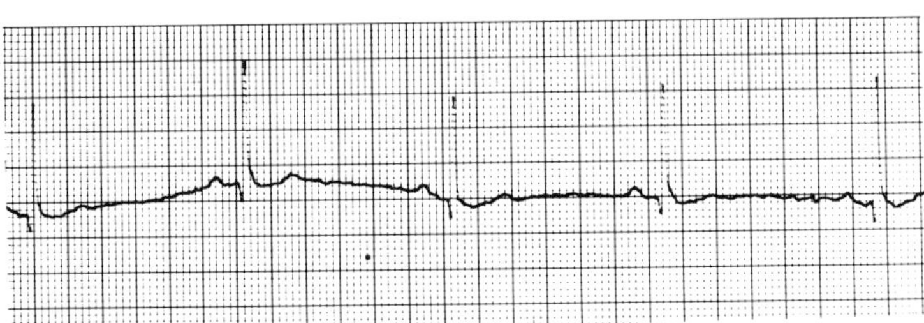

TRANSTELEPHONIC RECORDING DURING SYMPTOMS

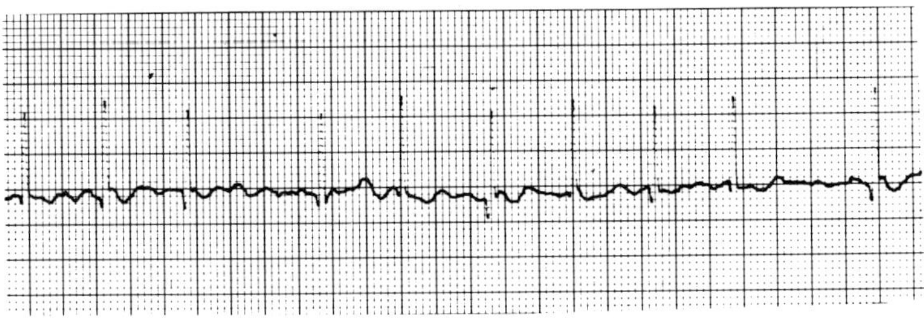

Figure 4-2 An example of the clinical value of transtelephonic ECG monitoring. These recordings were made from a 63-year-old male who complained of intermittent palpitations. A 24-hour ambulatory ECG recording failed to document the cause of his symptoms because no palpitations occurred during the recording period. The upper ECG strip shows a baseline recording sent by the patient that demonstrates only sinus bradycardia. One night during an episode of palpitations the patient transmitted the lower strip, which shows atrial fibrillation with a moderate ventricular response.

in a larger format for detailed interpretation. This type of system offers the advantages of the physician being able to review all the recorded ECG data while minimizing dependence on technician analysis. Such playback systems may require the generous use of expensive silver-containing photographic paper. The other major type of scanner unit permits a combination of visual and automatic analysis of the ECG signal, usually at 60-120 times real time. Standard real-time ECG rhythm strips are made of important arrhythmic events. Computer technology has complemented these systems and improved the accuracy of arrhythmia analysis significantly. All types of systems require close machine-operator interaction, and technicians scanning tapes must be knowledgeable in arrhythmia diagnosis and work closely with both the physician ordering the test and the physician interpreting the test. All systems provide a variety of data output formats. These typically include plots of heart rate vs. time, ventricular ectopic activity vs. time, and ST segment shifts vs. time. Ideally, these scanners should permit easy verification of all data presented in graphic or tabular form.

Esophageal Recordings

One technical problem with 24-hour ambulatory ECG recordings is that P wave identification can be difficult. Even when P waves are easily seen during baseline recordings of sinus rhythm, changes in the patient's body position or activity level may make them difficult to see in one or both of the monitored leads. During episodes of atrial tachyarrhythmia or during ventricular tachycardia P waves are frequently not seen at all. Distinguishing ventricular ectopic beats from supraventricular premature beats with aberration is similarly difficult. Recently, Arzbaecher (1978) described a technique for obtaining long-term esophageal ECG recordings using a small bipolar "pill" electrode that can be placed in a gelatin capsule, which the patient swallows (Figure 4-3). This electrode is connected to a small filtering device that eliminates the respiratory fluctuations that are commonly encountered in esophageal recordings. This system permits excellent continuous recording of atrial activity. By using one channel of the ambulatory ECG recorder for recording surface ECG activity and the other channel for recording esophageal (atrial) activity, the characterization of recorded arrhythmias is enhanced significantly (Figures 4-4 and 10-1). The pill electrodes are well tolerated by most patients over a 24-hour period, although we generally prescribe a soft diet during their use.

PATIENT DIARY

During the ambulatory ECG recording patients should record in a diary or log all activities such as exercise, sleep, and so on. They should also record any cardiac symptoms and the time medications are taken, especially antiarrhythmic drugs. These data are invaluable to the physician interpreting ECG data, enabling him or her to correlate cardiac rate and rhythm with the patient's activities and symptoms. Patients should be instructed to activate the event marker when symptoms or other events occur.

ARTIFACTS

To interpret the results of an ambulatory ECG recording properly, one must understand the types of artifacts that commonly occur on these

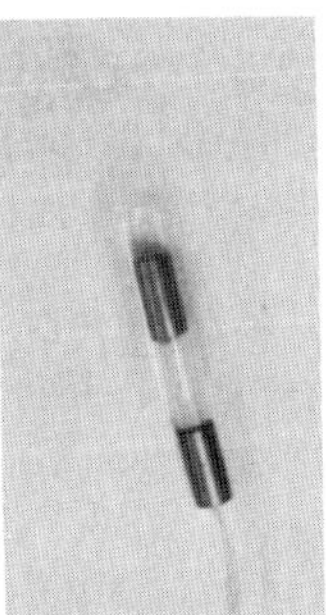

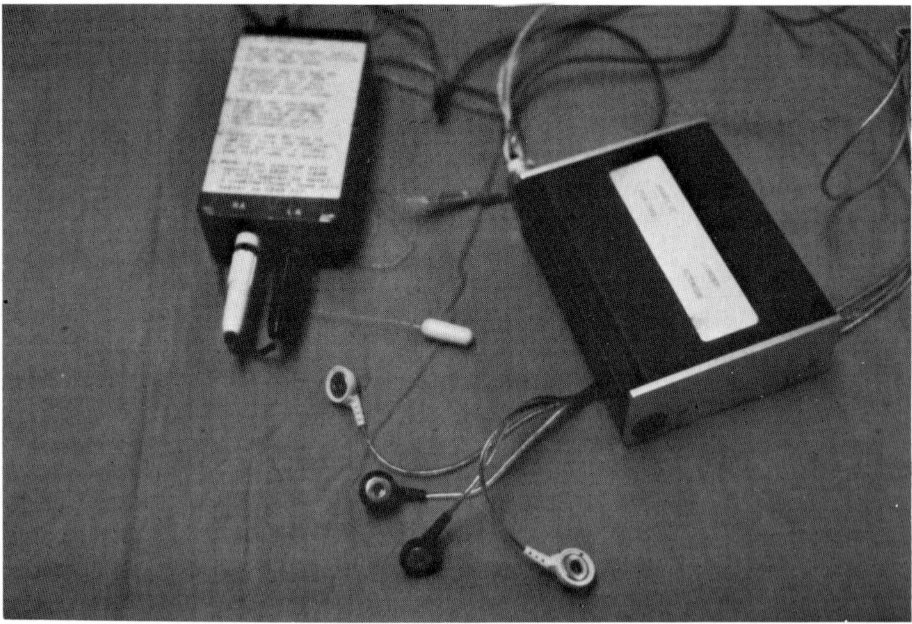

Figure 4-3 Twenty-four hour esophageal ambulatory ECG recording. Figure 4-3A shows the pill electrode, which is swallowed by the patient. This small electrode has two contacts that are 1 cm apart, and in this example it is encased in a clear gelatin capsule. The fine wire exiting from one end of the pill passes up the esophagus and out the corner of the patient's mouth. Figure 4-3B shows the same pill (in the center of the picture) in an opaque gelatin capsule. To the pill's left is the preprocessing box that is connected to one channel of a standard 24-hour ambulatory ECG recorder (which is on the right). Using this equipment it is possible to record 24-hour esophageal recordings and characterize atrial activity even when it is difficult to see P waves on the surface leads.

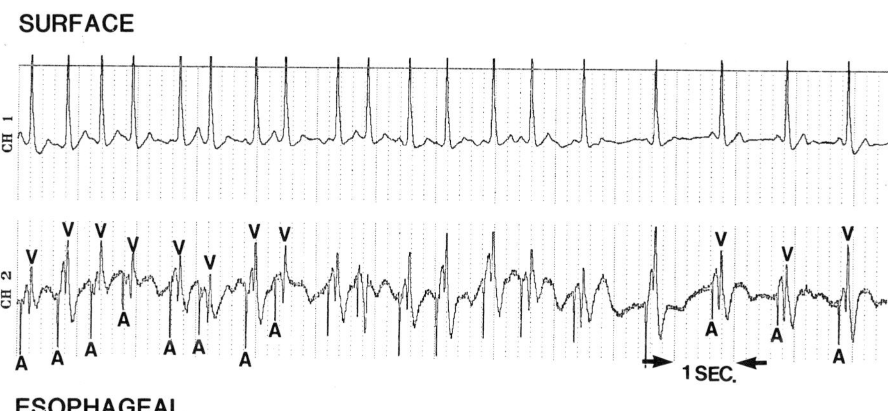

Figure 4-4 An example of the clinical utility of 24-hour esophageal recordings in a patient with arrhythmias. The upper channel shows the surface ECG and the lower channel shows the simultaneously registered esophageal recording. Note that the left-hand portion of the surface lead shows an irregularly irregular rhythm suggestive of atrial fibrillation. The last four QRS complexes show the resumption of normal sinus rhythm. The simultaneously recorded esophageal lead shows that each ventricular electrogram (labeled V) is preceded by a single discrete atrial electrogram (labeled A). This confirms that the arrhythmia was an irregular atrial tachycardia and not atrial fibrillation.

recordings (Krasnow and Bloomfield, 1976). Most artifacts result from improper skin preparation, poor electrode placement and securement, or recorder or playback malfunction. The use of two-channel recordings minimizes the problem, but artifacts can still mimic cardiac rhythm disturbances. Physicians who only see finished reports of ambulatory ECG monitoring data are unlikely to appreciate the variety of artifacts encountered during scanning because most scanning services eliminate artifacts from their final reports.

Artifacts may be classified as pseudoarrhythmias and nonarrhythmias. A variety of pseudoarrhythmias can create diagnostic difficulty for those who are scanning tapes. One common type of artifact probably occurs as a result of transient loss of electrode contact from the patient's skin. This transient loss of signal can mimic sinus pauses or heart block. It usually appears as a gradual diminution in signal followed by a return of the signal over several more beats. Sinus pauses and heart block can also be mimicked by transient slowing or sticking of the tape during playback (Kronzon, et al., 1975). Pseudotachycardias (Malek and Glushien, 1972; Hansmann and Sheppard, 1973) occur most frequently during battery failure at the end of the recording. These can, however, occur intermittently in the middle of a tape and mimic brief episodes of atrial tachycardia. At the end of a tape pseudotachycardias are recognized by the gradual progression of cardiac rate and often a slight diminution in amplitude or cessation of the signal. They show a proportional narrowing of PR interval, QRS duration, and QT interval. Isolated artifacts can mimic premature ventricular complexes or, on occasion, atrial premature beats. Broken leads or poor contact can create a small undulating baseline that can simulate atrial fibrillation or atrial flutter. Gross cyclical irregularities in the signal can sometimes be mistaken for ventricular tachycardia or ventricular flutter.

Nonarrhythmia artifacts generally create problems only because they obscure the normal signal, a problem that is especially severe during automated data analysis. Tapes may occasionally be scanned backward, a situation that is easily recognized by T waves preceding and P waves following the QRS complexes. If tapes are reused, they may be incompletely demagnetized, and two competing rhythms may appear on the tape. Changes in the patient's body position may also mimic ischemic ST-T changes.

MONITORING FOR SPECIFIC SYMPTOMS

Palpitations

Widespread experience with long-term ECG monitoring suggests that a majority of patients with abnormalities of cardiac rhythm are asymptomatic. However, many patients are aware of their rhythm disturbances, and physicians are frequently asked to determine the cause of a patient's palpitations. These palpitations are often brief and may be perceived as isolated skipped or heavy beats or as a sensation of the heart "flip-flopping" in the chest. Palpitations may also be felt as a sensation of the heart stopping and are commonly noted when patients are quiet or resting. Complaints of a rapid racing heart action may also require evaluation. Such symptoms may or may not be related to specific activities. Ambulatory ECG monitoring is ideally suited for evaluating the possible cardiac origin of such complaints (Figure 4-5). The frequency of occurrence and duration of the symptoms should dictate the type of ambulatory ECG monitoring to be employed (i.e., continuous, intermittent, or transtelephonic).

Little data exist regarding the prevalence with which symptoms of palpitation occur in the general population or in patients with specific cardiac diseases and the extent to which such symptoms are caused by cardiac rhythm disturbances. It is not uncommon to discover that symptoms, although highly suggestive of a cardiac origin, occur at a time when a patient has a normal rate and rhythm. Such symptoms are also often caused by isolated atrial or ventricular premature beats and, at

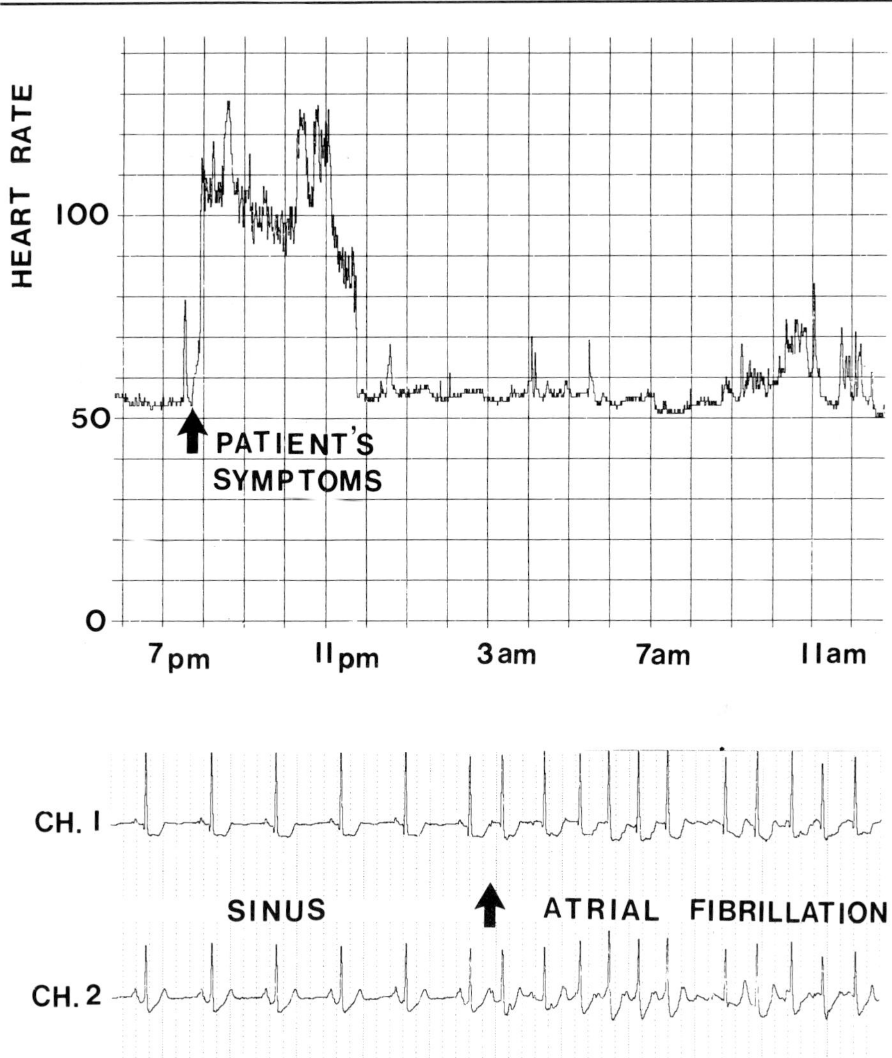

Figure 4-5 Use of ambulatory ECG recordings in symptomatic patients. This figure shows a recording from a female who complained of intermittent palpitations. The upper panel shows a graph of heart rate versus time obtained from an ambulatory ECG recording. At approximately 7:45 P.M. the patient's diary noted the onset of palpitations. These lasted until approximately 11:40 P.M. The heart rate graph illustrates that during this time there was an increase from approximately 55 beats/min to slightly over 100 beats/min. The lower panel shows two simultaneous channels of surface ECG recordings made at the time of onset of the patient's symptoms that document the onset of atrial fibrillation.

times, to more serious rhythm disturbances such as brief sinus pauses or short episodes of a tachyarrhythmia. Patients without symptoms during a period of monitoring may have a variety of asymptomatic arrhythmias recorded. Although such asymptomatic arrhythmias may give a clue as to the etiology of the patient's symptoms, they may be common in the general population. Therefore, serious diagnostic and therapeutic errors may be made if one attributes the patient's symptoms to these asymptomatic arrhythmias. To be of maximal value the ECG recording must be made during an episode of the patient's typical symptoms.

Dizziness and/or Syncope

While palpitations or an awareness of cardiac action may be distressing to the patient, the arrhythmias that cause these symptoms are rarely life-threatening. Symptoms of dizziness and/or syncope, however, can be caused by more serious and life-threatening rhythm disturbances. Patients may complain of dizziness, lightheadedness, a feeling that they are losing consciousness, or actual loss of consciousness. Although these symptoms may have a noncardiac origin or may have a cardiac origin that is unrelated to an arrhythmia, cardiac arrhythmias are one important and readily treated cause (Figure 4-6).

Many studies (Walter, et al., 1970; Goldberg, et al., 1975; Tzivoni and Stern, 1975; Van Durme, 1975; Golf, 1977; Johansson, 1977) have been conducted examining the value of ambulatory ECG monitoring in

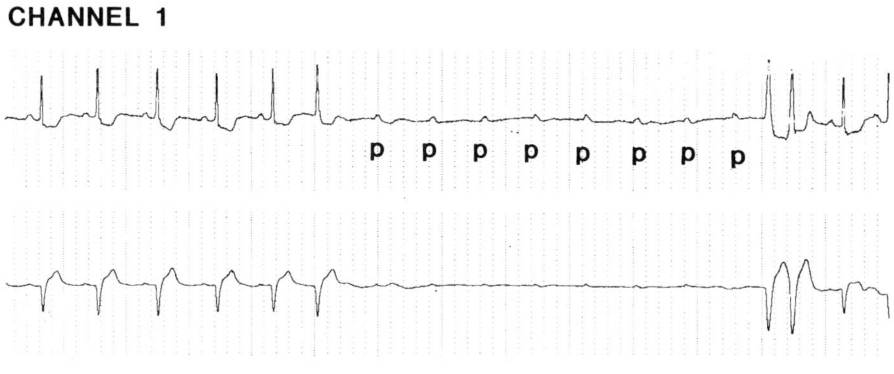

Figure 4-6 Ambulatory ECG recording made in a patient complaining of a vague sensation of intermittent dizziness. A complete neurologic workup had been unrewarding. The two simultaneously recorded surface ECG channels show a 7-second episode of complete heart block terminated by two ventriuclar escape beats. Implantation of a permanent pacemaker completely eliminated these symptoms.

patients with symptoms of dizziness and/or syncope. These studies have confirmed the value of the ambulatory ECG recording in such patients. Because the patient's symptoms may often occur without warning, the continuous type of ECG recording device is most appropriate. The following conclusions may be drawn with regard to ambulatory ECG monitoring in this patient population:

1. Asymptomatic arrhythmias are common in these patients and may not necessarily be the cause of the symptoms. Brief sinus pauses, short bursts of atrial and ventricular tachycardia, and transient first- or second-degree AV block may be recorded, but when the symptoms in question occur, the patient may only have sinus rhythm. One must require that symptoms and arrhythmias occur simultaneously to be certain that the two are causally related. If no symptoms occur, asymptomatic arrhythmias may sometimes give a clue as to the etiology of the patient's symptoms, and empiric therapy may be initiated.
2. A wide variety of cardiac arrhythmias are responsible for symptoms of dizziness and/or syncope. These rhythms include sinus pauses that may occur as a primary event or as post-tachycardia pauses, transient episodes of AV block without adequate escape rhythm, or runs of supraventricular or ventricular tachycardia.
3. Many patients will have their typical symptoms without significant arrhythmia, and important negative information will be obtained that prevents the institution of unnecessary and ineffective antiarrhythmic or pacemaker therapy.
4. Relatively long periods of monitoring may be required to record an episode of the symptom in question. The normal length of time until a cardiac arrhythmia can be confirmed or excluded ranges from several days to as long as several weeks. Given the expense of ambulatory ECG recording this may present a problem in a clinical setting. One valuable technique is to record several days of ECG recording but to not process the recorded ECG data unless symptoms occur.

Virtually all patients with unexplained dizziness, near-syncope, or syncope should have one or more ambulatory ECG recordings performed and ideally the patient should be monitored until symptoms occur. Depending on the patient population anywhere from 10% to 100% of individuals will have an arrhythmic origin of their symptoms confirmed or denied. Specific therapy can be instituted in those cases where an arrhythmia causes symptoms and avoided when symptoms occur during sinus rhythm. Physicians must use clinical judgment regarding a trial of therapy in a situation where asymptomatic arrhythmias are recorded that could account for the symptoms but in which no symptoms occur despite extensive periods of monitoring.

Seizure Disorders

Cardiac arrhythmias can result in generalized seizure activity, and the ambulatory ECG recording can be valuable in determining the etiology of these seizures (Stern and Tzivoni, 1976; Woodley, et al., 1977). No good data exist that estimate the frequency with which apparent epilepsy is caused by cardiac arrhythmias. One recent report found that 20% of patients referred to a neurologic department over a 6-month period had cardiac arrhythmias as the cause of their seizure disorders (Schott, et al., 1977). Long periods of ECG monitoring may be necessary to make this diagnosis. In such patients inappropriate anticonvulsant therapy may be avoided and appropriate antiarrhythmic treatment or pacemaker therapy initiated based on the findings of the ambulatory ECG recordings. Given the frequency with which epilepsy occurs in the general population, it may be unreasonable to recommend ambulatory ECG monitoring for all patients who have a diagnosis of epilepsy. However, any patient in whom other neurologic tests are not consistent with a diagnosis of epilepsy or in whom seizures are not easily controlled with anticonvulsive therapy should undergo prolonged ECG monitoring (Figure 4-7). Such recordings should be continuous unless the patients have auras before their seizures, which would permit activation of intermittent recorders.

ARRHYTHMIAS IN "NORMAL" SUBJECTS

Many studies have characterized the types of arrhythmias recorded on ambulatory ECG recordings in normal subjects, those who are free of obvious organic heart disease, or in a cross section of the population, including patients with and without cardiac diseases (Gilson, et al., 1964; Gilson, 1965; Hinkle, et al., 1969; Clarke, et al., 1976; Raftery and Cashman, 1976; Brodsky, et al., 1977; Glasser, et al., 1979). These studies documented a wide range of arrhythmias that had previously been considered as potentially serious, especially when they occurred in patients with organic heart disease.

Approximately 25%-50% of young healthy subjects will have occasional atrial or ventricular premature beats. Frequent and complex ectopic beats are unusual in this population, occurring in less than 5% of

Figure 4-7 Ambulatory ECG recording from a patient with a well documented seizure disorder that had been controlled for many years with anticonvulsant therapy. Recently, this patient began to develop a new type of seizure that was not manifested by tonoclonic movements but rather by a sensation of "graying out." Ambulatory ECG recording during one of these episodes indicated that the patient had sinus node dysfunction without an escape rhythm. The patient's symptoms were completely eliminated by implantation of a permanent-demand ventricular pacemaker. (*Source:* Reprinted by permission of the publisher from Winkle, R. November 23, 1982. "Indications for Ambulatory ECG Monitoring." *Cardiology Update: Reviews for Physicians.* Copyright 1981 by Elsevier Science Publishing Co., Inc.)

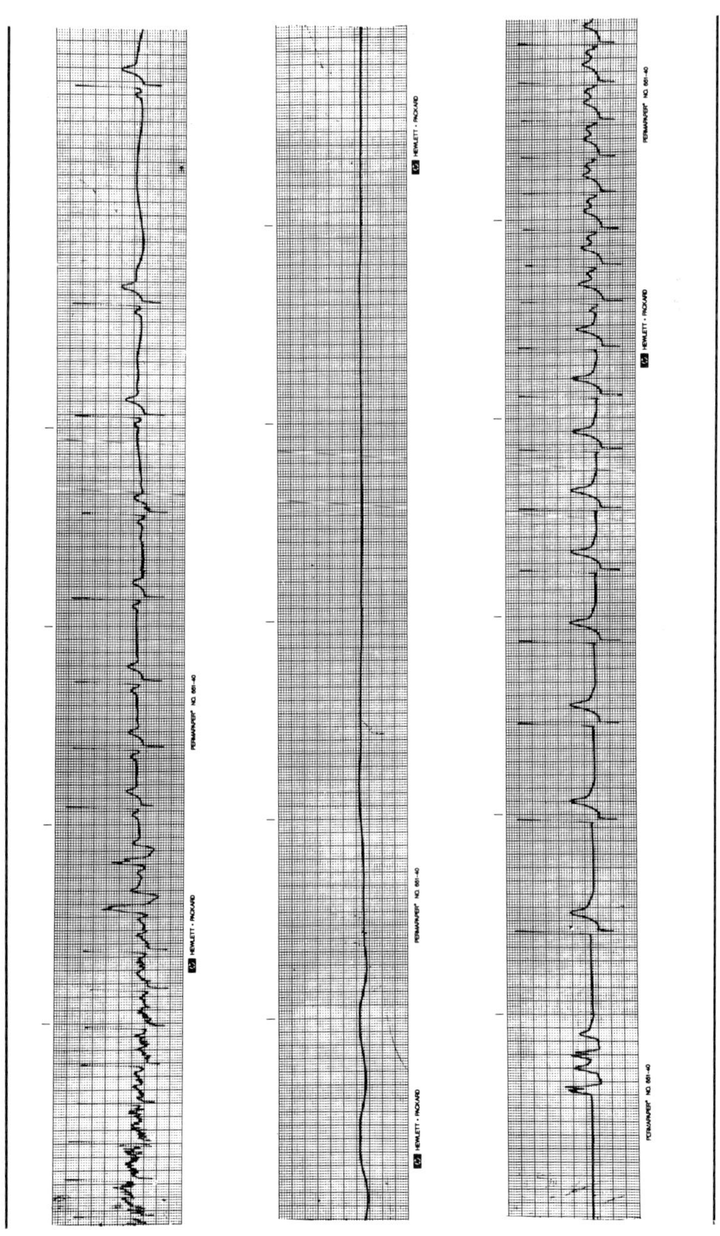

subjects. In a population of older subjects the number who have some premature beats increases to as many as 60% or 70%. Frequent and complex ventricular ectopic beats, including short runs of ventricular or supraventricular tachycardia, occur in up to 10% of middle-aged subjects. Although these more serious arrhythmias are often associated with hypertension or cardiopulmonary disease, they frequently occur in otherwise healthy individuals. Bradyarrhythmias, including marked sinus arrhythmia, brief sinus pauses, and transient nocturnal Wenckebach second-degree AV block, are common in young people and trained athletes but are apparently less frequent in older patient populations.

Thus, a wide range of cardiac conduction disturbances and arrhythmias will be observed when persons without evidence of organic heart disease undergo ambulatory ECG monitoring. Physicians obtaining ambulatory ECG recordings in asymptomatic subjects must interpret the findings carefully in light of these facts. It is important that potentially dangerous antiarrhythmic therapy not be initiated in the presence of ECG findings that have no known clinical significance. Very little information is available regarding the long-term prognostic significance of these arrhythmias, and it must be stressed that the presence of rhythm disturbances in an apparently healthy population does not necessarily make them normal. Only long-term follow-up of these patients (which has not yet been reported) can determine the importance of these arrhythmias.

AMBULATORY ECG RECORDINGS IN SPECIFIC CARDIAC CONDITIONS

Conduction System Disease

Patients with abnormalities of the cardiac conduction system are frequently encountered in clinical practice (see Chapter 6). Such abnormalities include first-degree AV block, second-degree Wenckebach or Mobitz II block, and abnormalities of His-Purkinje conduction, including various types of bundle branch block and bi- and trifascicular block. In most clinical situations the indications for permanent pacing are clear-cut, and short rhythm strips or inhospital monitoring will have already provided enough information. However, ambulatory ECG monitoring can often provide important additional clinical information in such patients. When patients with abnormalities of the conduction system short of complete AV block have symptoms such as dizziness, presyncope, or syncope on 12-lead ECG, ambulatory ECG recording is valuable in searching for higher degrees of AV block. Several recordings may be required to get ECG recordings while symptoms are occurring, especially when symptoms are infrequent. Although complete heart block may be responsible for the symptoms, the conduction abnormalities on the 12-lead ECG may have been a false clue, and other arrhythmias such as supraventricular or ventricular tachyarrhythmias may be causing the symptoms. Because many of these patients will be elderly and can have a variety of non-arrhythmic etiologies for their symptoms, their symptoms are frequently unrelated to any cardiac rhythm disturbance. In such patients unnecessary permanent pacing will be avoided by the use of ambulatory ECG monitoring.

The indications for ambulatory ECG recordings in asymptomatic patients with abnormalities of the cardiac conduction system on resting ECGs are less certain. If routine ambulatory ECG monitoring is performed in such patients and no advanced degrees of conduction system disease are found, the physician may feel confident in following the patient without permanent pacing. The role of sequential monitoring over time in such patients has not been completely defined, but it may be valuable. A more difficult situation arises when monitoring done in patients for reasons other than suspected conduction system disease uncovers asymptomatic episodes of transient second- or third-degree AV block such as those that may occur during sleep. For such patients physicians must make individual decisions as to the advisability of permanent pacing. It should be remembered that episodes of first-degree AV block or transient episodes of second-degree Wenckebach block may be recorded occasionally, especially in younger healthy persons, and should not necessarily be considered as representing cardiac pathology.

Sinus Node Disease

Abnormalities of sinus node function may present as sinus bradycardia, sinus pause or arrest, or marked sinus node suppression after termination of supraventricular tachycardias (see Chapter 6). For many patients the diagnosis of sinus node disease will be readily apparent, and the indications for pacing will be obvious. However, ambulatory ECG monitoring can be valuable in patients with sinus node disease (Crook, et al., 1973; Reiffel, et al., 1977; Lister, et al., 1978), especially those patients who show minor abnormalities of sinus node function on resting ECGs or short rhythm strips or during intracardiac electrophysiologic studies. When such patients have symptoms suggesting more severe sinus node abnormality, prolonged monitoring with ambulatory ECGs may help to confirm the etiology of their symptoms. Although intracardiac electrophysiologic evaluation of sinus node function can detect abnormalities in many patients, such evaluations sometimes reveal normal sinus node function in patients with symptomatic sinus node dysfunction during prolonged ambulatory ECG monitoring. Therefore, ambulatory ECG monitoring is often a useful adjunct to intracardiac evaluations of sinus node function. It should be recognized that sinus bradycardia and brief sinus pauses may both be frequently recorded in younger patient populations and should not be presumed either to represent sinus node disease or to be an indication for permanent pacing. When patients undergo ambulatory ECG recordings for other indications and are found to have evidence of asymptomatic sinus node disease, the physician must make an individual decision regarding the advisability of therapy. Sequential monitoring of such patients during prolonged follow-up may play a role in defining the natural history of the disease and indications for pacing in such patients. Ambulatory ECG monitoring can also be valuable in patients with the bradycardia-tachycardia syndrome when antiarrhythmic therapy is necessary to control the tachyarrhythmias by evaluating whether such therapy aggravates the bradyarrhythmia caused by sinus node disease (Lipski, et al., 1976). This is most common when using digitalis, beta blocking agents, and calcium antagonists for the control of the supraventricular arrhythmias but can also occur when using membrane-active agents that depress sinus node function.

Pacemaker Evaluation

In addition to detecting those patients who are candidates for permanent pacing, ambulatory ECG recording can be valuable in the patient who already has a permanent pacemaker (Bleifer, et al., 1974; Ward, et al., 1977). Ambulatory ECGs can be used to detect pacemaker malfunction, which should be suspected when the symptoms that prompted the pacemaker's initial use recur. Although standard ECGs, precise pulse-width and cycle-length measuring devices, and transtelephonic pacemaker-analysis systems can usually detect pacemaker failure or impending battery depletion, ambulatory electrocardiography sometimes plays a role in detecting such malfunctions (Figure 4-8). Prolonged recording periods may be required to detect intermittent pacemaker malfunction.

Ambulatory ECG recordings can also document and confirm that pacemakers are functioning normally with respect to capture, sensing, and pacing rate. They provide information about other atrial and ventricular tachyarrhythmias that may be occurring, as well. With the growing complexity of current pacemaker generator and lead systems, the documentation of normal pacemaker function is becoming increasingly important. Routine ambulatory ECG monitoring is especially valuable in establishing the proper functioning of antitachycardia pacemakers. These pacemakers can be either patient-activated or may automatically activate to terminate ventricular or supraventricular tachyarrhythmias. Because appropriate function can only be documented when a tachyarrhythmia occurs, ambulatory ECG monitoring has proved to be an excellent method for establishing proper function.

Cardiomyopathies

Patients with all types of cardiomyopathies experience a variety of conduction disturbances and arrhythmias and may die a sudden arrhythmic

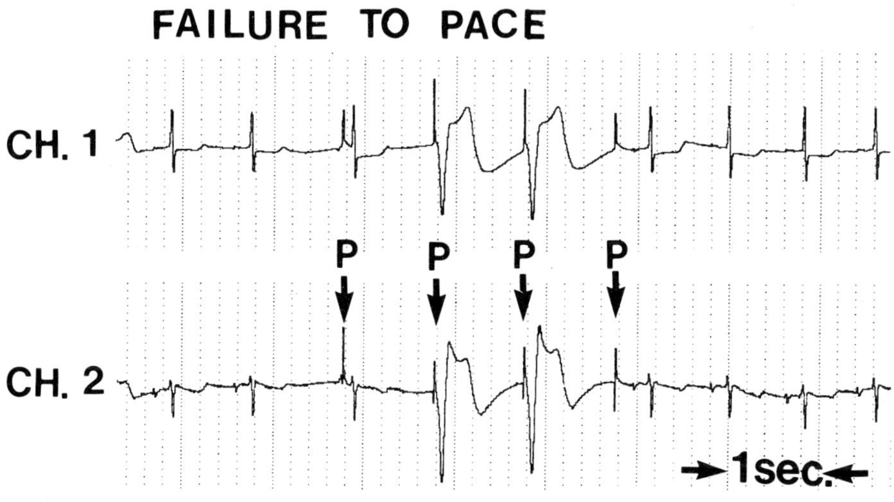

Figure 4-8 Example of pacemaker failure first detected by an ambulatory ECG recording. This shows two simultaneous surface ECG channels. There are four pacer spikes (labeled P). In this example the first and last pacer spike failed to capture the myocardium, indicating problems with the patient's pacemaker lead.

cardiac death. Patients with congestive cardiomyopathies are candidates for ambulatory ECG monitoring when resting ECGs reveal abnormalities of conduction and/or the patients suffer from symptoms that could be caused by cardiac arrhythmias. In such cases ambulatory electrocardiography can help to determine the need for specific antiarrhythmic and/or pacemaker therapy. Because little is known about the prognostic significance of asymptomatic arrhythmias recorded in such patients, decisions regarding the advisability of therapy must rest with the attending physician. Several systematic studies of the arrhythmias that occur in patients with hypertrophic cardiomyopathies have been conducted. One research team (Ingham, et al., 1975) found that 70% of patients have episodes of paroxysmal supraventricular tachycardia or atrial fibrillation. In many instances these are brief asymptomatic episodes, and their clinical significance is unknown. This same study also noted that 89% of patients had ventricular ectopic beats, including frequent premature ventricular beats in 25% and ventricular tachycardia in 7% of patients. Another study (Savage, et al., 1979) reported that 83% of patients had some ventricular arrhythmias and 28% had more than 100 ventricular ectopic beats in 24 hours. Complex arrhythmias were frequent, with 60% of patients having multiform premature ventricular complexes, 32% having pairs, and 19% having ventricular tachycardia.

Fifty-four percent of patients had atrial premature beats during the recording, and most patients with atrial ectopic beats had echocardiographic evidence of left atrial enlargement. Fifteen patients had paroxysms of supraventricular tachycardia during the monitoring. Twenty patients gave a prior history of syncope; however, arrhythmias were no different in these individuals than in the 80 patients who lacked a history of syncope. Ten of 18 patients complaining of palpitations during the ambulatory ECG recording had no arrhythmias at the time of their complaint; the others had only isolated ectopic beats. None of the 19 patients complaining of lightheadedness during the recording had serious arrhythmias at the time of symptoms. Both studies found that ambulatory ECG recordings were superior to exercise treadmill testing for the detection of cardiac arrhythmias in patients with hypertrophic cardiomyopathies.

Routine ambulatory ECG monitoring is not indicated for all patients with hypertrophic cardiomyopathies until more information becomes available about the prognostic value of detecting asymptomatic arrhythmias. The poor correlation between symptoms suggesting arrhythmia and the occurrence of major supraventricular or ventricular arrhythmias implies that all patients with symptoms should undergo ambulatory ECG monitoring before the initiation of antiarrhythmic therapy.

Mitral Valve Prolapse

The prevalence of arrhythmias in asymptomatic persons found to have mitral valve prolapse appears to be low. However, symptomatic (palpitations, chest pain, dyspnea, and presyncope or syncope) patients with mitral valve prolapse frequently have arrhythmias recorded on ambulatory ECG. In a Stanford study of 24 such patients we found that 90% had ventricular ectopic beats on a 24-hour ambulatory ECG recording and 50% had frequent ectopic beats (Winkle, et al., 1975). Twelve patients had pairs, nine had bigeminy, and five had brief episodes of ventricular tachycardia. Fifteen patients demonstrated atrial premature beats and seven had brief asymptomatic episodes of supraventricular tachycardia. There was a poor correlation between symptoms suggesting arrhythmias and the occurrence of serious cardiac arrhythmias. Another research team (DeMaria, et al., 1976) performed 10-hour ambulatory ECG recordings in 31 patients with mitral valve prolapse and noted premature ventricular beats in 58% of patients, most of whom had complex premature ventricular beats. Thirty-five percent of patients experienced supraventricular arrhythmias and 9% had bradyarrhythmias. Both our study and DeMaria's show that ambulatory ECG recordings are better than exercise treadmill tests for the detection of arrhythmias.

No information is available regarding the prognostic value of arrhythmias recorded on ambulatory ECGs in patients with mitral valve prolapse. Although sudden death can occur in this syndrome (Winkle, et al., 1976), the overall incidence is extraordinarily low considering the large number of patients with mitral valve prolapse and the frequency with which arrhythmias are recorded in symptomatic patients. Until more is known about the prognostic value of asymptomatic arrhythmias, we do not recommend routine ambulatory ECG recordings in all patients with mitral valve prolapse. However, because of the poor correlation between symptoms suggesting arrhythmias and the occurrence of cardiac arrhythmias requiring therapy, all patients who have symptoms suggesting a cardiac arrhythmia are candidates for ambulatory ECG monitoring. If arrhythmias are the cause of the symptoms, specific therapy can be initiated. If symptoms occur without cardiac arrhythmias, unnecessary therapy will be avoided.

Preexcitation Syndromes

Episodes of paroxysmal supraventricular tachycardia are uncommon on ambulatory ECG among asymptomatic patients who have only ECG findings of preexcitation (Isaeff, et al., 1972) but may be recorded in up to 25% of patients who have a history that suggests episodes of supraventricular tachycardia (Hindman, et al., 1973). When symptoms suggest an arrhythmia but no arrhythmias have been previously documented, we recommend ambulatory or transtelephonic ECG monitoring before consideration of specific therapy because the palpitations may be unrelated to cardiac arrhythmias. When symptoms are documented to be caused by an arrhythmia, further investigation, including invasive electrophysiologic studies, can be performed (see Chapters 2 and 9). If no arrhythmias are found at the time of palpitations, unnecessary therapy may be avoided.

Chronic Obstructive Pulmonary Disease

Patients with chronic obstructive pulmonary disease (COPD) have a variety of cardiac arrhythmias. Most studies have focused on arrhythmias occurring during acute respiratory failure in hospitalized patients and show frequent supraventricular arrhythmias, including sinus tachycardia atrial premature beats, multifocal atrial tachycardia, and atrial fibrillation. Ventricular arrhythmias are less common but do occur in such patients. In hospitalized patients on-line continuous ECG monitoring is the most appropriate method for arrhythmia evaluation.

Ambulatory ECGs in outpatients with COPD have shown a high prevalence of ventricular arrhythmias (Kleiger and Senior, 1974). Although sudden cardiac death does occur in patients with COPD, it is not known whether such deaths can be predicted by the finding of asymptomatic complex ventricular ectopy on ambulatory ECG recordings. For this reason routine ambulatory ECG recordings are not indicated for all patients with COPD. However, any patient with symptoms suggesting arrhythmias is a candidate for monitoring. Patients who have COPD take a variety of medications with the potential for cardiac stimulation, and ambulatory ECG monitoring may be valuable in those individuals with known ventricular arrhythmias or in those who have organic heart disease. Clinicians must judge the advisability of performing such recordings for each individual patient. Because ventricular arrhythmias can occur sporadically and nonreproducibly, physicians should be certain that any apparent worsening of arrhythmias by medication given for the pulmonary disease occurs reproducibly before assuming a definite cause-and-effect relationship.

Coronary Artery Disease

All patients with coronary heart disease who have symptoms suggesting a cardiac arrhythmia are candidates for ambulatory ECG monitoring. In contrast to other cardiac conditions, considerable knowledge exists about the prognostic value of asymptomatic ventricular arrhythmias occurring on ambulatory ECG recordings in patients with coronary artery disease, especially those who have had a recent acute myocardial infarction (Moss, et al., 1971; Kotler, et al., 1973; Moss, et al., 1974; Moss, et al., 1975; Schulze, et al., 1975; Vismara, et al., 1975; Wenger, et al., 1975; Luria, et al., 1976; Rehnqvist, 1976; Ruberman, et al., 1976; Moss, et al., 1977; Rehnqvist and Sjogren, 1977; Ruberman, et al., 1977; Schulze, et al., 1977; Bigger, et al., 1978; DeSoyza, et al., 1978; Rehnqvist, 1978; DeBusk, et al., 1980; Moss, et al., 1980). Although the many studies examining the prognostic value of these arrhythmias have varied considerably in terms of patient population, duration of ambulatory ECG recordings, definitions of frequent and complex ventricular ectopic beats, and definitions of end points and cardiac events, certain conclusions can be drawn from them. They all suggest that premature ventricular beats occur frequently in the postinfarction period, ranging from 52% of patients in studies using only 1-hour ECG recordings to 88% of patients in studies using 24 hours of recording with careful detailed scanning of the tapes. Frequent ventricular ectopic beats (defined as more than approximately 10-20 beats/hr) occur in from 7% to 26% of patients, and complex ventricular ectopic beats are even more frequent. Studies comparing ambulatory ECG recordings to exercise treadmill tests for arrhythmia detection have consistently found the ambulatory ECG to be superior (Crawford, et al., 1974; Ryan, et al., 1975; DeSoyza, et al., 1977; Problete, et al., 1978). However, these studies do show a small subset of patients whose arrhythmias only show up on exercise treadmill tests.

The majority of studies examining the prognostic importance of asymptomatic ventricular ectopic beats recorded in postinfarction patients have indicated that they identify patients at risk for subsequent death. These ectopic beats have prognostic value when they are frequent and complex. It is difficult to provide exact cutoff frequencies above which patients are at risk, because not all studies examined the frequency of ventricular ectopic beats independent of complexity and the ones that did used varying definitions. However, a commonly used cutoff frequency for identifying high-risk patients is 10 ventricular ectopic beats/hr. Similarly, it is not possible to state exactly which type of complex ventricular ectopic beat is most important in identifying patients at risk for sudden death because not all studies examined each category of complex beat, some used arbitrary classification schemes that provide information only about the highest grades of arrhythmias achieved, and the occurrence of one type of complex ectopic beat is not independent from the occurrence of other types. However, most investigators consider pairs and salvos (the repetitive forms) to be the most predictive of subsequent mortality. Studies examining multiple factors that may be predictive of subsequent cardiac death have generally found that, in addition to complex and frequent ectopic beats on ambulatory ECG recordings, a variety of factors relating to ventricular function (i.e., ejection fraction, functional class, history of congestive heart failure, diuretic therapy, blood urea nitrogen levels, and heart size) also have prognostic value. Ventricular ectopic beats have predictive value that is independent of that given by poor ventricular function. Most studies examining the predictive value of ventricular arrhythmias on ambulatory ECG used less than 24 hours of ambulatory ECG recording and were done several years ago when scanning techniques were less accurate than they are now. With longer periods of ambulatory ECG monitoring and more accurate methods of detection, very infrequent complex ectopic beats will be detected, which may not have the same prognostic value as when they occur more frequently.

Although arrhythmias on ambulatory ECG monitoring identify patients at increased risk of subsequent death, it remains controversial whether all patients with a recent infarction should undergo ambulatory ECG monitoring prior to or shortly after hospital discharge. Although many physicians prefer to treat coronary disease patients who have complex and frequent ectopic beats with antiarrhythmic therapy, the benefit to the patient is unproved. If it can ever be confirmed that pharmacologic suppression of ventricular ectopic beats in these patients prevents sudden death, widespread use of ambulatory ECG monitoring will clearly be indicated. Although some advocates of ambulatory ECG monitoring recommend sequential Holter monitoring for postinfarction patients, one study (Moss, et al., 1977) found that recordings made 5 months after infarction have no value in predicting subsequent mortality.

TREATING CHRONIC VENTRICULAR ARRHYTHMIAS

When patients with palpitations have isolated ventricular ectopic beats or brief runs of ventricular tachycardia as the cause of their symptoms and antiarrhythmic therapy seems justified, ambulatory ECG monitoring permits objective evaluation of the response of the arrhythmia to antiarrhythmic therapy. Although the clinical benefit of suppressing asymptomatic chronic ventricular arrhythmias with antiarrhythmic drugs remains unproved (see Chapter 10), the ambulatory ECG is the most objective method for judging drug efficacy.

When using ambulatory ECG recordings to document the suppression of chronic ventricular ectopic beats, one must consider the variability in numbers and complexity of chronic ventricular arrhythmias in untreated individuals (Figure 4-9). Misner and colleagues (1978) studied 40 ambulatory adult subjects with 6-hour recordings on two subsequent days and repeated the recordings after 6 weeks to 18 months, noting significant long-term variation in the number of ventricular ectopic beats in some individual patients. This study concluded that despite some underlying level of consistency, PVC frequency can exhibit considerable variation over time and emphasized "the danger of attributing effects on PVCs to environment, exercise, or therapeutic intervention on the basis of case histories outside a context of strong clinical and statistical control." In a Stanford study involving 20 patients with frequent ventricular premature beats we demonstrated the real nature of this danger (Winkle, 1978). We examined a 6-hour ECG recording simulating the conditions of acute antiarrhythmic drug testing and found that spontaneous variation in ventricular arrhythmias frequently mimicked antiarrhythmic drug effect if a criterion of drug efficacy of only 50%-80% PVC suppression were used. In that study a reasonable criterion of drug efficacy would have been 1 hour or more of 90% or greater ventricular ectopic beat reduction compared with a half-hour control period.

Morganroth and colleagues (1978) examined the variation in PVC frequencies in 15 patients undergoing repeated ambulatory ECG monitoring. That study noted that 48% of the variation in ectopic beat frequencies was hour-to-hour variation, 23% was day-to-day, and 37% occurred over longer periods. Using statistical techniques these researchers established criteria for separating spontaneous decline in arrhythmias from antiarrhythmic drug effect. For the usual 24-hour recording obtained on antiarrhythmic drug therapy, one would have needed to observe an 83% reduction in ectopic beats compared to a 24-hour control to attribute the reduction to drug response. In our study we estimated a similar figure of 90% based on two 24-hour ambulatory ECG recordings obtained 1 month apart (Winkle, et al. 1978). Another study (Engler, et al., 1979) found a similar figure of 78% based on two 24-hour recordings done 2 days apart. Because of differences in patient populations, duration of monitoring, and the time elapsing between recordings, it is difficult to assign an arbitrary percentage reduction for 24-hour ECG recordings that will define drug effect for all patients and patient populations. However, currently available data suggest that approximately 80% reductions are

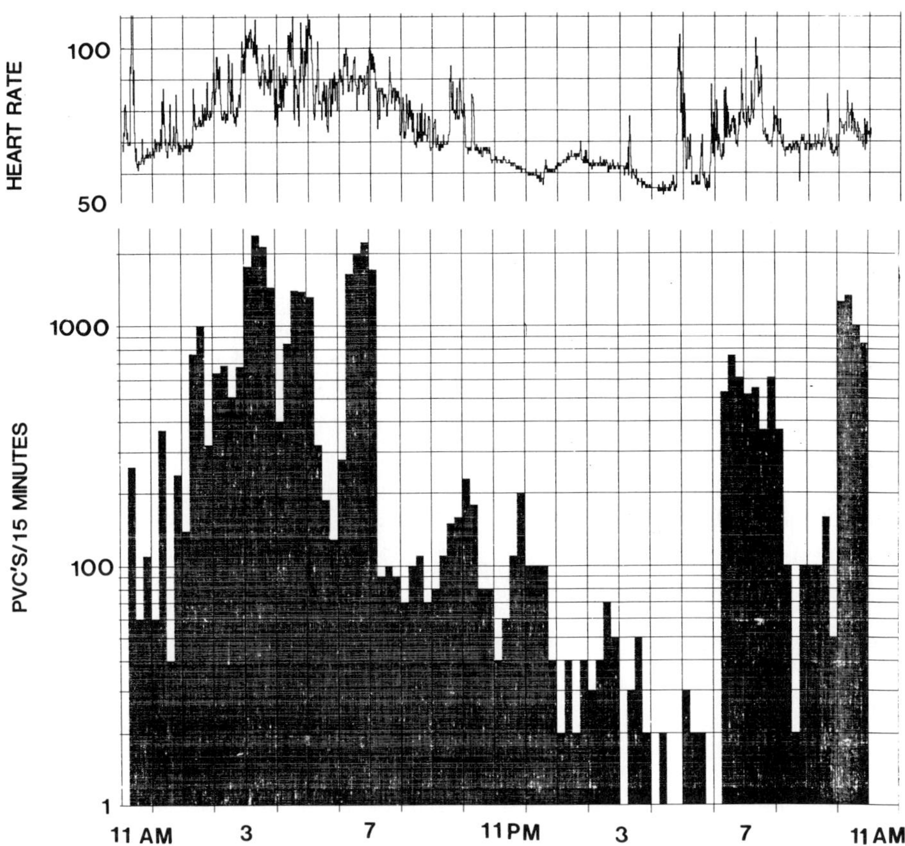

Figure 4-9 Relationship between spontaneous fluctuation of ventricular arrhythmias and changes in the underlying heart rate. Although for many patients there is no apparent cause for the marked spontaneous variation in ventricular ectopic beat frequency, the patient in this figure showed changes in heart rate that seemed to account for the variation in PVC frequency. The upper panel shows the heart rate over a 24-hour period, and the lower portion shows the number of PVCs per 15 minutes over the same 24-hour period. When heart rate increases so does PVC frequency, and when heart rate diminishes PVC frequency also diminishes. (*Source:* Winkle, R. A. 1982. The relationship between ventricular ectopic beat frequency and heart rate. *Circulation* 66:439-446.)

necessary to be confident of drug effect rather than spontaneous decline in arrhythmias. There is a similar significant variability in the occurrence of couplets and salvos that must be considered when judging drug efficacy (Michelson and Morganroth, 1980).

The value of documenting the suppression of asymptomatic ventricular ectopic beats using ambulatory ECG monitoring in patients with recurrent episodes of ventricular tachycardia and/or fibrillation is controversial. Graboys, et al., (1982) reported only a 2.3% annual mortality in a group of 98 patients with prior ventricular fibrillation or ventricular tachycardia in whom drugs were given to suppress advanced grades of asymptomatic ventricular ectopic beats as detected by ambulatory ECG monitoring and exercise and psychologic stress tests. However, another study (Myerburg, et al., 1979) suggested that drug therapy can prevent sudden death caused by ventricular fibrillation without suppressing complex ventricular ectopy on ambulatory ECG recording. Antiarrhythmic drug selection based on the inducibility of sustained ventricular tachycardia during intracardiac electrophysiologic studies may minimize the need to obtain ambulatory ECG recordings in patients with recurrent sustained ventricular tachycardia (Mason and Winkle, 1978 and 1980) or in patients resuscitated from out-of-hospital cardiac arrest (Ruskin, et al., 1980) (see Chapter 10).

REFERENCES

Arzbaecher, R. 1978. A pill electrode for the study of cardiac arrhythmia. *Med. Instrum.* 12:277-281.

Bigger, J. T., Jr.; Heller, C. A.; Wenger, T. L., et al. 1978. Risk stratification after acute myocardial infarction. *Am. J. Cardiol.* 42:202-210.

Bleifer, S. B.; Bleifer, D. J.; Hansmann, D. R., et al. 1974. Diagnosis of occult arrhythmias by Holter electrocardiography. *Prog. Cardiovasc. Dis.* 16:569-599.

Brodsky, M.; Wu, D.; Denes, P., et al. 1977. Arrhythmias documented by 24-hour continuous electrocardiographic monitoring in 50 male medical students without apparent heart disease. *Am. J. Cardiol.* 39:390-395.

Clarke, J. M.; Hamer, J.; Shelton, J. R., et al. 1976. The rhythm of the normal human heart. *Lancet* 1:508-512.

Crawford, M.; O'Rourke, R.; Ramakrishna, N., et al. 1974. Comparative effectiveness of exercise testing and continuous monitoring for detecting arrhythmias in patients with previous myocardial infarction. *Circulation* 50:301-305.

Crook, B. R. M.; Cashman, P. M. M.; Stott, F. D., et al. 1973. Tape monitoring of the electrocardiogram in ambulant patients with sinoatrial disease. *Br. Heart J.* 35:1009-1013.

DeBusk, R. F.; Davidson, D. M.; Houston, N., et al. 1980. Serial ambulatory electrocardiography and treadmill exercise testing following uncomplicated myocardial infarction. *Am. J. Cardiol.* 45:547-554.

DeMaria, A. N.; Amsterdam, E. A.; Vismara, L. A., et al. 1976. Arrhythmias in the mitral valve prolapse syndrome: prevalence, nature, and frequency. *Ann. Intern. Med.* 84:656-660.

DeSoyza, N.; Murphy, M. L.; Bissett, J. K., et al. 1977. Detecting ventricular arrhythmia after myocardial infarction: comparison of Holter monitoring and treadmill exercise. *South. Med. J.* 70:403-404.

DeSoyza, N.; Bennett, F. A.; Murphy, M. L., et al. 1978. The relationship of paroxysmal ventricular tachycardia complicating the acute phase and ventricular arrhythmia during the late-hospital phase of myocardial infarction to long-term survival. *Am. J. Med.* 64:377-381.

Engler, R.; Ryan, W.; LeWinter, M., et al. 1979. Assessment of long-term antiarrhythmic therapy: studies on the long-term efficacy and toxicity of tocainamide. *Am. J. Cardiol.* 43:612-618.

Gilson, J. S. 1965. Electrocardiocorder-AVSEP patterns in 37 normal adult men: a four-year experience. *Am. J. Cardiol.* 16:789-793.

Gilson, J. S.; Holter, N. J.; and Glasscock, W. R. 1964. Clinical observations using the Electrocardiocorder-AVSEP continuous electrocardiographic system: tentative standards and typical patterns. *Am. J. Cardiol.* 14:204-217.

Glasser, S. P.; Clark, P. I.; and Applebaum, H. J. 1979. Occurrence of frequent complex arrhythmias detected by ambulatory monitoring: findings in an apparently healthy asymptomatic elderly population. *Chest* 75:565-568.

Goldberg, A. D.; Raftery, E. B.; and Cashman, P. M. M. 1975. Ambulatory electrocardiographic records in patients with transient cerebral attacks or palpitation. *Br. Med. J.* 4:569-571.

Golf, S. 1977. Swallowing syncope. *Acta Med. Scand.* 201:585-586.

Graboys, T. B.; Lown, B.; Podrid, P. J., et al. 1982. Long-term survival of patients with malignant ventricular arrhythmia treatment with antiarrhythmic drugs. *Am. J. Cardiol.* 50:437-443.

Grodman, R. S.; Capone, R. J.; and Most, A. S. 1979. Arrhythmia surveillance by transtelephonic monitoring: comparison with Holter monitoring in symptomatic ambulatory patients. *Am. Heart J.* 98:459-464.

Hansmann, D. R.; and Sheppard, J. J. 1973. ECG-monitor artifacts (letter to the editor). *Ann. Intern. Med.* 78:619.

Hasin, Y.; David, D.; and Rogel, S. 1976. Diagnostic and therapeutic assessment by telephone electrocardiographic monitoring of ambulatory patients. *Br. Med. J.* 2:609-612.

Hindman, M. C.; Last, J. H.; and Rosen, K. M. 1973. Wolff-Parkinson-White syndrome observed by portable monitoring. *Ann. Intern. Med.* 79:654-663.

Hinkle, L. E.; Carver, S. T.; and Stevens, M. 1969. The frequency of asymptomatic disturbances of cardiac rhythm and conduction in middle-aged men. *Am. J. Cardiol.* 24:629-650.

Ingham, R. E.; Rossen, R. M.; Goodman, D. J., et al. 1975. Ambulatory electrocardiographic monitoring in idiopathic hypertrophic subaortic stenosis (abstract). *Circulation* 51 and 52 (*Suppl.* II):II-93.

Isaeff, D. M.; Gaston, J. H.; and Harrison, D. C. 1972. Wolff-Parkinson-White syndrome. Long-term monitoring for arrhythmias. *J.A.M.A.* 222: 449-453.

Johansson, B. W. 1977. Long-term ECG in ambulatory clinical practice. *Eur. J. Cardiol.* 5:39-48.

Juson, P.; Holmes, D. R.; and Baker, W. P. 1979. Evaluation of outpatient arrhythmias utilizing transtelephonic monitoring. *Am. Heart J.* 97:759-761.

Kleiger, R. E.; and Senior, R. M. 1974. Long-term electrocardiographic monitoring of ambulatory patients with chronic airway obstruction. *Chest* 65:483-487.

Kotler, M. N.; Tabatznik, B.; Mower, M. M., et al. 1973. Prognostic significance of ventricular ectopic beats with respect to sudden death in the late postinfarction period. *Circulation* 47:959-966.

Krasnow, A. Z.; and Bloomfield, D. K. 1976. Artifacts in portable electrocardiographic monitoring. *Am. Heart J.* 91:349-357.

Kronzon, I.; Schloss, M.; and Bear, G. 1975. Malfunctioning electrocardiographic monitor simulating sinus arrest. *Chest* 68:582-583.

Lipski, J.; Cohen, L.; Espinoza, J., et al. 1976. Value of Holter monitoring in assessing cardiac arrhythmias in symptomatic patients. *Am. J. Cardiol.* 37:102-107.

Lister, J. W.; Gosseline, A. J.; and Swaye, P. S. 1978. Obscure syncope and the sick sinus syndrome. *PACE* 1:68-79.

Luria, M. H.; Knoke, J. D.; Margolis, R. M., et al. 1976. Acute myocardial infarction: prognosis after recovery. *Ann. Intern. Med.* 85:561-565.

Malek, J.; and Glushien, A. 1972. Artifacts in portable ECG monitoring. *Ann. Intern. Med.* 77:1004.

Mason, J. W.; and Winkle, R. A. 1978. Electrode-catheter arrhythmia induction in the selection and assessment of antiarrhythmic drug therapy for recurrent ventricular tachycardia. *Circulation* 58:971-985.

Mason, J. W.; and Winkle, R. A. 1980. Accuracy of the ventricular tachycardia-induction study for predicting long-term efficacy and inefficacy of antiarrhythmic drugs. *N. Engl. J. Med.* 303:1073-1077.

Michelson, E. L.; and Morganroth, J. 1980. Spontaneous variability of complex ventricular arrhythmias detected by long-term electrocardiographic recording. *Circulation* 61:690-695.

Misner, J. E.; Imrey, P. B.; Smith, L., et al. 1978. Secular variation in frequency of premature ventricular contractions in untreated individuals. *J. Lab. Clin. Med.* 92:117-125.

Morganroth, J.; Michelson, E. L.; Horowitz, L. N., et al. 1978. Limitations of routine long-term electrocardiographic monitoring to assess ventricular ectopic frequency. *Circulation* 58:408-414.

Moss, A. J.; Schnitzler, R.; Green, R., et al. 1971. Ventricular arrhythmias 3 weeks after acute myocardial infarction. *Ann. Intern. Med.* 75:837-841.

Moss, A. J.; DeCamilla, J. J.; Engstrom, F., et al. 1974. The posthospital phase of myocardial infarction: identification of patients with increased mortality risk. *Circulation* 49:460-466.

Moss, A. J.; DeCamilla, J. J.; Mietlowski, W., et al. 1975. Prognostic grading and significance of ventricular premature beats after recovery from myocardial infarction. *Circulation* 51 and 52 (*Suppl.* III):III, 204-210.

Moss, A. J.; DeCamilla, J. J.; Davis, H. P., et al. 1977. Clinical significance of ventricular ectopic beats in the early posthospital phase of myocardial infarction. *Am. J. Cardiol.* 39:635-640.

Moss, A. J.; Davis, H. P.; DeCamilla, J. J., et al. 1980. Ventricular ectopic beats and their relation to sudden and nonsudden cardiac death after myocardial infarction. *Circulation* 60:998-1003.

Myerburg, R. J.; Conde, C.; Sheps, D. S., et al. 1979. Antiarrhythmic drug therapy in survivors of prehospital cardiac arrest: comparison of effects on chronic ventricular arrhythmias and recurrent cardiac arrest. *Circulation* 59:855-863.

Problete, P. F.; Kennedy, H. L.; and Caralis, D. G. 1978. Detection of ventricular ectopy in patients with coronary heart disease and normal subjects by exercise testing and ambulatory electrocardiography. *Chest* 74:402-407.

Raftery, E. B.; and Cashman, P. M. M. 1976. Long-term recording of the electrocardiogram in a normal population. *Postgrad. Med. J.* 52:32-38.

Rehnqvist, N. 1976. Ventricular arrhythmias prior to discharge after acute myocardial infarction. *Eur. J. Cardiol.* 4:63-70.

Rehnqvist, N. 1978. Ventricular arrhythmias after an acute myocardial infarction. *Eur. J. Cardiol.* 7:169-187.

Rehnqvist, N.; and Sjogren, A. 1977. Ventricular arrhythmias prior to discharge and one year after acute myocardial infarction. *Eur. J. Cardiol.* 5:425-442.

Reiffel, J. A.; Bigger, J. T., Jr.; Cramer, M., et al. 1977. Ability of Holter electrocardiographic recording and atrial stimulation to detect sinus nodal dysfunction in symptomatic and asymptomatic patients with sinus bradycardia. *Am. J. Cardiol.* 40:189-194.

Ruberman, W.; Weinblatt, E.; Frank, C. W., et al. 1976. Prognostic value of one hour of ECG monitoring of men with coronary heart disease. *J. Chron. Dis.* 29:497-512.

Ruberman, W.; Weinblatt, E.; Goldberg, J., et al. 1977. Ventricular premature beats and mortality after myocardial infarction. *N. Engl. J. Med.* 297:750-757.

Ruskin, J. N.; DiMarco, J. P.; and Garan, H. 1980. Out-of-hospital cardiac arrest electrophysiologic observations and selection of long-term antiarrhythmic therapy. *N. Engl. J. Med.* 303:607-613.

Ryan, M.; Lown, B.; and Horn, H. 1975. Comparison of ventricular ectopic activity during 24-hour monitoring and exercise testing in patients with coronary heart disease. *N. Engl. J. Med.* 292:224-229.

Savage, D. D.; Seides, S. F.; Maron, B. J., et al. 1979. Prevalence of arrhythmias during 24-hour electrocardiographic monitoring and exercise testing in patients with obstructive and nonobstructive hypertrophic cardiomyopathy. *Circulation* 59:866-875.

Schott, G. D.; McLeod, A. A.; and Jewitt, D. E. 1977. Cardiac arrhythmias that masquerade as epilepsy. *Br. Med. J.* 1:1454-1457.

Schulze, R. A., Jr.; Rouleau, J.; Rigo, P., et al. 1975. Ventricular arrhythmias in the late-hospital phase of acute myocardial infarction: relation of left ventricular function detected by gated cardiac blood pool scanning. *Circulation* 52:1006-1011.

Schulze, R. A., Jr.; Strauss, H. W.; and Pitt, B. 1977. Sudden death in the year following myocardial infarction. *Am. J. Med.* 62:192-199.

Stern, S.; and Tzivoni, D. 1976. Atrial and ventricular asystole for 19 seconds without syncope. *Isr. J. Med. Sci.* 12:28-33.

Tzivoni, D.; and Stern, S. 1975. Pacemaker implantation based on ambulatory ECG monitoring in patients with cerebral symptoms. *Chest* 67:274-278.

Van Durme, J. P. 1975. Tachyarrhythmias and transient cerebral ischemic attacks. *Annotations* 89:538-540.

Vismara, L. A.; Amsterdam, E. A.; and Mason, D. T. 1975. Relation of ventricular arrhythmias in the late-hospital phase of acute myocardial infarction to sudden death after hospital discharge. *Am. J. Med.* 59:6-12.

Walter, P. F.; Reid, S. D.; and Wenger, N. K. 1970. Transient cerebral ischemia due to arrhythmia. *Ann. Intern. Med.* 72:471-474.

Ward, D. E.; Camm, A. J.; and Spurrell, A. J. 1977. Ambulatory monitoring of the electrocardiogram: an important aspect of pacemaker surveillance. *Biotelemetry* 4:109-114.

Wenger, T. L.; Bigger, J. T., Jr.; and Merrill, G. S. 1975. Ventricular arrhythmias in the late hospital phase of acute myocardial infarction. *Circulation* 51 and 52 (*Suppl.* II):II-110.

Winkle, R. A. 1978. Antiarrhythmic drug effect mimicked by spontaneous variability of ventricular ectopy. *Circulation* 57:1116-1121.

Winkle, R. A. 1982. The relationship between ventricular ectopic beat frequency and heart rate. *Circulation* 66:439-446.

Winkle, R. A.; Lopes, M. G.; Fitzgerald, J. W., et al. 1975. Arrhythmias in patients with mitral valve prolapse. *Circulation* 52:73-81.

Winkle, R. A.; Lopes, M. G.; Popp, R. L., et al. 1976. Life-threatening arrhythmias in the mitral valve prolapse syndrome. *Am. J. Med.* 60: 961-967.

Winkle, R. A.; Gradman, P. H.; and Fitzgerald, J. W. 1978. Antiarrhythmic drug effect assessed from ventricular arrhythmia reduction in the ambulatory electrocardiogram and treadmill test: comparison of propranolol, procainamide, and quinidine. *Am. J. Cardiol.* 42:473-480.

Woodley, D.; Chambers, W.; Starke, H., et al. 1977. Intermittent complete atrioventricular block masquerading as epilepsy in the mitral valve prolapse syndrome. *Chest* 72:369-372.

5 Exercise Testing in the Diagnosis and Management of Cardiac Arrhythmias

Robert F. DeBusk, M.D.
Associate Professor Clinical Medicine
Stanford University School of Medicine
Stanford, California

This chapter was supported in part by Grant HL 18907 from the National Heart, Lung, and Blood Institute, National Institutes of Health, Bethesda, Maryland.

Cardiac arrhythmias are a cause of concern for at least three reasons: (1) they may cause symptoms such as palpitations, dizziness, and syncope; (2) they may lead to sudden cardiac death in the absence of symptoms; and (3) they may indicate underlying cardiac disease. Cardiac arrhythmias present the following management difficulties:

1. They are very common and their prevalence increases with age even in persons without evidence of cardiovascular disease.
2. They are often transient and not easily detected.
3. They simulate many other organic conditions such as cerebrovascular insufficiency.
4. They are a common feature of functional cardiac disorders, and are often associated with anxiety.
5. A firm causal connection between symptoms and cardiac arrhythmias can only be established when they are recorded simultaneously.
6. Their independent prognostic significance in patients with organic heart disease is difficult to establish: the nature of the underlying heart disease is often more important prognostically than the nature of the arrhythmias associated with the heart disease.

Therefore, the selection of patients to receive antiarrhythmic therapy is often difficult to make. Practical clinical guidelines are needed to deal with these complex disorders. This chapter emphasizes the role of exercise testing in the detection and treatment of arrhythmias, especially those of ventricular origin.

MECHANISMS OF EXERCISE-INDUCED CARDIAC ARRHYTHMIAS

Although the precise mechanisms underlying exercise-induced ventricular ectopic activity remain uncertain, several general features of these arrhythmias have been described. Increased sympathetic tone may lead to enhanced phase 4 depolarization and to triggered rhythms (Cranefield, 1977). Myocardial ischemia caused by an increase in myocardial oxygen requirements resulting from increased heart rate, systolic pressure, and cardiac contractility predisposes to nonhomogeneous impulse conduction. This is especially true in the presence of underlying myocardial fibrosis resulting from prior myocardial infarction. This may result in local block and in reentrant arrhythmias (Watanabe and Dreifus, 1968). Depression of wall motion may result from local tissue hypoxia and acidosis. Regional myocardial ischemia predisposes to both enhanced ventricular automaticity and to reentrant tachyarrhythmias (Bigger, et al., 1977). Offsetting these mechanisms that enhance ventricular ectopic activity during exercise is the tendency of rapid heart rates to suppress ectopic pacemakers (overdrive suppression), which partly accounts for the greater frequency of ventricular ectopic activity during recovery than during exercise.

INCREASED YIELD OF EXERCISE COMPARED TO REST FOR ARRHYTHMIA DETECTION

The characteristics of exercise-induced ventricular ectopic activity vary according to the population undergoing evaluation. Jelinek and Lown (1974) performed exercise testing in a population in which 44% of patients had coronary heart disease, 44% had possible heart disease, and 12% were clinically normal. In 1000 exercise tests carried out by these 625 patients the prevalence of exercise-induced supraventricular premature complexes was 33%. Exercise increased the prevalence of nonrepetitive supraventricular ectopic activity threefold and the prevalence of repetitive atrial tachyarrhythmias, including atrial flutter, atrial fibrillation, supraventricular tachycardia, and junctional tachycardia nearly twofold. The detection of supraventricular ectopic activity was enhanced to a greater extent for isolated forms than for repetitive forms. Because supraventricular ectopic activity detected with exercise testing or ambulatory ECG recording has not been associated with an increase in mortality from coronary heart disease, it will not be discussed further in this chapter.

The prevalence of exercise-induced ventricular ectopic activity was 61% in this series, occurring during the 3-minute control period in approximately 40% of tests, during exercise in approximately 60% of tests, and during recovery in approximately 80% of tests. The number of tests demonstrating premature ventricular complexes (PVCs) of any description was more than doubled by exercise as compared to rest. The occurrence of ventricular couplets and ventricular tachycardia increased by factors of 7.6 and 7.7, respectively, while detection of infrequent PVCs increased with exercise by a factor of only 1.7. Exercise, therefore, preferentially enhanced the appearance of more advanced, repetitive forms of ventricular ectopic activity.

THE IMPORTANCE OF THE MAXIMAL HEART RATE

The maximal heart rate attained during exercise has a major influence on the occurrence of ventricular ectopic activity in individuals without manifest heart disease. Blackburn and colleagues (1973) found that the frequency of exercise-induced PVCs, the total number of PVCs, and the proportion of individuals with PVCs increased during a progressive treadmill exercise test in middle-aged high-risk men who were free of manifest coronary heart disease. The proportion of men with any ventricular ectopic activity increased from 3% at standing rest to 30%

at maximal effort and from less than 3% at heart rates of 73-102 beats/min to over 50% at heart rates exceeding 170 beats/min. The yield of exercise-induced PVCs during and following exercise increased by over one-third when exercise was carried to a symptom-limited maximum as opposed to a predetermined submaximal heart rate. The proportion of men with runs and multiform complexes increased as the heart rate increased, and the cumulative frequency of runs and multifocal complexes was approximately twice as great for maximal as for submaximal effort (heart rate of 150 beats/min).

In patients with manifest coronary heart disease the prevalence of exercise-induced PVCs is also related to the maximal heart rate. The maximal attainable heart rate is strongly influenced by the presence or absence of angina pectoris. Among patients with coronary heart disease the prevalence of premature ventricular complexes was 25% in those patients who stopped because of angina pectoris and 42% in those individuals who stopped because of fatigue (Jelinek and Lown, 1974). When these two patient subgroups were matched for maximal heart rate, however, the prevalence of ventricular ectopic activity, especially of complex forms, remained higher in patients with angina pectoris. This was also true when the two subgroups were matched for age. This underscores the importance of underlying myocardial ischemia in the genesis of ventricular ectopic activity. Despite the association between exercise-induced ventricular ectopic activity and coronary artery obstruction (see the section on prognostic stratification in patients with coronary heart disease in this chapter), the occurrence of ventricular ectopic activity usually correlates poorly with the appearance of ischemic ST segment depression developing during or following exercise testing (Jelinek and Lown, 1974).

REPRODUCIBILITY OF VENTRICULAR ECTOPIC ACTIVITY

The clinical utility of ventricular ectopic activity recorded by any technique depends on its reproducibility, that is, the extent to which the response noted on one test will be present on another test performed under similar circumstances. The reproducibility of exercise-induced ventricular ectopic activity has been regarded as poor (Faris, et al., 1976; DeBacker, et al., 1978), but these reports appear to present an unduly pessimistic view of the potential of exercise testing to disclose ventricular ectopic activity (Sami, et al., 1979b). A major methodological problem has been the lack of a suitable method for expressing reproducibility. For example, many authors have considered only the tendency for a test response (i.e., the presence of PVCs) to be observed on a second test: they have evaluated only unidirectional changes, from positive to negative. But it is also important to know that a patient without PVCs on a first test remains free of PVCs on subsequent testing. The optimal method for expressing the reproducibility of discrete responses is the kappa coefficient (Spitzer and Fleiss, 1974), which permits evaluation of bidirectional changes, that is, negative to positive *and* positive to negative, within the entire population. The kappa coefficient considers changes in response from test to test in relation to changes expected by chance alone. This method has the further advantage of expressing reproducibility as a single number from 0 (chance level) to 1 (perfect reproducibility). Levels of reproducibility have been established for many clinical and laboratory methods and in general range from values of a kappa of 0.3 to 0.6 (Koran, 1975). When we used this method, we found reproducibility to be statistically significant in several studies in which the reproducibility of exercise-induced PVCs had been considered poor. Of course, statistical significance and clinical significance are not synonymous, and the clinician must judge whether PVCs are significantly reproducible to be valuable in an individual patient.

In evaluating the reproducibility of PVCs following myocardial infarction, we found the presence of PVCs to be more reproducible than their absence: 85% and 76%, respectively, when the two tests were performed 1-5 days apart during the eleventh week after myocardial infarction (kappa 0.44). The degree of reproducibility was not further enhanced by classifying PVCs into discrete categories of simple or complex, even when various definitions for simple and complex were compared (Sami, et al., 1979b). We found a substantially higher reproducibility for continuous measures of PVCs, such as mean frequency, than for discrete measures such as presence or absence. The clinician should, therefore, use continuous measures, especially when evaluating the response to antiarrhythmic therapy, as is discussed in the section on monitoring antiarrhythmic drug efficacy at the end of this chapter.

The reproducibility of exercise-induced PVCs is also critically related to the manner in which the test is performed. It is important to maintain consistency in the mode of testing, that is, bicycle versus treadmill, the exercise protocol, including end points, the time of day, and the relation of the test to meals, smoking, and drugs. When exercise tests were carefully standardized, we found the reproducibility (r) of exercise-induced PVCs to be similar to that observed for PVCs recorded on ambulatory ECGs: r = 0.86 for the mean frequency of exercise-induced PVCs per minute, and r = 0.94 for the mean frequency of PVCs recorded on ambulatory ECGs per hour (Sami, et al., 1980).

TYPES OF EXERCISE TESTING FOR THE DETECTION OF VENTRICULAR ARRHYTHMIAS

In patients with advanced left ventricular dysfunction static or isometric exercise, such as handgrip, may be more sensitive than dynamic effort, such as treadmill or bicycle exercise, for the detection of ventricular ectopic activity (Atkins, et al., 1976). Most other studies conducted in patients with less severe left ventricular dysfunction have demonstrated the diagnostic superiority of dynamic over static effort (Jelinek and Lown, 1974). In our study we noted PVCs in only 11 of 32 patients with coronary heart disease who performed handgrip or forearm lifting, yet 21 of these same 32 patients demonstrated PVCs during dynamic arm or leg cranking (DeBusk, et al., 1978). The incidence of PVCs was similar with arm and with leg cranking. When static effort (forearm lifting) was added to dynamic (treadmill) exercise, neither the prevalence, frequency, nor grade of PVCs was increased above that noted for dynamic effort alone (DeBusk, et al., 1979). In the detection of ventricular ectopic activity, therefore, dynamic testing is preferred over static testing. Bicycle and treadmill exercise are equally effective in eliciting ventricular ectopic activity.

INDICATIONS FOR TERMINATING EXERCISE

In general, symptom-limited exercise testing is preferable to heart rate-limited testing because the diagnostic yield of PVCs is nearly one-third greater with symptom-limited than with heart rate-limited testing. The risk of exercise testing is more closely related to the nature of the patient undergoing evaluation than to the nature of the protocol used to test the patient. In general, frequent or complex ventricular ectopic activity, that is, multifocal PVCs, pairs, or ventricular tachycardia, are observed more frequently in patients with manifest coronary heart disease than in apparently normal individuals. On the other hand, the disappearance of complex ventricular ectopic activity with continued exercise is a relatively frequent occurrence in patients with manifest coronary heart disease and does not exclude the presence of even severe coronary artery obstruction (Goldschlager, et al., 1973).

In many laboratories ventricular ectopic activity occurring at rest that becomes more frequent or ominous is used as an end point for exercise testing. However, we have used only exercise-induced ventricular tachycardia, that is, three or more consecutive PVCs, as an absolute indication to terminate exercise testing, even in patients 3 weeks after myocardial infarction. There is no safe heart rate below which complex PVCs are absent during exercise (DeBusk, et al., 1980). If exercise is terminated because of PVCs occurring prior to the onset of limiting symptoms, potentially important information may be lost. Because of its greater diagnostic sensitivity and reproducibility and its equivalent safety record, we, therefore, favor symptom-limited exercise testing over heart rate-limited testing.

EXERCISE-INDUCED ARRHYTHMIAS IN THE MITRAL VALVE PROLAPSE SYNDROME

Palpitation is a characteristic feature of mitral valve prolapse and often leads to the diagnosis of this disorder. On the other hand, palpitation is relatively uncommon in unselected individuals with mitral valve prolapse in whom PVCs and palpitation are often poorly correlated. Winkle and colleagues (1975) found 24-hour ambulatory ECGs to be more sensitive than exercise or resting ECGs for the detection of PVCs in 24 unselected patients with mitral valve prolapse. The frequency of any PVC for these tests was 90%, 85%, and 40%, respectively. A close relationship existed between the frequency of PVCs during and following exercise and that recorded on ambulatory ECGs. All of 12 patients with one or more PVCs on the exercise ECG demonstrated frequent PVCs on ambulatory ECGs, whereas 10 of 12 patients with none or only one PVC on the exercise ECG demonstrated none or only infrequent PVCs on ambulatory ECGs. The frequency and complexity (bigeminy, pairs, ventricular tachycardia) of PVCs recorded on ambulatory ECGs were highly correlated. Similar findings were reported in another study (DeMaria, et al., 1976) in which a higher prevalence of ventricular arrhythmias was noted in 31 patients with mitral valve prolapse than in 40 normal individuals. In this study patients with mitral valve prolapse PVCs were detected with 24-hour ambulatory ECGs, exercise ECGs, and resting ECGs in 58%, 45%, and 35% of patients, respectively (DeMaria, et al., 1976) (see Chapter 4). From a practical standpoint, therefore, most patients with exercise-induced PVCs do not require ambulatory ECG recording for the detection of frequent or complex PVCs.

EXERCISE-INDUCED ARRHYTHMIAS IN HYPERTROPHIC CARDIOMYOPATHIES

In the most definitive study of this relationship available to date Savage and colleagues (1979) noted exercise-induced PVCs in 73% of 74 patients with documented hypertrophic cardiomyopathy. By contrast, ambulatory ECG recording detected 98% of PVCs in these same patients. Of the patients with PVCs of grade 3 or higher on ambulatory ECGs, only 43% demonstrated exercise-induced PVCs. While the absence of exercise-induced PVCs did not ensure their absence on ambulatory ECGs, patients with frequent or complex PVCs caused by exercise also demonstrated frequent and complex PVCs on ambulatory ECGs. Ambulatory ECG recording, therefore, appears to be superior to exercise ECG monitoring for the detection of PVCs in patients with hypertrophic cardiomyopathy.

VALUE OF EXERCISE-INDUCED ARRHYTHMIAS FOR THE DETECTION OF CORONARY HEART DISEASE IN ASYMPTOMATIC INDIVIDUALS

Exercise-induced ventricular ectopic activity is more frequently noted in patients with definite or suspected coronary heart disease than in apparently healthy individuals (McHenry, et al., 1976). The heart rate at the onset of ventricular ectopic activity is generally lower in patients with coronary heart disease than in apparently healthy men. Thirty-nine percent of men with PVCs occurring at a heart rate less than or equal to 150 beats/min had possible or definite coronary heart disease, as compared with 11% of men whose PVCs occurred at a heart rate exceeding 150 beats/min (McHenry, et al., 1976). Another study (Vedin, et al., 1972) also noted a higher prevalence of exercise-induced ventricular ectopic activity in patients with definite or probable coronary heart disease than in apparently normal individuals. In this study 13.5% of patients with definite or probable coronary heart disease had PVCs that appeared or were aggravated with exercise, whereas only 3% of normal subjects demonstrated such ventricular ectopic activity (a more than fourfold difference).

There is little doubt that the prevalence of exercise-induced ventricular ectopic activity in populations of patients with coronary heart disease is higher than in populations of apparently healthy individuals. But are exercise-induced PVCs sufficiently specific for coronary heart disease to constitute a clinically useful screening test for this condition in individuals without manifest disease? Two types of studies, follow-up study and coronary angiography, have addressed this question.

Follow-up Studies

Froelicher and colleagues (1974) examined the prognostic value of treadmill exercise testing in 1390 asymptomatic men, fewer than 12% of whom had definite or probable coronary heart disease. The prevalence of any exercise-induced ventricular ectopic activity was 35% and was 2% for ominous or complex patterns. During a mean follow-up of 6.3 years, 46 patients (3%) experienced angina pectoris (23 patients), myocardial infarction (7 patients), or sudden cardiac death (16 patients). The sensitivity of ominous patterns of PVCs was 6.5%, that is, only 6.5% of patients who developed cardiac events had such PVCs. The more clinically relevant issue is the predictive accuracy, that is, the number of patients with complex PVCs who actually experienced a cardiac event. In this study only 10% of patients with complex PVCs developed cardiac events. A related issue is the risk ratio, which is the extent to which a cardiac event is likely to occur in individuals with complex PVCs compared to patients without such PVCs. The risk ratio in this study was 3.4. In contrast, other treadmill test parameters, especially exercise-induced ST segment depression, had higher sensitivities, predictive accuracy, and risk ratios. In Froelicher's study the sensitivity of an ischemic ST segment response was 61%, the predictive accuracy was 20%, and the risk ratio was 14.3. These figures are substantially similar to those found in other follow-up studies (Bruce and McDonough, 1969; Aronow, 1973). It is apparent that exercise-induced ventricular ectopic activity is such a poor predictor of coronary events in asymptomatic individuals that it should not be used for this purpose.

Coronary Angiographic Studies

Because of its inherent risks, coronary angiography is not performed in persons without suspected heart disease. This selection factor limits conclusions regarding the relationship between PVCs and coronary anatomy in the general population. From a population of 62 asymptomatic, apparently healthy people who were incidentally found to have frequent and complex ventricular ectopic activity, Kennedy and colleagues (1980) selected 25 individuals for cardiac catheterization and coronary angiography. In 20 of these patients the indication for study was the presence of one or more risk factors of cigarette smoking, hypertension, or hypercholesterolemia. Five other individuals without risk factors required confirmation of normal cardiac status to remain on active military duty. None of these 25 patients had abnormal Q or QS waves or ST segment or T wave abnormalities on the resting ECG. Coronary arteriography revealed normal coronary arteries in 14 of these subjects. Five subjects had luminal narrowing of less than 50% of a major coronary artery (noncritical disease), and six patients showed luminal narrowing greater than or equal to 50% (significant disease). Of the six individuals with significant coronary artery disease, two had three-vessel disease and four had two-vessel disease. No ischemic ST segment abnormalities or angina pectoris was noted during testing in any patients. Further, maximal treadmill exercise testing revealed no significant differences in mean functional aerobic impairment or in peak heart rate, systolic pressure, or maximal pressure-rate product according to the presence or absence of coronary artery disease. Abolition of all ventricular ectopic activity at maximal exercise was noted in 17 of 24 subjects, including five of the six patients with significant coronary artery disease. Individuals with and without coronary artery disease could not be distinguished on the basis of the mean frequency of ectopic beats per hour recorded on ambulatory ECGs.

Kennedy's study indicates that most apparently healthy subjects with frequent and complex ventricular ectopic activity do not have significant coronary artery disease. Only 24% of the individuals who were evaluated demonstrated significant disease, and this percentage would undoubtedly have been less in a general population of subjects with a lesser prevalence of coronary risk factors. No mortality was noted during an average follow-up period of 34 months (range 1-60 months). The authors of this study suggested that ventricular ectopic activity was not an independent risk factor for sudden cardiac death in apparently healthy persons. Therefore, the presence of complex and frequent ventricular ectopic activity does not appear to constitute an adequate indication for the performance of coronary angiography in asymptomatic individuals.

EXERCISE-INDUCED ARRHYTHMIAS AND PROGNOSTIC STRATIFICATION IN PATIENTS WITH CORONARY HEART DISEASE

Chronic Coronary Heart Disease

In patients with clinical coronary heart disease prognosis is often poorly related to the severity of angina pectoris. The clinician is, therefore, interested in tests that help to identify individuals who are at particularly high risk for cardiac events. This is a complex issue because exercise-induced ventricular ectopic activity, like that recorded on ambulatory ECGs, is closely related to the extent of coronary artery narrowing and left ventricular dysfunction, abnormalities which themselves are major prognostic determinants (Schulze, et al., 1977). Goldschlager and colleagues (1973) found that patients with coronary heart disease and exercise-induced ventricular ectopic activity had a significantly greater incidence of prior myocardial infarction, abnormal ventricular contraction patterns, and double or triple coronary artery disease than patients with coronary heart disease who did not demonstrate exercise-induced ventricular ectopic activity. This was particularly true of patients whose ventricular ectopic activity appeared during the recovery period rather than during exercise. The patients selected for this study were those undergoing coronary angiography, generally to evaluate disabling angina pectoris. Because of this selection factor the results cannot be extended to all patients with coronary heart disease, particularly those who have fewer symptoms. The authors of this study concluded that exercise-induced ventricular ectopic activity might be a clinically useful marker for severe anatomic involvement in patients with clinical coronary heart disease. Another research team (Helfant, et al., 1974) also noted a strong relationship between exercise-induced ventricular ectopic activity and coronary angiographic abnormalities. Patients with PVCs that appeared or increased during exercise had a high incidence of angiographic coronary artery disease. Of the 22 patients in this category, 20 of whom had exercise-induced ischemic ST segment depression of 0.2 mV or more, 12 had three-vessel disease, six had two-vessel disease, and four had single-vessel disease. In contrast, of 38 patients with PVCs that decreased in frequency, only six had coronary artery disease (two-vessel disease in two patients and single-vessel disease in four patients) and none demonstrated exercise-induced ischemic ST segment depression. These results suggest that exercise-induced PVCs, like exercise-induced ischemic ST segment depression, may be a diagnostically and prognostically important marker for severe coronary artery disease.

Udall and Ellestad (1977) further investigated this association in a follow-up study of patients who underwent treadmill exercise testing for the evaluation of chest pain. These investigators found a higher rate of cardiac events (myocardial infarction, angina pectoris, and sudden cardiac death) in patients with exercise-induced PVCs than in patients without exercise-induced PVCs, regardless of whether exercise-induced ischemic ST segment depression was present. In 6500 patients undergoing treadmill exercise testing 1327 (20%) exhibited ventricular ectopic activity before, during, or following exercise. Within this population the incidence of cardiac events was 1.7% per year in patients with neither exercise-induced ischemic ST segment depression nor ventricular ectopic activity, 6.4% in those with exercise-induced ventricular ectopic activity only, 9.5% in those with exercise-induced ST segment depression only, and 11.4% in patients who had both abnormalities. The presence of exercise-induced ventricular ectopic activity increased the risk of cardiac events by more than four times. Further, complex ventricular ectopic activity conferred additional prognostic information. For example, among patients with nonischemic test responses the incidence of cardiac events was 29% in those with ominous patterns (multiform, bigeminal, repetitive, and ventricular tachycardia) as compared to 15% in patients with lower grades of exercise-induced ventricular ectopic activity. This study suggests that exercise-induced ventricular ectopic activity may have prognostic significance that is independent of its association with the extent of coronary heart disease. This issue is not resolved, however, because ventricular ectopic activity recorded by ambulatory ECG recording is closely related to the anatomic severity of coronary artery disease and left ventricular dysfunction (Schulze, et al., 1977; Califf, et al., 1978). Further, when sensitive techniques have been used to characterize ventricular function, PVCs recorded on ambulatory ECGs appear to have little or no prognostic significance independent of their association with left ventricular dysfunction (Borer, et al., 1980).

Following Myocardial Infarction

Exercise testing has been performed safely in large numbers of patients within 2-3 weeks of acute myocardial infarction. In our patients without clinical heart failure or S_3 gallops 3 weeks after myocardial infarction we have found by multivariate analysis techniques that PVCs recorded on treadmill exercise tests or on ambulatory ECGs were not prognostically important. In contrast, exercise-induced ischemic ST segment depression of 0.2 millivolts or more or a low maximal treadmill workload (i.e., less than 4 METs or multiples of resting energy expenditure) were prognostically important. Thus, ambulatory ECG monitoring and treadmill exercise testing are not merely redundant techniques for detecting ventricular ectopic activity. In some populations subsequent coronary events may be more strongly reflected by other treadmill test variables than by ventricular ectopic activity (DeBusk, et al., 1980). Another study (Ivanova, et al., 1980) noted similar results in a population of patients with established coronary heart disease who underwent exercise testing and ambulatory ECG recordings. In general, a diminished maximal heart rate of 115 beats/min, especially when associated with exercise-induced ST segment depression, was a powerful determinant of prognosis, regardless of whether PVCs were present during exercise testing or during ambulatory ECG monitoring. As noted by Weld and Bigger (1978), in patients with severe left ventricular dysfunction, exercise-induced PVCs and a low treadmill workload 2 weeks following a myocardial infarction may be more important than exercise-induced ST segment depression in the prediction of subsequent cardiac events. Ventricular ectopic activity recorded on ambulatory ECGs also had prognostic significance within the population. In a study of a similar population Granath and colleagues (1977) found exercise-induced PVCs 3 and 9 weeks after infarction to be significantly more frequent in patients who died within the next 2-5 years than in patients who were free of ventricular ectopic activity. Thus, the prognostic utility of an exercise test is closely dependent on the characteristics of the population to which it is applied.

Exercise-induced PVCs recorded soon after myocardial infarction may predict subsequent cardiac events other than sudden cardiac death. One study (Kentala, et al., 1975) found that the coronary death rate was greater in patients with exercise-induced PVCs, but the study failed to indicate whether the deaths were sudden or gradual. We found in our study that patients who experienced recurrent, nonfatal myocardial infarction within 2 years of their index infarctions had a higher prevalence of exercise-induced ventricular arrhythmias on serial treadmill tests performed 3 and 11 weeks after infarction than patients without recurrent events (Sami, et al., 1979a). The timing of the exercise test has an important bearing on the prognostic utility of the test. Three of four cardiac arrests in our patients occurred within 1 month of infarction, and all were predicted by the presence of ischemic ST segment depression of 0.2 millivolts or more 3 weeks after infarction.

THE ROLE OF EXERCISE-INDUCED VENTRICULAR ECTOPIC ACTIVITY IN MONITORING ANTIARRHYTHMIC DRUG EFFICACY

Ambulatory ECG recording is generally preferred to exercise testing for monitoring the response to antiarrhythmic therapy, but when ventricular ectopic activity is sufficiently frequent, these methods are equally useful. We have compared the efficacy of ambulatory ECGs and treadmill exercise testing for monitoring antiarrhythmic response (Sami, et al., 1980). In our study we used two ambulatory ECGs and two exercise tests, performed 2 weeks apart while the patients received no antiarrhythmic therapy, to establish the limits of spontaneous variability of PVCs. Figure 5-1 shows the regression of average PVC frequency of the second test on the average PVC frequency of baseline tests for exercise-induced ventricular ectopic activity. Once this regression line and confidence

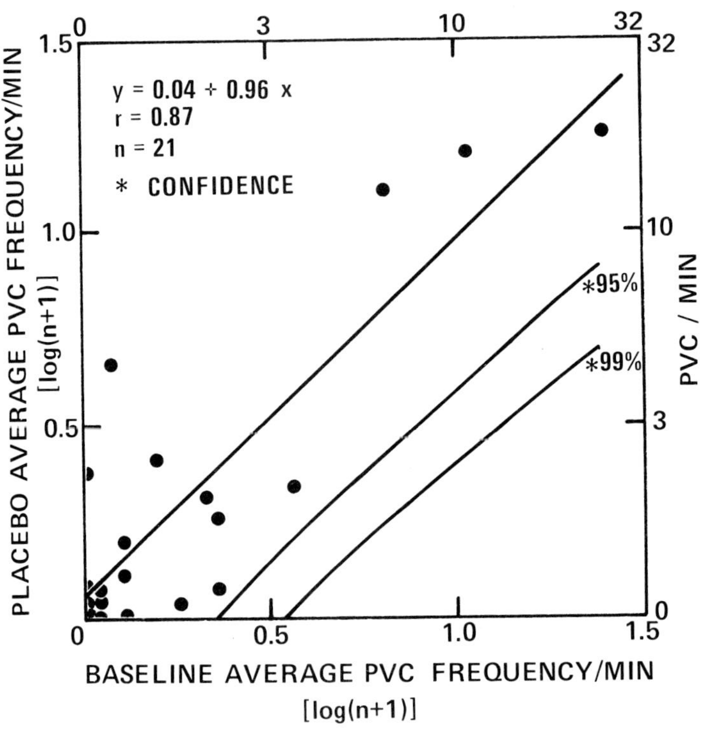

Figure 5-1 Linear regression analysis with determination of 95% confidence intervals of variability for baseline vs. placebo measurements of average PVC frequency/minute of treadmill exercise test. Analysis was performed on the log (PVC frequency + 1). The corresponding absolute values are shown on the opposing scales. The 95% confidence line represents the one-tailed lower confidence interval for individual data points. The point at which the confidence line crosses the baseline axis determines the sensitivity threshold, below which even total PVC suppression cannot be distinguished from spontaneous variability.

interval is established for the population of patients, the response of individual patients can be determined by plotting a single point that describes the baseline and postdrug PVC frequency. If this point falls below the 95% confidence interval, patients are said to have a drug effect. The minimal PVC frequency on a baseline treadmill exercise test that permits the evaluation of antiarrhythmic drug efficacy is a mean frequency of 1.2 PVCs/min. In patients with a lesser frequency of PVCs on the baseline test antiarrhythmic drug efficacy cannot be evaluated.

A similar analysis was performed using ambulatory ECG monitoring. The minimal mean frequency of PVCs on ambulatory ECGs required to establish antiarrhythmic drug efficacy was 2.2 PVCs/hr. Significantly, all patients exceeded this sensitivity threshold with ambulatory ECG recording, whereas only 29% of these same patients had sufficiently frequent PVCs on their baseline treadmill exercise tests to permit evaluation of their response to antiarrhythmic drugs. The proportion of patients exceeding the sensitivity threshold with exercise testing may be artificially low because patients were accepted into the study primarily on the basis of demonstrating a sufficient PVC frequency on ambulatory ECG monitoring. As the baseline frequency of PVCs increased above the sensitivity threshold, the percentage reduction in the baseline frequency of PVCs required to establish antiarrhythmic drug efficacy declined from 100% at the sensitivity threshold of 2.2 PVCs/hr for ambulatory ECG recordings and 1.2 PVCs/min for treadmill exercise testing to stable minimal values of 65% and 68% at baseline frequencies of 30 PVCs/hr and 9 PVCs/min, respectively (Table 5-1).

Table 5-1 Relationship of baseline PVC frequency to the percent reduction in PVCs required to establish antiarrhythmic efficacy with 95% confidence

AE average PVC/hr	TM average PVC/min	PVC reduction*
2.2†	<1.2†	—
2.2-3.0	1.2-1.5	100%-90%
3.0-5.5	1.5-2.5	90%-80%
5.5-11	2.5-5.5	80%-70%
11-20	5.5-9	70%-68%
—	9 or more	68%‡
20-30	—	65%-68%
30 or more	—	65%§

*Percent reduction from baseline PVC frequency is necessary to establish drug efficacy with 95% confidence.

†Sensitivity threshold is the frequency below which an antiarrhythmic drug response cannot be assessed with 95% confidence.

‡Minimal percent reduction to TM average PVCs/min.

§Minimal percent reduction for AE average PVCs/hr.

Abbreviations: PVC = premature ventricular complex; AE = 24-hour ambulatory electrocardiography; TM = treadmill exercise testing.

(*Source:* Sami, M.; Kraemer, H.; Harrison, D. C., et al. 1980. A new method for evaluating antiarrhythmic drug efficacy in individual patients. *Circulation* 62:1172-1179.)

From a practical standpoint ambulatory ECG monitoring is the superior technique for evaluating antiarrhythmic drug efficacy because it permits evaluation of all patients with ventricular ectopic activity. In contrast, only patients with relatively frequent exercise-induced PVCs can be evaluated with treadmill exercise testing. If a patient being considered for antiarrhythmic drug efficacy has had neither test, ambulatory ECG recording is a logical first step. On the other hand, if a patient has had a treadmill exercise test in which PVCs were relatively frequent, it appears that his or her response to antiarrhythmic medication can be adequately assessed by repeat treadmill exercise testing after a suitable treatment interval.

REFERENCES

Aronow, W. S. 1973. Thirty-month follow-up of maximal treadmill stress test and double Master's test in normal subjects. *Circulation* 47: 287-290.

Atkins, J. M.; Matthews, O. A.; Blomqvist, C. G., et al. 1976. Incidence of arrhythmias induced by isometric and dynamic exercise (abstract). *Br. Heart J.* 38:465.

Bigger, J. T., Jr.; Dresdale, R. J.; Heissenbuttel, R. H., et al. 1977. Ventricular arrhythmias in ischemic heart disease: mechanism, prevalence, significance, and management. *Prog. Cardiovasc. Dis.* 19:255-300.

Blackburn, H.; Taylor, H. L.; Hamrell, B., et al. 1973. Premature ventricular complexes induced by stress testing. Their frequency and response to physical conditioning. *Am. J. Cardiol.* 31:441-449.

Borer, J. S.; Rosing, D. R.; Miller, R. H., et al. 1980. Natural history of left ventricular function during 1 year after acute myocardial infarction: comparison with clinical, electrocardiographic, and biochemical determinations. *Am. J. Cardiol.* 46:1-12.

Bruce, R. A.; and McDonough, J. R. 1969. Stress testing in screening for cardiovascular disease. *Bull. N.Y. Acad. Med.* 45:1288-1305.

Califf, R. M.; Burks, J. M.; Behar, V. S., et al. 1978. Relationships among ventricular arrhythmias, coronary artery disease, and angiographic and electrocardiographic indicators of myocardial fibrosis. *Circulation* 57: 725-732.

Cranefield, P. F. 1977. Action potentials, afterpotentials, and arrhythmias. *Circ. Res.* 41:415-423.

DeBacker, G.; Jacobs, D.; Prineas, R., et al. 1978. Ventricular premature beats. Reliability in various measurement methods at rest and during exercise. *Cardiol.* 63:53-63.

DeBusk, R.; and Haskell, W. 1980. Symptom-limited vs. heart rate-limited exercise testing soon after myocardial infarction. *Circulation* 61:738-743.

DeBusk, R. F.; Valdez, R.; Houston, N., et al. 1978. Cardiovascular responses to dynamic and static effort soon after myocardial infarction. Application to occupational work assessment. *Circulation* 58:368-375.

DeBusk, R. F.; Pitts, W.; Haskell, W. L., et al. 1979. A comparison of cardiovascular responses to combined static-dynamic and dynamic effort alone in patients with chronic ischemic heart disease. *Circulation* 59: 977-984.

DeBusk, R.; Davidson, D.; Houston, N., et al. 1980. Serial ambulatory electrocardiography and treadmill exercise testing following uncomplicated myocardial infarction. *Am. J. Cardiol.* 45:547-554.

DeMaria, A. N.; Amsterdam, E. A.; Vismara, L. A., et al. 1976. Arrhythmias in the mitral valve prolapse syndrome. Prevalence, nature, and frequency. *Ann. Intern. Med.* 84:656-660.

Faris, J. V.; McHenry, P. L.; Jordan, J. W., et al. 1976. Prevalence and reproducibility of exercise-induced ventricular arrhythmias during maximal exercise testing in normal men. *Am. J. Cardiol.* 37:617-622.

Froelicher, V. F., Jr.; Thomas, M. M.; Pillow, C., et al. 1974. Epidemiologic study of asymptomatic men screened by maximal treadmill testing for latent coronary artery disease. *Am. J. Cardiol.* 34:770-776.

Goldschlager, N.; Cake, D.; and Cohn, K. 1973. Exercise-induced ventricular arrhythmias in patients with coronary artery disease. *Am. J. Cardiol.* 31:434-440.

Granath, A.; Sodermark, T.; Winge, T., et al. 1977. Early work load tests for evaluation of long-term prognosis of acute myocardial infarction. *Br. Heart J.* 39:758-763.

Helfant, R. H.; Pine, R.; Kabde, V., et al. 1974. Exercise-related ventricular premature complexes in coronary heart disease. Correlations with ischemia and angiographic severity. *Ann. Intern. Med.* 80:589-592.

Ivanova, L. A.; Mazur, N. A.; Smirnova, T. M., et al. 1980. Electrocardiographic exercise testing and ambulatory monitoring to identify patients with ischemic heart disease at high risk of sudden death. *Am. J. Cardiol.* 45:1132-1138.

Jelinek, M. V.; and Lown, B. 1974. Exercise stress testing for exposure of cardiac arrhythmia. *Prog. Cardiovasc. Dis.* 16:497-522.

Kennedy, H. L.; Pescarmona, J. E.; Bouchard, R. J., et al. 1980. Coronary artery status of apparently healthy subjects with frequent and complex ventricular ectopy. *Ann. Intern. Med.* 92:179-185.

Kentala, E.; Pyorala, K.; Heikkila, J., et al. 1975. Factors related to long-term prognosis following acute myocardial infarction. Importance of left ventricular function. *Scand. J. Rehab. Med.* 7:118-124.

Koran, L. M. 1975. The reliability of clinical methods, data, and judgments (part II). *N. Engl. J. Med.* 293:695-701.

McHenry, P. L.; Morris, S. N.; Kavalier, M., et al. 1976. Comparative study of exercise-induced ventricular arrhythmias in normal subjects and patients with documented coronary artery disease. *Am. J. Cardiol.* 37: 609-616.

Sami, M.; Kraemer, H.; and DeBusk, R. F. 1979a. The prognostic significance of serial exercise tests soon after myocardial infarction. *Circulation* 60:1238-1246.

Sami, M.; Kraemer, H.; and DeBusk, R. F. 1979b. Reproducibility of exercise-induced ventricular arrhythmia after myocardial infarction. *Am. J. Cardiol.* 43:724-730.

Sami, M.; Kraemer, H.; Harrison, D. C., et al. 1980. A new method for evaluating antiarrhythmic drug efficacy in individual patients. *Circulation* 62:1172-1179.

Savage, D. D.; Seides, S. F.; Maron, B. J., et al. 1979. Prevalence of arrhythmias during 24-hour electrocardiographic monitoring and exercise testing in patients with obstructive and nonobstructive hypertrophic cardiomyopathy. *Circulation* 59:866-875.

Schulze, R. A., Jr.; Humphries, J. O.; Griffith, L. S. C., et al. 1977. Left ventricular and coronary angiographic anatomy. Relationship to ventricular irritability in the late-hospital phase of acute myocardial infarction. *Circulation* 55:839-843.

Spitzer, R. L.; and Fleiss, J. L. 1974. Re-analysis of the reliability of psychiatric diagnosis. *Br. J. Psychiatry* 125:341-347.

Udall, J. A.; and Ellestad, M. H. 1977. Predictive implications of ventricular premature contractions associated with treadmill stress testing. *Circulation* 56:985-989.

Vedin, J. A.; Wilhelmsson, C. E.; Wilhelmsen, L., et al. 1972. Relation of resting and exercise-induced ectopic beats to other ischemic manifestations and to coronary risk factors. *Am. J. Cardiol.* 30:25-31.

Watanabe, Y.; and Dreifus, L. S. 1968. Newer concepts in the genesis of cardiac arrhythmias. *Am. Heart J.* 76:114-135.

Weld, F. M.; and Bigger, J. T., Jr. 1978. Risk stratification by exercise testing and 24-hour ambulatory electrocardiogram two weeks after acute myocardial infarction (abstract). *Circulation* 58 and 59 (*Suppl.* II):II-198.

Winkle, R. A.; Lopes, M. G.; Fitzgerald, J. W., et al. 1975. Arrhythmias in patients with mitral valve prolapse. *Circulation* 52:73-81.

6 Sinus Node Disease and Heart Block

David L. Ross, M.B., F.R.A.C.P.

Staff Specialist (Cardiology)
Cardiology Unit
Westmead Hospital
Westmead, Australia

This chapter was supported in part by Grant No. 79 N110A of the American Heart Association, California affiliate.

Many defects in cardiac impulse formation and conduction can occur either acutely or chronically (Figure 6-1). The end result may be a ventricular bradyarrhythmia with consequent decrease in cardiac output. If severe enough, this condition produces cardiac symptoms or even death. The clinical recognition of the problem and precise definition of the type of impaired impulse formation or conduction usually permit effective treatment with appropriate pacing systems. This chapter considers sinus node disease, acute and chronic atrioventricular (AV) block, and chronic bundle branch block.

SINUS NODE DISEASE

Sinus node disease has many synonyms, which are usually descriptive of some of the salient clinical features. The two most commonly used alternative terms are the sick sinus syndrome and the brady-tachy syndrome.

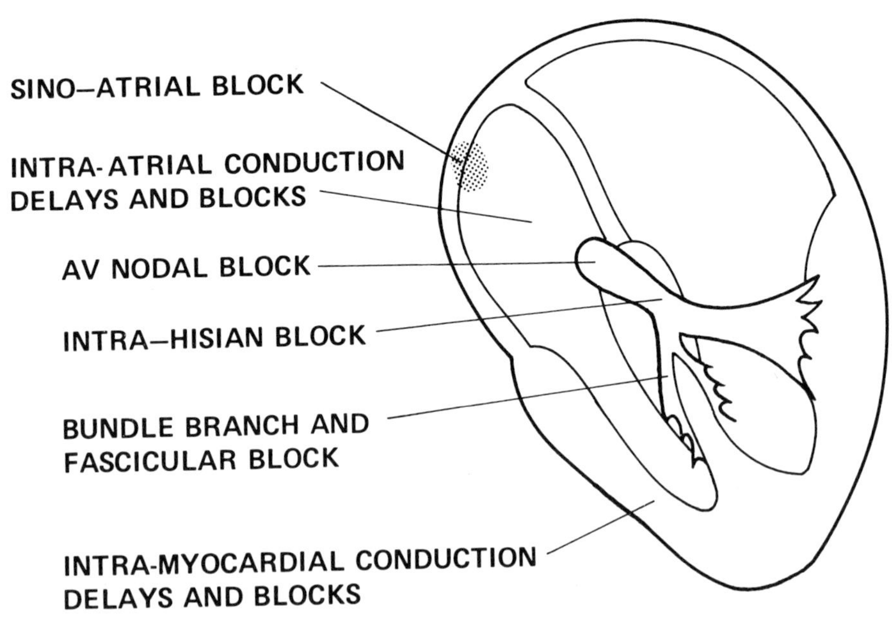

Figure 6-1 Major sites of conduction delays and blocks in AV conduction. Although intra-atrial and intramyocardial conduction delays are common, they rarely lead to clinically significant impairment of AV conduction.

Clinical Features

Sinus node disease usually occurs in the elderly (over 60 years) (Moss and Davis, 1974) but can also affect young people, including children. A wide variety of presenting symptoms are related to the underlying rhythm disturbance. Dizzy spells, syncope, transient cerebral ischemic attacks, and, in rare cases, sudden death may occur as a result of cardiac asystole or profound bradycardias. Palpitations caused by associated tachycardias may be the predominant symptom in some cases. Persistent sinus bradycardia can present as cardiac failure, angina, or effort intolerance. Thromboembolism may occur in patients with alternating tachycardias and bradycardias. Some form of associated cardiovascular disease (usually coronary artery disease, valvular heart disease, cardiomyopathy, hypertension, or congenital heart disease) is present in more than 70% of cases (Moss and Davis, 1974). The remaining 30% of patients have no other identifiable cardiovascular disease.

Pathologic Findings

Pathologic examination usually shows nonspecific changes of atrophy, fibrosis, and fatty infiltration of the sinus node area in association with the typical hallmarks of any associated cardiovascular disease. In those cases with idiopathic sinus node disease the sinus node can have a wide variety of appearances, ranging from normal to atrophied, fibrotic, or showing amyloid infiltration (Evans and Shaw, 1977). The sinus node arterial supply is usually normal in these cases.

Pathophysiology and ECG Manifestations

The functional defects in sinus node disease are a slow rate of impulse formation and/or impaired sinus node and sinoatrial (SA) conduction. The dominant pacemaker fibers may fire slowly, irregularly, or not at all because of impaired automaticity. The clinical counterparts are sinus bradycardia and sinus arrest or standstill (Figure 6-2). Impaired SA conduction is usually only apparent with second- or third-degree SA block causing irregular sinus cycles (SA Wenckebach) or sinus pauses equal to a multiple of the basic sinus cycle (sinus node exit block). In experimental preparations complete SA block may occur despite regular discharge of the dominant sinus node pacemaker cells. Whatever the mechanism, the end result in all cases is a decrease in effective sinus node discharge. The degree of symptoms depends on the length of the pauses and the efficiency of the subsidiary pacemakers that should take over the cardiac rhythm (the escape mechanisms). In sinus node disease the escape mechanisms usually originate in the atrium or AV junction. In about 60% of

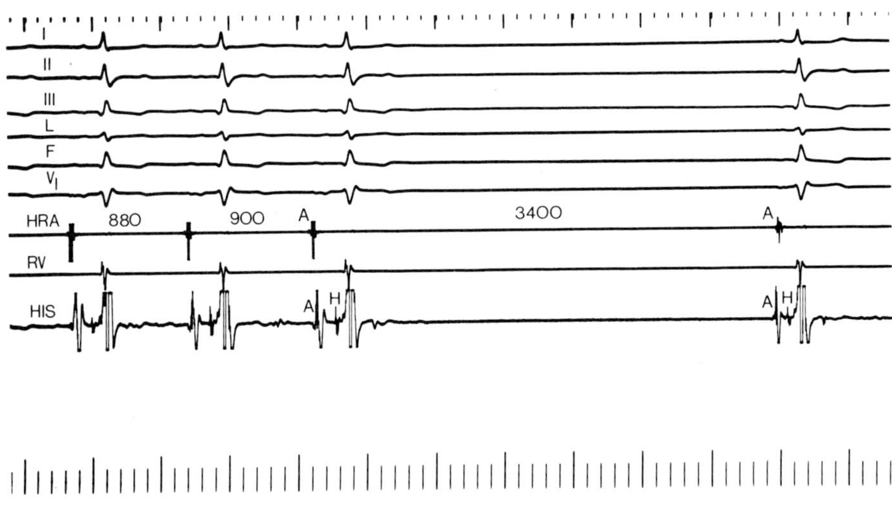

Figure 6-2 Surface ECG leads I, II, III, aVL, aVF, and V_1 with intracardiac electrograms from the high right atrium (HRA), right ventricle (RV), and His bundle region (His) are shown. The measured intervals are in milliseconds. Sinus arrest occurs spontaneously during sinus rhythm of 880-900 milliseconds. The pause is terminated by an escape beat of atrial origin (note that the atrial electrogram in the His lead precedes the HRA). Other abbreviations: A = atrial electrogram and H = His bundle electrogram.

cases sinus node disease is associated with impairment of other components of the conduction system (Narula, 1971). This associated impairment compromises the normal escape mechanisms that should take over during sinus pauses and may cause the periods of ventricular asystole that bring the disease to clinical attention.

The combination of slow conduction and block in the sinus node area sets the scene for reentrant arrhythmias. However, sustained sinus node reentrant arrhythmias are rare. Atrial arrhythmias, such as atrial fibrillation or flutter, are much more common. Intra-atrial and AV junctional tachycardias also occur. Termination of these tachyarrhythmias is often associated with a prolonged sinus node pause (Figure 6-3), sometimes causing post-tachycardia syncope. This combination of fast and slow atrial rhythms is alluded to in the term brady-tachy syndrome. The use of antiarrhythmic drugs (especially beta blockers, quinidine-like drugs, and verapamil) in treating tachyarrhythmias frequently exacerbates the bradyarrhythmias by further depressing sinus node function.

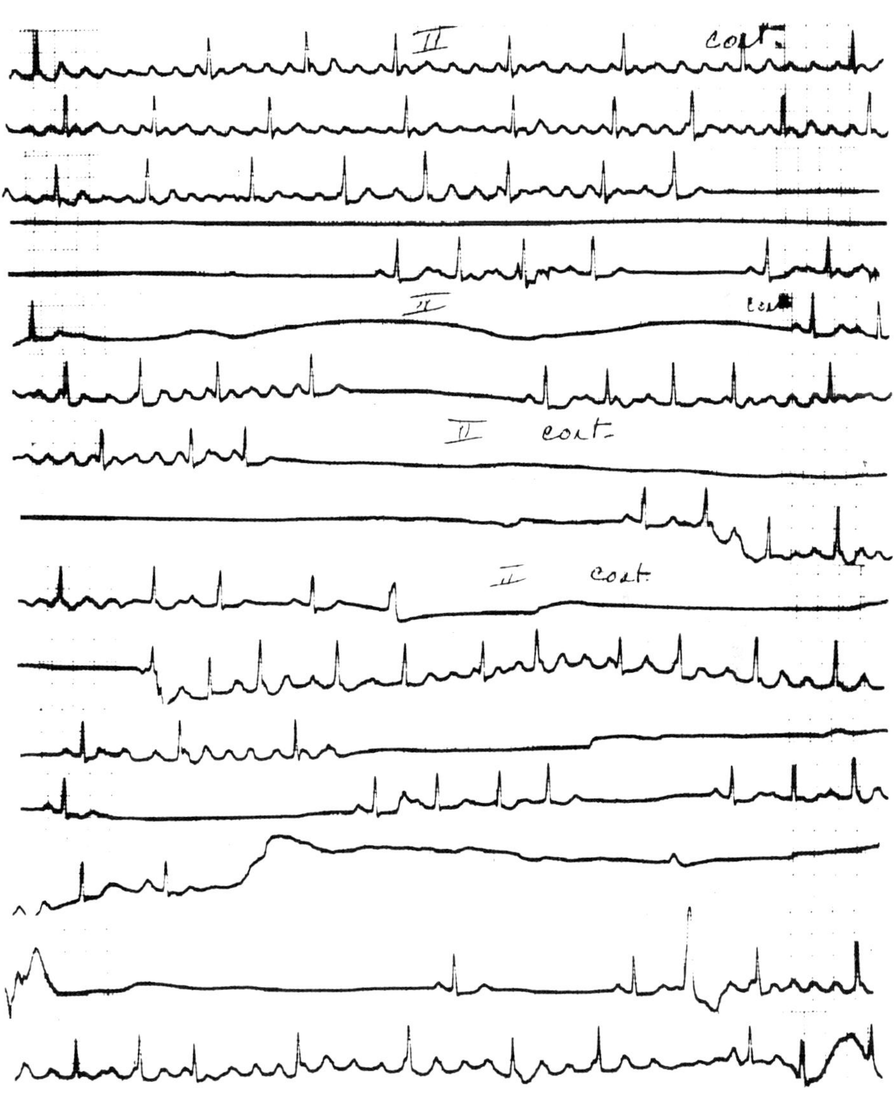

Figure 6-3 Continuous ECG lead II rhythm strips are shown. Terminations of paroxysms of atrial flutter-fibrillation are followed by varying periods of sinus arrest. Escape mechanisms of subsidiary cardiac pacemakers are also impaired, but occasional escape beats of atrial or ventricular origin occur.

Diagnosis

The mainstay of diagnosis remains continuous ECG recordings with documentation of excessive sinus node pauses. Definitely pathologic pauses can usually be identified in patients who are symptomatic from sinus node disease (i.e., pauses longer than 3-4 seconds with impaired lower escape mechanisms). The clinician should always confirm that symptoms coincide with the periods of bradycardia. It is noteworthy that sinus pauses can occur in normal people during Holter recordings, especially in young persons during sleep. Such pauses usually last less than 2.5 seconds (Brodsky, et al., 1977). Pauses of this magnitude are, therefore, not necessarily pathologic, underscoring the need to correlate symptoms with the ECG. Trained athletes may also have a significant resting bradycardia with occasional junctional escape beats, and in such persons this finding should not be considered pathologic. Carotid sinus massage may be helpful on occasions in inducing sinus node pauses if these are not already apparent. The results of carotid massage should be interpreted cautiously in elderly patients, but pauses lasting more than 3 seconds suggest sinus node disease (Mandel, et al., 1972). Carotid sinus massage in patients with syncopal symptoms caused by sinus node disease may precipitate a long symptomatic period of asystole and, therefore, full resuscitative facilities should be available. The Valsalva maneuver is rarely helpful as a diagnostic test. Exercise, atropine, or isoproterenol may have a beneficial effect on sinus rate. Patients with sinus node disease have a reduced response to intravenous atropine (the normal response is a greater than 50% increase in heart rate compared to baseline conditions following 0.04 mg/kg of intravenous atropine). The effects of exercise and isoproterenol on sinus rate are variable in patients with sinus node disease; some studies show impaired responses while others do not. The inability to respond to these agents with an increase in rate does, however, suggest sinus node disease.

Electrophysiologic studies are beneficial in some patients in whom the diagnosis remains unclear (see Chapter 2). Sinus node recovery times are determined by measuring the time it takes the sinus node to discharge after rapid atrial pacing (Mandel, et al., 1971; Narula, et al., 1972) and allow definition of abnormal and normal responses to overdrive pacing. An example of an abnormal sinus node recovery time is shown in Figure 6-4. Sinus node recovery times following cessation of pacing are usually corrected for the underlying sinus rate. This is done by either subtracting the baseline sinus cycle length from the postpacing pause (normal values <525 milliseconds) (Narula, et al., 1972) or taking the ratio of the pause to the sinus cycle length (normal value <125%-150%). The sensitivity and specificity of this type of measurement are difficult to determine because no definitive all-inclusive marker exists for sinus node dysfunction. A normal sinus node recovery time does not exclude sinus node

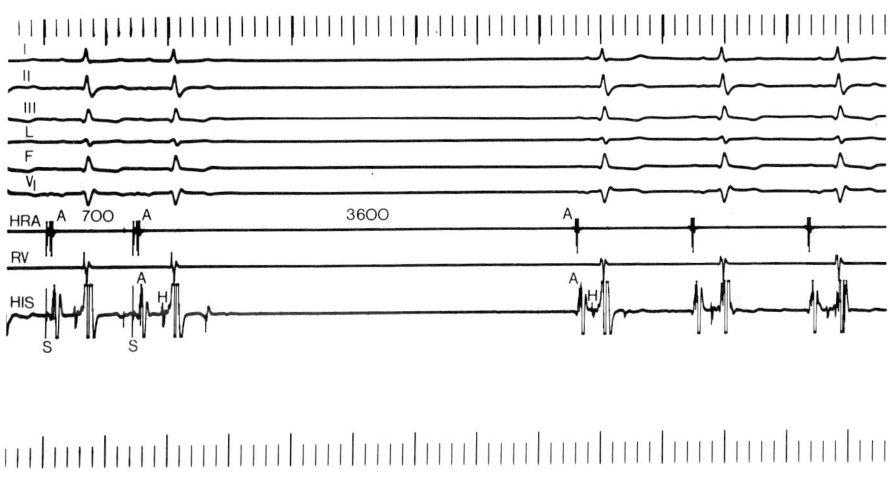

Figure 6-4 This figure has the same format as Figure 6-2. Cessation of atrial pacing at a cycle length of 700 milliseconds is followed by a prolonged sinus pause (3600 milliseconds) before sinus rhythm resumes. This sinus node recovery time is abnormal and indicates sinus node disease.

disease and occurs in approximately one-third of patients with documented spontaneous sinus pauses. A prolonged sinus node recovery time may not correlate with ambulatory or other ECG monitoring evidence of sinus node disease. The use of both prolonged ECG monitoring (see Chapter 4) and intracardiac electrophysiologic evaluation probably increases diagnostic accuracy (Reiffel, et al., 1977). The longest sinus pause is occasionally not the first sinus cycle after pacing is terminated but several cycles later. These sinus pauses are called secondary pauses and also suggest sinus node disease (Benditt, et al., 1976). Estimations of SA conduction time can be made using atrial stimulation (Strauss, et al., 1973; Narula, et al., 1978). More recently, direct recordings of SA nodal electrograms using catheter techniques have allowed the direct measurement of SA conduction times in humans (Hariman, et al., 1980; Reiffel, et al., 1980; Gomes, et al., 1982). These values are often abnormal in patients with sinus node dysfunction, especially if ECG evidence of SA block exists (Breithardt, et al., 1977). However, these tests are usually not of much clinical value if the diagnosis is in doubt, and they remain largely a research tool. Electrophysiologic study is of considerable value in assessing the function of the remainder of the conduction system and identifying the site of origin and mechanism of associated tachycardias. The effects of intravenous antiarrhythmic drugs on suppression of tachycardias and any adverse effects of drugs on sinus node function or AV conduction can also be determined during these studies. These data are useful in deciding whether the patient needs a permanent pacing system and what sort of system (i.e., atrial, ventricular, or AV sequential) should be used.

Treatment

Treatment is indicated when symptoms are present. The diseased sinus node generally responds poorly to pharmacologic agents that are aimed at increasing sinus rate, and long-term therapy with these agents is usually of little benefit. The treatment of choice is permanent cardiac pacing. Further details about the specifics of cardiac pacing are reviewed in Chapter 7. Should patients with asymptomatic sinus bradycardia or sinus pauses be paced? Because sudden death as a result of sinus node disease alone is rare and asymptomatic sinus bradycardia is relatively common, there is little justification for prophylactic pacing. Long, asymptomatic sinus pauses are more difficult to deal with. If these pauses are longer than 3-4 seconds without a reasonable escape rhythm, a prophylactic pacemaker is probably indicated on the basis that significant symptoms are likely to develop and that evidence already exists of an impaired escape mechanism.

ATRIOVENTRICULAR BLOCK

Atrioventricular (AV) blocks can be classified on a pathophysiologic basis into proximal and distal blocks. This is a very useful distinction for clinical management. Proximal block is defined as block above the level of the His bundle. Distal block includes blocks distal to the His bundle and intra-Hisian block. Intra-Hisian block is uncommon, and for practical purposes (i.e., the risk of Stokes-Adams attacks) it is best considered with the distal blocks. The clinical and functional differences of proximal and distal complete heart block are summarized in Table 6-1. In most cases the level of block can be inferred from the ECG by using the criteria in Table 6-1. Rosen and colleagues (1973) found that narrow QRS escape rhythms were caused by AV nodal block in more than 80% of cases and intra-Hisian block in less than 20% of cases. It is exceptionally rare for a ventricular escape rhythm in distal heart block to have a narrow QRS configuration. The ECG is less specific for wide QRS escape rhythms. These are caused by distal block in approximately 70% of cases and intra-Hisian and AV nodal blocks in the remaining 30% of patients (Rosen, et al., 1973). Definitive localization of the level of AV

Table 6-1 Comparative features of proximal and distal complete heart block

Feature	Proximal block	Distal block
Level of block	AVN	Intra-Hisian or distal
Preceding type of second-degree heart block	Mobitz I (Wenckebach)	Mobitz II
Usual level of escape pacemaker	AV junction	Distal HPS or ventricle
QRS duration	<0.12 seconds	<0.12 seconds
Ventricular rate (beats/min)	40-60	0-30
Stability of escape mechanism	Stable	Less stable
Response to autonomic stimulants	Moderate	Poor
Stokes-Adams attacks	Rare	Common

Abbreviations: AVN = atrioventricular node; HPS = His-Purkinje system.

block may be obtained by His bundle ECG recording. A normal His bundle ECG is illustrated in Figure 6-5. The PA interval is measured from the onset of the P wave to the onset of local atrial activity in the His bundle lead. The PA interval is a measure of intra-atrial conduction time. The AH interval (measured as shown) is a measure of AV nodal conduction time, and the HV interval represents His-Purkinje system conduction time. Prolongation of the AH or HV interval with 1:1 AV conduction at normal atrial rates represents first-degree proximal or distal AV block, respectively. In second- or third-degree AV block some or all atrial complexes fail to activate the ventricles. In proximal block the atrial impulse fails to conduct to the His bundle (Figure 6-6). Periods of Wenckebach (second-degree or Mobitz Type I) block often precede complete block at the level of the AV node. However, exceptions do occur. In distal block (Figure 6-7) atrial activity crosses the AV node and depolarizes the His bundle but is not conducted to the ventricle. This type of block may be preceded by occasional dropped beats without a preceding change in the PR interval (Mobitz type II block). Conducted beats in these patients usually have a wide QRS interval reflecting underlying disease in the His-Purkinje system. In complete AV block atrial and ventricular activities become dissociated. In proximal block atrial and His bundle activities are dissociated. In distal block His bundle and ventricular activities are dissociated. However, occasional conducted beats during complete heart block are not uncommon if long strips are examined. It is interesting that V-A conduction may be preserved despite the presence

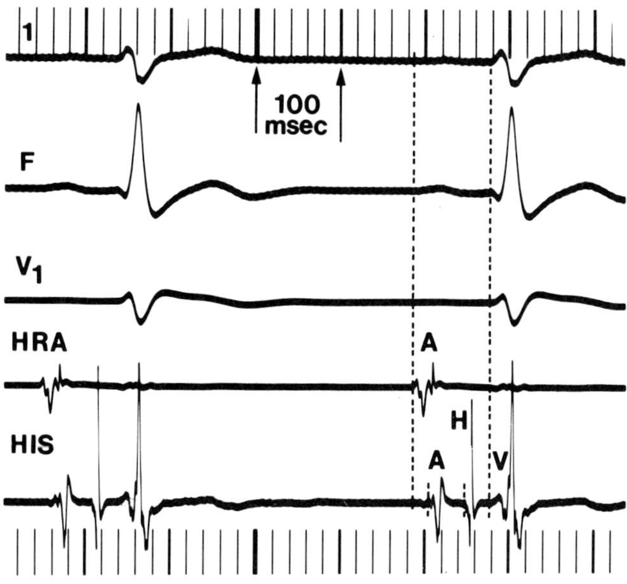

Figure 6-5 Surface ECG leads I, aVF, V, and intracardiac leads from the high right atrium (HRA) and His bundle area (His) are displayed. Note that atrial activity in the HRA occurs simultaneously with the onset of the P wave in the surface leads. A, H, and V are atrial, His bundle, and ventricular electrograms, respectively. The dotted lines on the right show the points from which PA, AH, and HV intervals are measured in the His bundle electrogram.

of complete AV block (Schuilenburg, 1976). Intra-Hisian block is diagnosed by the appearance of a split His potential in the His bundle ECG. In high-degree intra-Hisian block these two His bundle potentials may be dissociated.

Acute Heart Block

The most common circumstance associated with acute heart block is acute myocardial infarction (AMI). However, acute myocarditis, drug intoxication, electrolyte imbalances, and trauma may also cause acute heart block.

Figure 6-6 Surface ECG leads I, II, III, aVL, aVF, V_1, and intracardiac His bundle ECG (His) are shown. Two-to-one AV block at the level of the AV node is present because every second atrial complex fails to conduct to the His bundle. Note that the QRS width and HV interval of conducted beats are normal.

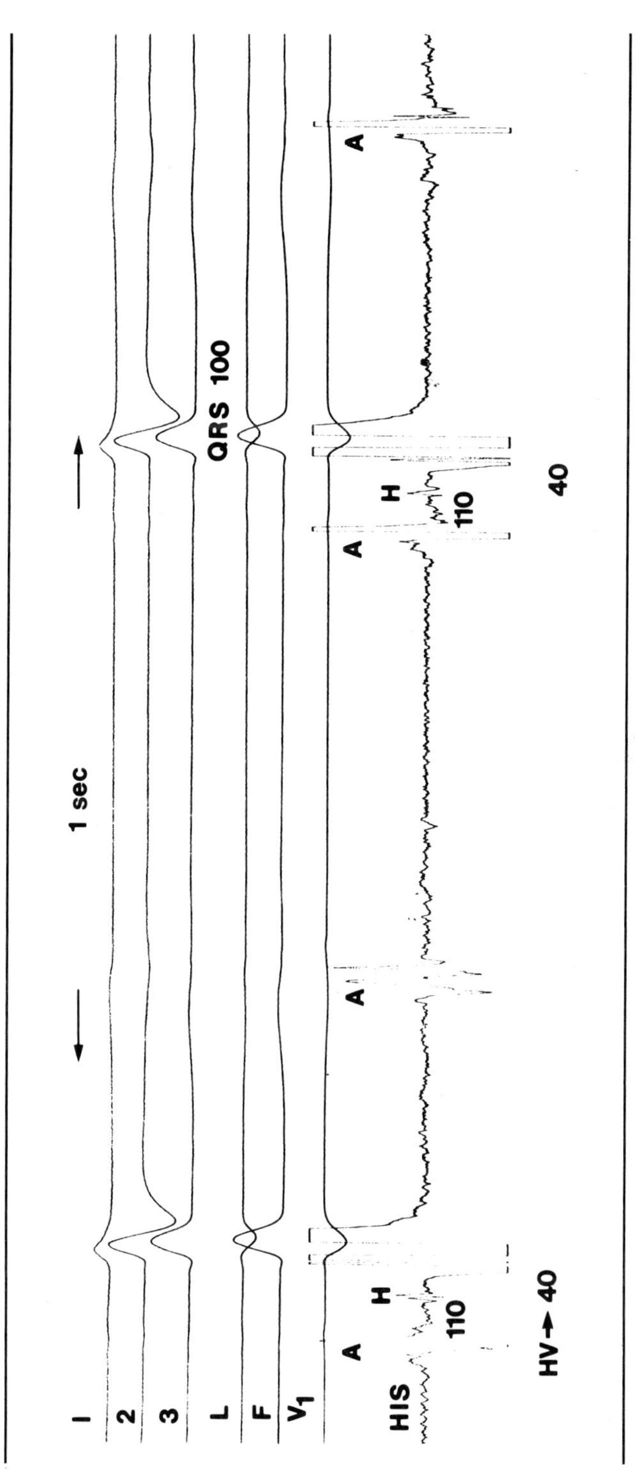
I
2
3
L
F
V_1
HIS
A
H
110
HV→ 40
1 sec
A
H
110
40
QRS 100
A
A

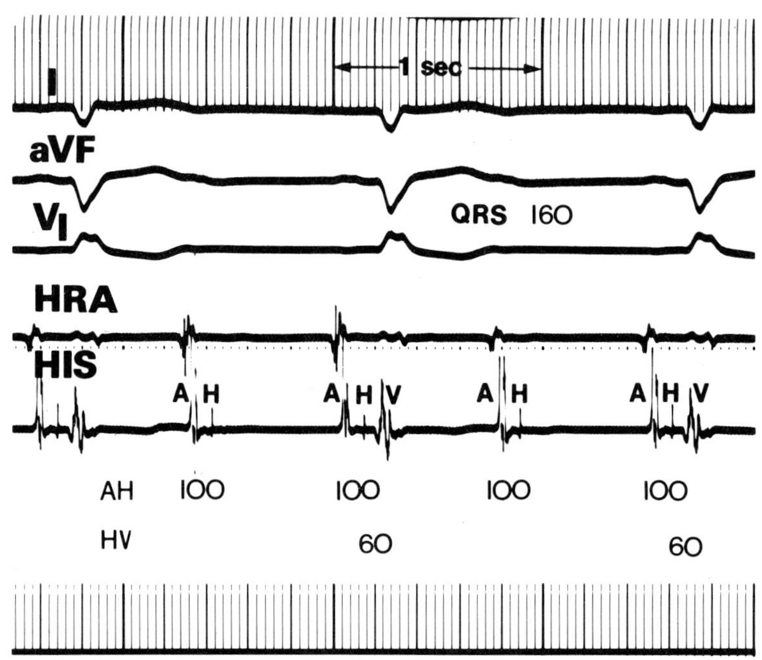

Figure 6-7 Surface ECG leads I, aVF, V_1, and intracardiac leads from the high right atrium (HRA) and His bundle region (His) are shown. Two-to-one AV block distal to the His bundle is present because every second His bundle depolarization fails to conduct to the ventricles. Note that the QRS duration and HV interval of conducted beats are both prolonged (compare with Figure 6-6). The AV nodal conduction times (AH) are within normal limits.

Heart block caused by acute myocardial infarction An understanding of the vascular supply to the conduction system is essential to understand the consequences of acute infarction on the AV node, His bundle, and bundle branches. Two main arterial sources supply the conduction system: the AV nodal artery (a branch of the right coronary artery in 90% of human hearts) and the septal branches (especially the first) of the left anterior descending coronary artery (LAD) (Frink and James, 1973). The AV node is almost completely supplied by the AV nodal artery except for a small amount of blood that comes from an anterior interatrial branch. The His bundle usually has a dual blood supply (i.e., both AV nodal artery and the first septal branch of the LAD). The proximal bundle branches also tend to have a dual blood supply but to a lesser extent than the His bundle. In hearts where only one main arterial source supplies the proximal bundle branches the right bundle branch and left anterior fascicle of the left bundle branch are supplied by the septal branches of the LAD, and the left posterior fascicle of the left bundle branch is supplied by the AV nodal artery and branches of the posterior descending coronary artery. Anterior myocardial infarction is generally caused by left coronary artery obstruction and, therefore, exerts its main effects on the distal conduction system, which tends to spare the AV node. Inferior infarction is generally caused by obstructions in the right coronary arterial system. It is, therefore, often associated with AV nodal ischemia but has less effect on the distal conduction system (His bundle and its branches) unless extensive left coronary disease is also present. It has been postulated that inferior infarction also causes increases in parasympathetic tone, which may be an additional factor contributing to sinus node and AV nodal dysfunction (see also Chapter 12).

Atrioventricular block in inferior acute myocardial infarction Prolongation of the PR interval, Wenckebach AV block, and high-degree AV block are the usual preceding stages observed with continuous ECG monitoring. The level of block is usually the AV node, and it behaves as a proximal block (see Table 6-1). High-degree AV block during inferior AMI is associated with increasing age, larger size of MI, and increased mortality (Tans and Lie, 1976). In about 50% of cases complete AV block is present on hospital admission so that the type of preceding lower-degree AV block (i.e., Wenckebach vs. Mobitz Type II) is not observed. If second-degree AV block is present soon after admission, about 50% of these patients progress to complete AV block. Most episodes (60%) of high-degree block resolve within 24 hours of onset. Almost all high-degree blocks resolve within 10 days. The time of onset and duration of high-degree block are not related to mortality, in contrast to the situation that one sees with anterior infarction. It is noteworthy that the escape rhythm has a broad QRS complex (greater than 0.12 seconds) in about 40% of cases. This is frequently caused by a junctional escape rhythm with a bradycardia-dependent left bundle branch block (Lie, et al., 1976). If the escape QRS complex has a right bundle branch block morphology, it usually originates in the distal conduction system. This type of rhythm is less stable than that seen with a junctional focus. Because the type of AV block seen in inferior infarction is usually proximal with a satisfactory escape rhythm pacing is indicated only if there are bradycardia-related symptoms (syncope, hypotension, power failure, angina, and arrhythmias). Atropine should be administered while the patient is prepared for the insertion of a temporary pacemaker. Isoproterenol may increase ventricular irritability and should only be used as second-line treatment when atropine has been unsuccessful. Administration of these drugs usually results in an increase in ventricular rate by increasing sinus rate or decreasing the degree of AV block or by acceleration of the escape junctional rhythm. If, in the absence of symptoms, a wide QRS complex escape rhythm exists that does not have a left bundle branch block configuration, a His bundle electrogram is helpful in determining the level of block. Patients with distal heart block should have a temporary pacemaker inserted even in the absence of symptoms because the escape focus may be unstable. Power failure associated with the onset of high-degree block usually resolves with temporary cardiac pacing. The persistence of power failure despite the commencement of pacing is an ominous sign with a poor prognosis. Development of nonbradycardia-dependent bundle branch block in the course of an inferior infarction is very uncommon and its natural history is unknown. Permanent pacing is rarely indicated for conduction disturbances occurring during inferior AMI (see Chapter 12).

Atrioventricular block in anterior acute myocardial infarction AV block in anterior infarction is almost always predominantly distal block. It is usually preceded by the development of bundle branch block and bifascicular block. Bundle branch block may be preexistent or occur acutely as a result of the AMI. Most investigators agree that fresh bundle branch block has a more malignant prognosis. Previous ECGs should be reviewed in all patients with bundle branch block in the course of AMI to determine the time of onset. In about 25%-50% of cases it is not possible to determine whether bundle branch block is old or new. When in doubt, the bundle branch block should be regarded as new. New-onset bundle branch block in anterior AMI is almost always right bundle branch block. Left bundle branch block is uncommon and leads to high-degree block less frequently. The natural history of fresh right bundle branch block in anterior AMI was carefully studied by Lie and colleagues (1976). Preceding incomplete right bundle branch block develops gradually. Complete right bundle branch block develops abruptly within one beat. Additional hemiblock develops gradually and may precede or follow the onset of right bundle branch block. Complete heart block occurs in more than one-third of patients who develop a new right bundle branch block with associated hemiblock (i.e., bifascicular block). Using tape recorders and multiple ECG leads, Lie and colleagues showed that bifascicular block always developed before the onset of complete heart block. Most coronary care units monitor only a single ECG lead, and, consequently, the onset of associated hemiblock may be missed. If complete AV block occurs, its onset is nearly always within 3 days of the onset of AMI. Preceding Mobitz Type II block is infrequently observed, but when it does occur it generally indicates the need for temporary pacing. Right bundle branch block that is transient and lasts less than 6 hours rarely leads to complete heart block. Recording of a His bundle ECG in a patient developing bifascicular block is a useful indicator of those patients who will develop complete AV block. In Lie's study 12 of 16 patients with bifascicular block and prolonged HV interval developed complete heart block, as compared to one patient of 14 with a normal HV interval.

The occurrence of high-degree distal block during anterior AMI is associated with a poor escape mechanism that is unstable and slow. Emergency temporary pacing is necessary. Prophylactic temporary pacing for patients with anterior AMI and bifascicular block is usually recommended. One rational approach to the patient with new bifascicular block is to insert a temporary pacing catheter via the femoral vein. The HV interval can be measured using this catheter, and, if normal, the pacer may be left in place for 24 hours and then removed. If the HV interval is prolonged, the catheter may be left in for several days and the HV interval remeasured during removal. Although prophylactic pacing may be life-saving in individual cases, it does not generally lower group mortality because development of complete heart block and bundle branch block during anterior AMI carries a bad prognosis, and most patients die subsequently from power failure or ventricular arrhythmias. However, when complete AV block occurs, the transition to a paced rhythm is smooth and less disturbing to the patient. Prophylactic temporary pacing is sometimes associated with pacemaker sensing problems that may precipitate pacemaker-induced arrhythmias. If sensing problems occur, change from bipolar to unipolar pacing by using a skin electrode as the indifferent electrode is sometimes useful. Another approach is to turn the pacer off but leave it connected so that it can be switched on if high-degree block occurs. Continuous ECG monitoring and vigilant staff are required for the latter approach.

Permanent cardiac pacing is required for the few patients with persistent high-degree AV block who survive their AMI. Some investigators have recommended permanent cardiac pacing in all patients surviving anterior AMI complicated by transient complete heart block (Waugh, et al., 1973; Mullens and Atkins, 1976; Hindman, et al., 1978). These recommendations are based on suggestive data; no definitive studies are currently available. Further research is needed before this approach can be completely endorsed. Patients who revert to 1:1 AV conduction but who have a grossly prolonged (>75 milliseconds) HV interval may also benefit from permanent pacing. Confirmatory data for this recommendation are also not currently available.

Patients who develop bundle branch block during the course of anterior AMI have a high incidence of ventricular fibrillation occurring 2-6 weeks after infarction (Lie, et al., 1978). This arrhythmia does not appear to be based on poor left ventricular function. All such patients should be monitored in a hospital setting where full resuscitative facilities are readily available for a longer period than usual. Routine prophylactic arrhythmic drug treatment has been recommended in these patients (Norris and Woo, 1978).

Other causes of acute heart block Iatrogenic administration of drugs may be associated with heart block. Digoxin and its analogues, beta-adrenergic blocking drugs, and edrophonium may precipitate proximal AV block. Type I antiarrhythmic drugs (quinidine, procainamide, disopyramide) may cause distal AV block. Overdose of these and other drugs (i.e., tricyclic antidepressants) may also cause severe cases of high-degree heart block. Treatment consists of stopping the offending drug and employing temporary pacing if there are symptoms or if the site of block is distal. Cardiac catheterization may traumatize the conduction system, causing heart block. This is usually transient but if sustained may require temporary pacing until AV conduction resumes. Cardiac surgical procedures may also cause high-degree heart block. This is frequently transient and requires only temporary pacing. If there is any doubt about the stability of 1:1 AV conduction when conduction returns, electrophysiologic study should be performed to determine conduction intervals and the response of the AV conduction system to atrial pacing at increasing heart rates. Distal AV block at rates of less than 130 beats/min or a grossly prolonged HV interval are indications for permanent pacing. Hyperkalemia, usually in patients with renal impairment, may cause high-degree AV block. Treatment consists of standard measures to lower serum potassium levels. Temporary pacing may be required.

Chronic Heart Block

Congenital atrioventricular block The underlying etiology of heart block depends on the age group in which it occurs. Congenital heart block is usually a proximal type of block with a stable junctional escape rhythm. In the usual case with no associated congenital heart disease it is often asymptomatic and compatible with normal development. If associated congenital heart disease exists, corrected transposition of the great vessels is one of the most frequent associations. Complete AV block in corrected transposition may not be present in infancy but may develop later in life. Cardiac pacing is indicated only if the heart block causes symptoms. Surgically induced heart block complicating repair of congenital heart defects often requires permanent pacing.

Acquired atrioventricular block *Etiology* Possible causative factors are identified in about 50% of patients. Coronary artery disease or other vascular disease is the most common association. Cardiomyopathy, valvular heart disease, myocarditis, cardiac surgery, hypertension, or diabetes may also occur. In the remaining patients no etiology is identified. These cases are classed as idiopathic heart block or primary conduction system disease.

Clinical findings The presenting symptoms of sudden onset are cardiac arrest or Stokes-Adams attacks. Symptoms of gradual onset include cardiac failure, effort intolerance, fatigue, and angina. Some patients are entirely asymptomatic. Physical examination reveals bradycardia, cannon waves in the neck veins, and variable intensity of the first heart sounds. An ECG confirms the diagnosis.

Management Symptomatic chronic high-degree AV block requires permanent pacing irrespective of the level of the block. Intravenous atropine should be used in patients with hemodynamically significant heart block presenting as an emergency. If this is unsuccessful, intravenous isoproterenol should be used. A temporary pacemaker should be inserted as soon as possible. After appropriate investigation to exclude cases of acute heart block the physician may elect to implant a permanent pacemaker. In asymptomatic cases the level of block should be determined, as outlined earlier in this chapter. Asymptomatic high-degree distal AV block requires permanent pacing because of the likelihood of potentially fatal Stokes-Adams attacks (Rosen, et al., 1973). Syncopal episodes develop less frequently in patients with high-degree proximal AV block who are initially asymptomatic. These patients may be observed until the onset of symptoms. The problem of possible paroxysmal AV block in patients with syncope who lack documented evidence of high-degree AV block is discussed in the next section. Complete heart block may occasionally cause profound prolongation of the QT interval, ventricular ectopy, and ventricular tachyarrhythmias of the torsade de pointes type. Although syncope is caused by tachyarrhythmias in this context, control is usually achieved by correction of the underlying bradycardia with pacing.

CHRONIC BUNDLE BRANCH BLOCK

Chronic bundle branch block, especially bifascicular block, frequently precedes the onset of high-degree distal AV block. Although this field has been extensively studied, the natural history of chronic bundle branch block has only recently become clearer. The conclusions of some of these studies have been contradictory, and the medical management of chronic bundle branch block remains controversial (Scheinman, et al., 1973; Narula, et al., 1975; Vera, et al., 1976; Scheinman, et al., 1977; McAnulty, et al., 1978; Altschuler, et al., 1979; Dhingra, et al., 1979). Careful review of these studies suggests that most differences in findings can be explained by differences in the study populations. Chronic bundle branch block is best considered by division into two groups: symptomatic and asymptomatic.

Symptomatic Bundle Branch Block

Symptomatic bundle branch block refers to transient neurologic manifestations that might be caused by a transient cardiac bradyarrhythmia.

This includes dizzy spells, syncope, and epilepsy. Patients in whom these symptoms are dramatic or recurrent should undergo prolonged continuous ECG monitoring in an attempt to document a rhythm disturbance (tachycardia or bradycardia). Other causes of syncope should be systematically searched for and excluded. The workup generally includes a thorough history and physical examination, noninvasive cardiac testing (ECG, chest x-ray, and echocardiogram), and EEG and other appropriate neurologic tests. If all investigations are negative, electrophysiologic study may be helpful. Evidence may exist of severe sinus node or AV node disease. Programmed stimulation of the atria or ventricles may cause high-grade AV block. Atrial pacing at rates less than 130 beats/min may cause a block that is distal to the His bundle. Premature atrial beats at long coupling intervals may be blocked distal to the His bundle. The significance of a prolonged HV interval alone is controversial (Scheinman, et al., 1973; Narula, et al., 1975; Vera, et al., 1976; Scheinman, et al., 1977; McAnulty, et al., 1978; Altschuler, et al., 1979; Dhingra, et al., 1979). Some data suggest that a prolonged HV interval in symptomatic patients detects a subset of individuals who are at high risk for developing complete AV block if other causes of syncope are systematically excluded (Altschuler, et al., 1979). If any of the above findings occur during electrophysiologic study, permanent pacing is indicated. Recent data suggest that pacing reduces symptoms but does not significantly reduce overall mortality or the incidence of sudden death (Scheinman, et al., 1980). These findings emphasize the importance of underlying heart disease in determining mortality in patients with bundle branch block.

Asymptomatic Bundle Branch Block

The incidence of progression to complete heart block in asymptomatic bundle branch block is very low (<1% in U.S. Air Force personnel in 10 years of follow-up) (Rotman and Triebwasser, 1975). Studies of older populations and hospital-based populations with significant associated cardiac disease confirm the low incidence of progression to complete heart block (Kulbertus, et al., 1978; McAnulty, et al., 1978; Dhingra, et al., 1979). Electrophysiologic study or prophylactic pacing are, therefore, not indicated. Patients with asymptomatic bundle branch block do not have a significantly increased risk of heart block during general anesthesia or when taking antiarrhythmic drugs that depress conduction in the His-Purkinje system (Scheinman, et al., 1974; Hirschfeld, et al., 1977; Pastore, et al., 1978; Desai, et al., 1979). Thus, prophylactic pacing is not usually required in these circumstances. The presence of asymptomatic bundle branch block may be an indicator of associated cardiac disease. The predictive value depends on the age group of the patient and whether heart disease is already apparent at the time of examination. Associated cardiovascular disease occurs in more than 50% of adults with right bundle branch block and in an even higher percentage in patients with left bundle branch block. Newly acquired bundle branch block has a high incidence of associated heart disease, which if not present at the time of detection, often becomes apparent on follow-up (Schneider, et al., 1979; Schneider, et al., 1980). The prognosis in patients with bundle branch block and associated heart disease is significantly impaired. In contrast, young persons (<30 years) with right or left bundle branch block and no evidence of associated heart disease have an excellent prognosis (Rotman and Triebwasser, 1975).

REFERENCES

Altschuler, H.; Fisher, J. D.; and Furman, S. 1979. Significance of isolated H-V interval prolongation in symptomatic patients without documented heart block. *Am. Heart J.* 97:19-26.

Benditt, D. G.; Strauss, H. C.; Scheinman, M. M., et al. 1976. Analysis of secondary pauses following termination of rapid atrial pacing in man. *Circulation* 54:436-441.

Breithardt, G.; Seipel, L.; and Loogen, F. 1977. Sinus node recovery time in normal subjects and in patients with sinus node dysfunction. *Circulation* 56:43-50.

Brodsky, M.; Wu, D.; Denes, P., et al. 1977. Arrhythmias documented by 24-hour continuous electrocardiographic monitoring in 50 male medical students without apparent heart disease. *Am. J. Cardiol.* 39:390-395.

Desai, J. M.; Scheinman, M. M.; Peters, R. W., et al. 1979. Electrophysiological effects of disopyramide in patients with bundle branch block. *Circulation* 59:215-225.

Dhingra, R. C.; Wyndham, C. R.; Amat-y-Leon, F., et al. 1979. Incidence and site of atrioventricular block in patients with chronic bifascicular block. *Circulation* 59:238-246.

Evans, R.; and Shaw, D. B. 1977. Pathological studies in sinoatrial disorder (sick sinus syndrome). *Br. Heart J.* 39:778-786.

Frink, R. J.; and James, T. N. 1973. Normal blood supply to the human His bundle and proximal bundle branches. *Circulation* 47:8-18.

Gomes, J. A. C.; Kang, P. S.; El-Sherif, N. 1982. The sinus node electrogram in patients with and without sick sinus syndrome: techniques and correlation between directly measured and indirectly estimated sinoatrial conduction time. *Circulation* 66:864-873.

Hariman, R. J.; Krongrad, E.; Boxer, R. A., et al. 1980. Method for recording electrical activity of the sinoatrial node and automatic atrial foci during cardiac catheterization in human subjects. *Am. J. Cardiol.* 45:775-781.

Hindman, M. C.; Wagner, G. S.; Atkins, J. M., et al. 1978. The clinical significance of bundle branch block complicating acute myocardial infarction. 2. Indications for temporary and permanent pacemaker insertion. *Circulation* 58:689-699.

Hirschfeld, D. S.; Ueda, C. T.; Rowland, M., et al. 1977. Clinical and electrophysiological effects of intravenous quinidine in man. *Br. Heart J.* 39:309-316.

Kulbertus, H. E.; deLaval-Rutten, F.; Dubois, M., et al. 1978. Prognostic significance of left anterior hemiblock with right bundle branch block in mass screening. *Am. J. Cardiol.* 41:385.

Lie, K. I.; Wellens, H. J. J.; Schuilenburg, R. M., et al. 1974. Mechanism and significance of widened QRS complexes during complete A-V block in acute inferior myocardial infarction. *Am. J. Cardiol.* 33:833-839.

Lie, K. I.; Wellens, H. J. J.; and Schuilenburg, R. M. 1976. Bundle branch block and acute myocardial infarction. In *The conduction system of the heart: structure, function, and clinical implications.* H. J. J. Wellens; K. I. Lie; and M. J. Janse, editors. Philadelphia: Lea & Febiger. pp. 662-672.

Lie, K. I.; Liem, K. L.; Schuilenburg, R. M., et al. 1978. Early identification of patients developing late in-hospital ventricular fibrillation after discharge from the coronary care unit. A 5½ year retrospective and prospective study of 1897 patients. *Am. J. Cardiol.* 41:674-677.

Mandel, W. J.; Hayakawa, H.; Danzig, R., et al. 1971. Evaluation of sino-atrial node function in man by overdrive suppression. *Circulation* 44: 59-66.

Mandel, W. J.; Hayakawa, H.; Allen, H. N., et al. 1972. Assessment of sinus node function in patients with sick sinus syndrome. *Circulation* 46:761-769.

McAnulty, J. H.; Rahimtoola, S. H.; Murphy, E. S., et al. 1978. A prospective study of sudden death in "high risk" bundle branch block. *N. Engl. J. Med.* 299:209-215.

Moss, A. J.; and Davis, R. J. 1974. Brady-tachy syndrome. *Prog. Cardiovasc. Dis.* 16:439-454.

Mullens, C. B.; and Atkins, J. M. 1976. Prognosis and management of ventricular conduction blocks in acute myocardial infarction. *Mod. Conc. Cardiovasc. Dis.* 45:129-133.

Narula, O. S. 1971. Atrioventricular conduction defects in patients with sinus bradycardia: analysis by His bundle recordings. *Circulation* 44: 1096-1110.

Narula, O. S.; Samet, P.; and Javier, R. P. 1972. Significance of sinus node recovery time. *Circulation* 45:140-158.

Narula, O. S.; Gann, D.; and Samet, P. 1975. Prognostic value of H-V intervals. In *His bundle electrocardiography and clinical electrophysiology.* O. S. Narula, editor. Philadelphia: F. A. Davis Co. p. 437.

Narula, O. S.; Shantha, N.; Vasquez, M., et al. 1978. A new method for measurement of sinoatrial conduction time. *Circulation* 58:706-714.

Norris, R. M.; and Woo, K. S. 1978. Bundle branch block after myocardial infarction: short and long-term effects. In *Advances in the management of arrhythmias.* D. T. Kelly, editor. Sydney, Australia: Telectronics. pp. 364-373.

Pastore, J. O.; Yurchak, P. M.; Janis, K. M., et al. 1978. The risk of advanced heart block in surgical patients with right bundle branch block and left axis deviation. *Circulation* 57:677-680.

Reiffel, J. A.; Bigger, J. T., Jr.; and Cramer, M. 1977. Ability of Holter electrocardiogram recording and atrial stimulation to detect sinus nodal dysfunction in symptomatic and asymptomatic patients with sinus bradycardia. *Am. J. Cardiol.* 40:189-194.

Reiffel, J. A.; Gang, E.; Gliklich, J., et al. 1980. The human sinus node electrogram: a transvenous catheter technique and a comparison of directly measured and indirectly estimated sinoatrial conduction time in adults. *Circulation* 62:1324-1334.

Rosen, K. M.; Dhingra, R. C.; Loeb, H. S., et al. 1973. Chronic heart block in adults: clinical and electrophysiological observations. *Arch. Intern. Med.* 131:663-672.

Rotman, M.; and Triebwasser, J. H. 1975. A clinical and follow-up study of right and left bundle branch block. *Circulation* 51:477-484.

Scheinman, M. M.; Weiss, A.; and Kunkel, F. 1973. His bundle recordings in patients with bundle branch block and transient neurologic symptoms. *Circulation* 48:322-330.

Scheinman, M. M.; Weiss, A. N.; Benowitz, N., et al. 1974. Electrophysiologic effects of procainamide in patients with intraventricular conduction delay. *Circulation* 49:522-529.

Scheinman, M. M.; Peters, R. W.; Modin, G., et al. 1977. Prognostic value of infranodal conduction time in patients with chronic bundle branch block. *Circulation* 56:240-244.

Scheinman, M. M.; Goldschlager, N. F.; and Peters, R. W. 1980. Bundle branch block. In *Cardiovascular arrhythmias: mechanisms and management.* A. Castellanos, editor. Cardiovascular Clinics 11, no. 1, Philadelphia: F. A. Davis Co. pp. 57-80.

Schneider, J. F.; Thomas, H. E.; Kreger, B. E., et al. 1979. Newly acquired left bundle branch block: the Framingham study. *Ann. Intern. Med.* 90: 303-310.

Schneider, J. F.; Thomas, H. E.; Kreger, B. E., et al. 1980. Newly acquired right bundle branch block: the Framingham study. *Ann. Intern. Med.* 92:37-44.

Schuilenburg, R. M. 1976. Patterns of V-A conduction in the human heart in the presence of normal and abnormal A-V conduction. In *The conduction system of the heart: structure, function, and clinical implications.* H. J. J. Wellens; K. I. Lie; and M. J. Janse, editors. Philadelphia: Lea & Febiger. pp. 485-503.

Strauss, H. C.; Saroff, A. L.; and Bigger, J. T., Jr. 1973. Premature atrial stimulation as a key to the understanding of sinoatrial conduction in man. *Circulation* 47:86-93.

Tans, A. C.; and Lie, K. I. 1976. AV nodal block in acute myocardial infarction. In *The conduction system of the heart: structure, function, and clinical implications.* H. J. J. Wellens; K. I. Lie; and M. J. Janse, editors. Philadelphia: Lea & Febiger. pp. 655-661.

Vera, Z.; Mason, D. T.; Fletcher, R. D., et al. 1976. Prolonged His-Q interval in chronic bifascicular block. Relation to impending complete heart block. *Circulation* 53:46-55.

Waugh, R. A.; Wagner, G. S.; Haney, T. L., et al. 1973. Immediate and remote prognostic significance of fascicular block during acute myocardial infarction. *Circulation* 47:765-775.

7 Advances in Cardiac Pacing

Jerry C. Griffin, M.D.

Director of Pacing Programs
Baylor College of Medicine and The Methodist Hospital
Houston, Texas

Since the implantation of the first electronic device for artificial stimulation of the heart in 1959 by Elmquist and Senning (1960), many advances have occurred in the understanding and application of artificial pacemakers in the treatment of cardiac rhythm abnormalities. Pacing has broadened from its original role as a treatment for complete heart block to include the management of the sinus node dysfunction syndrome, tachyarrhythmias, and a variety of other conditions. Advances in engineering technology have increased both the reliability and complexity of pacing systems. In 1978, in over 2500 hospitals in the United States alone, nearly 100,000 pacemakers were implanted. Presently, over 300,000 patients in the United States have cardiac pacemakers (Parsonnet, 1979).

The second decade of cardiac pacing has proved to be one of great advancement and innovation. Great improvements have been made in pacemaker design and function. The combination of the lithium power cell and digital integrated circuitry has led to the development of small, light, reliable pacemakers that are capable of complex functions. Programmability, the noninvasive alteration of pacemaker function, has increased greatly in scope thanks to such design improvements. Programmability is useful in the modification of pacemaker function at the time of implant, at the time of follow-up evaluation, and throughout the pacemaker's life and in the prevention of operative revision for the correction of problems.

These technical advances have led to the development of pacemakers that may effectively coordinate atrial and ventricular events, providing appropriate pacing and sensing function for both chambers. The clinical application of this technology is currently being investigated and will undoubtedly increase. Finally, pacemakers designed for the specific purpose of terminating tachycardias have begun to see limited clinical application. These complex devices are fully programmable, automatically detect tachycardias, and provide an appropriate sequence of pacing stimuli designed to interrupt the reentrant circuit and restore normal rhythm.

ENGINEERING ADVANCES

Perhaps the most important development in cardiac pacing in the 1970s was the discovery of new and more reliable power sources for implantable pacemakers. Mercury-zinc batteries were the most commonly used power source prior to 1972. Although with continued refinement improved reliability and longevity were attained, mercury-zinc pacemakers remained disappointing for several reasons. The mercury-zinc cell generates gas during its chemical reaction, making hermetic sealing difficult, allows significant internal energy losses, decreasing the amount of energy available for external work, and displays irregular and sometimes unpredictable failure modes, making follow-up difficult (Parsonnet, 1977).

The Lithium Battery

In 1971 Greatbatch and colleagues introduced the lithium-polymer iodine cell as a pacemaker power source. Although at present cells with this chemistry are the most commonly used, lithium batteries with other cathode materials have also been designed. The lithium battery has several attributes that make it superior to other available power sources. It has a high energy density (stored energy/volume). Because of the nature of the chemical reaction, its internal energy losses are minimal, resulting in a long shelf life. The chemical reaction is a self-sealing process, increasing battery reliability and making primary premature battery failure rare. The batteries using lithium iodide and some others may be hermetically sealed (completely enclosed in moisture-proof metal cases). However, some lithium batteries, such as the silver chromate cell, use a liquid electrolyte and cannot be hermetically sealed (Parsonnet, 1977; Tyers and Brownlee, 1978). Thus, the lithium power source permits small, light, reliable pacemakers having greater longevity and reliability than their mercury-zinc predecessors.

Unfortunately, not all of the initial expectations of the lithium battery have been met. After 8 years' experience with a variety of lithium chemistries it now seems clear that significant differences exist between cells, and certain initial predictions were inaccurate. A particular problem has been the battery's failure to deliver all of its stored charge, resulting in pacemakers with significantly less than expected longevity. Some manufacturers have used a number of different power sources in their various models of pacemaker, which makes it difficult to follow patients with lithium pacemakers. At the present time, follow-up of lithium pacemakers must be individualized on the basis of both manufacturer and power source, and the clinician must rely on manufacturers' recommendations and published follow-up data such as those of Hauser and Giuffre (1979); Welti (1980); Bilitch (1980); and Hurzeler and colleagues (1980).

Digital Integrated Circuits

The availability of a reliable and relatively large-capacity power source prompted the second major engineering development during the 1970s: the incorporation of digital integrated circuits into pacemaker design. Integrated circuits have decreased power consumption, improved reliability, and greatly increased the complexity of the functions of which modern pacemakers are now capable. This combination has finally made extensive programmability and dual-chamber pacing an obtainable goal.

PROGRAMMABILITY

Programmability may be defined as the noninvasive, persistent, alteration of one or more variables of pacemaker function within a predetermined range. Although not a new concept, programmability has enjoyed a rapidly increasing popularity over the past 5 years. Currently, pacemakers are available that offer programmability of a wide range of operating characteristics (Table 7-1).

Applications

At least four applications of programmability are available in managing patients with cardiac pacemakers: (1) the pacemaker may be adjusted to suit each patient's exact requirements at the time of implantation; (2) programmability allows the physician to adjust the pacemaker for a specific application, such as atrial pacing. This decreases the need for a large variety of custom-designed pacemakers; (3) programmability combined with telemetry, which is available in some pacemakers, allows for a more thorough and exacting follow-up evaluation than can be done with nonprogrammable models; (4) some evidence exists that programmability may allow the physician to adjust pacemaker function to compensate for any departure from the patient's initial condition at the time of implant, thus helping to preserve the functional life of the pacemaker system and reduce the likelihood of operative intervention and generator replacement prior to battery depletion.

Rate was one of the first features to be made programmable. The most important use of rate programmability is the facilitation of sinus rhythm in patients who are not totally pacemaker-dependent. This is achieved by reducing the pacemaker escape interval to correspond to a rate below the patient's usual minimum sinus rate. This causes fewer changes from sinus to paced rhythm, decreasing the likelihood of symptoms of pacemaker syndrome (see the section on the hemodynamics of pacing in this chapter). It also increases the longevity of the pacing system by reducing current drain. Occasional patients with concomitant coronary artery disease will experience less angina pectoris at slower-paced rates. Although less commonly used, pacing rates greater than 80 beats/min are important for pediatric patients, for the overdrive suppression of tachyarrhythmias, and possibly for the improvement of cardiac output in certain patients (see the section on the hemodynamics of pacing in this chapter).

Rate hysteresis programmability is the capability of the pacemaker to vary its escape interval independent of its pacing interval. A pacemaker with this capability might allow itself to be inhibited by sinus rhythm as slow as 50 beats/min, but whenever pacing is initiated it will occur at 70 pulses/min. This facilitates sinus rhythm but provides a faster ventricular pacing rate should pacing be required.

The threshold for excitation is related to both the amplitude and duration of the stimulating pulse (Figure 7-1). For this reason either or both of these variables may be used to provide output programmability.

Table 7-1 Spectrum of available programmability

Feature	Capability
Rate	30-150 pulses/min
Output	
Amplitude	1.3-7.5 volts
Impulse duration	0.5-2.3 milliseconds
Input sensitivity	0.6-8 millivolts
Refractory period	180-450 milliseconds
Hysteresis	0-60 pulses/min
Mode	Asynchronous, inhibited, triggered

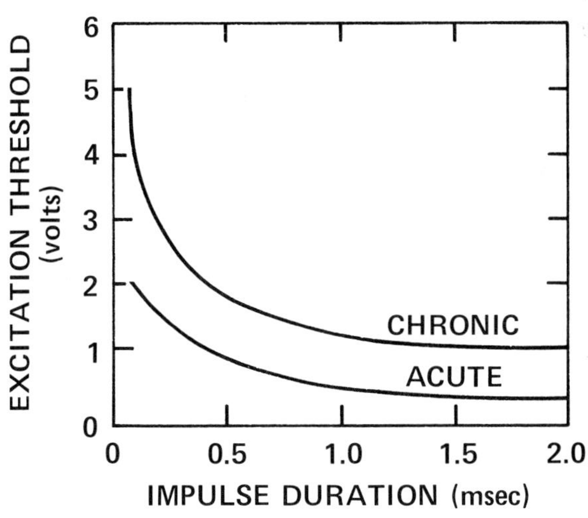

Figure 7-1 This figure shows the strength-interval curve, which is the relationship between the voltage required for myocardial excitation and impulse duration. At the time of electrode placement (acute) the voltages are lower than those seen later (chronic), probably because of the development of fibrosis between the electrode surface and viable myocardium.

Pulse duration alteration is most applicable in the range of 0.1-1 milliseconds where its influence on the strength-interval curve is greatest. Pulse duration adjustment is, therefore, most effective for reducing current drain while maintaining adequate safety margins. Amplitude programmability is more useful when dealing with that portion of the curve beyond 1 millisecond in pulse duration, such as when attempting to correct for high excitation thresholds. Especially useful for this purpose are several new pacemakers that can be programmed to outputs above the nominal 5 volts.

Decreasing pulse amplitude and/or duration results in increased longevity of the pacemaker, as well as decreasing the likelihood of stimulating noncardiac tissues such as diaphragm and pectoral muscle. Increasing pulse duration and/or amplitude may allow the maintenance of reliable pacing in the face of increased excitation threshold.

Sensitivity programmability allows the pacemaker to be made more or less sensitive to incoming signals from the electrode. The pacemaker may be made more sensitive to detect smaller amplitude electrograms such as from the atria, from a ventricular electrode demonstrating less than optimal performance, or from a PVC having electrogram characteristics that are different from those of the accompanying sinus beats. The pacemaker may be made less sensitive to screen out unwanted electrical signals, either extrinsic, such as electromagnetic interference from the environment, or intrinsic, such as skeletal muscle activity, or T waves.

The ability to alter pacemaker function (Figure 7-2) from inhibited mode to R-wave synchronous (i.e., triggered) mode may be useful in circumstances in which false inhibition occurs because of either intrinsic or extrinsic electromagnetic interference. In this circumstance if noise was sensed in the inhibited mode, there would be no pacemaker output, a situation that could be dangerous in patients without spontaneous ventricular activity. In the R-wave synchronous mode the ventricle is paced each time activity is sensed; therefore, noise would cause pacing to occur. The asynchronous mode may be used occasionally to reduce current drain in those patients with complete heart block and no ventricular ectopy.

Refractory period programmability enables one to shorten the refractory period to detect very early premature beats or lengthen the refractory period to prevent T wave sensing in ventricular pacemakers

Figure 7-2 Ventricular pacing modes. These recordings were made in a patient with a programmable pacemaker. The pacer spikes are labeled P. In the top strip the pacemaker is programmed to asynchronous (VOO) pacing at a rate of 50 beats/min. In this mode pacer spikes occur at a rate of 50 beats/min regardless of the patient's own rhythm. Pacer spikes falling during the absolute refractory period of the patient's own sinus beats (see the first QRS interval) will fail to

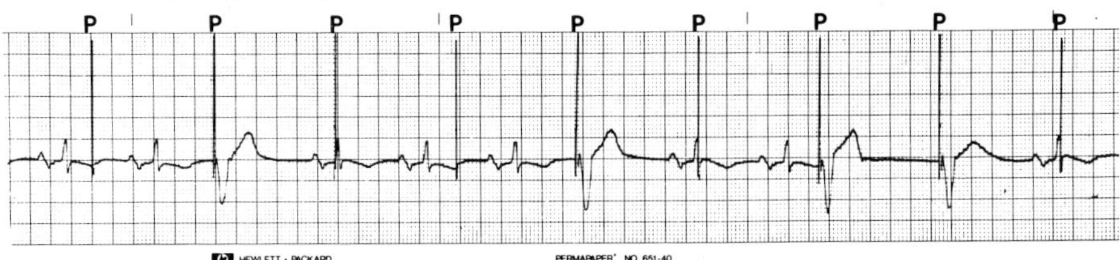

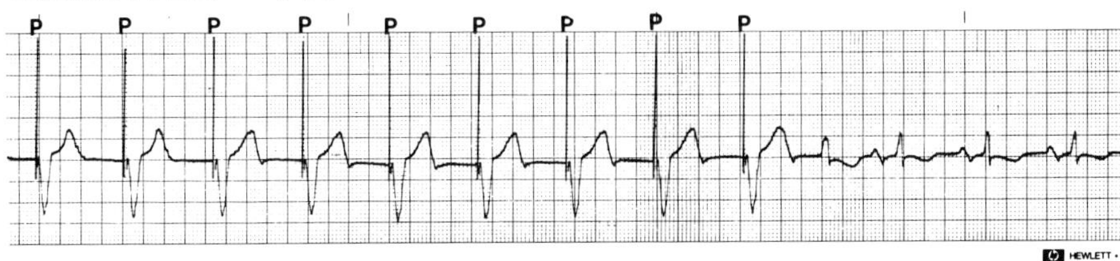

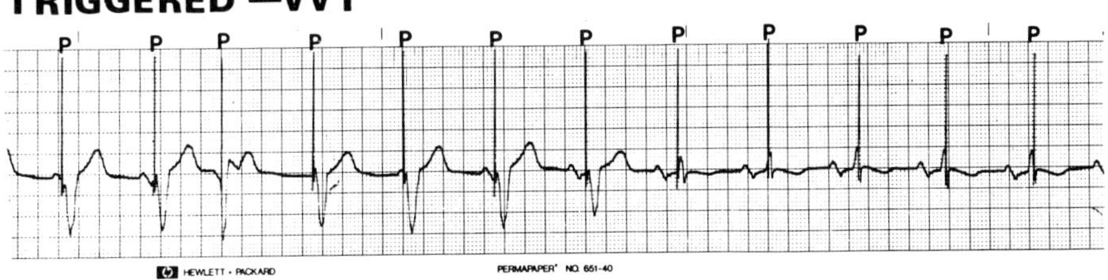

pace. Pacing on the T wave in this mode can initiate ventricular tachyarrhythmias. This pacing mode is rarely used today except during magnet testing of pacemaker function. The middle strip shows ventricular inhibited pacing (VVI) at a rate of 70 beats/min. When the patient's own rhythm is less than this rate, ventricular pacing occurs. When the patient's own rhythm occurs, such as at the right of the strip, pacing is inhibited. This is also known as demand pacing. The bottom strip shows ventricular triggered pacing (VVT) at a rate of 66 beats/min. Whenever the patient's own rhythm is less than this, the pacemaker paces the ventricle. However, in the triggered mode sinus rhythm (right-hand portion of strip) causes a pacer spike to occur in each QRS interval rather than inhibiting pacemaker function as it did in the inhibited mode. Note that the spontaneous premature ventricular beat (third QRS interval from the left) is sensed by the pacemaker and causes a pacemaker spike to occur. Although the triggered mode results in more rapid battery depletion, it is valuable for patients with myopotential inhibition in the VVI mode.

or QRS interval sensing in atrial pacemaker systems. The latter is particularly important if the coronary sinus is used for electrode placement for atrial pacing.

Follow-up Testing with Programmability

In addition to the permanent applications of programmability described in the previous section temporary alteration of pacemaker function can be utilized to provide more thorough follow-up evaluation. The pulse duration threshold can be measured, and in those patients with pacemakers that have both amplitude and pulse duration programmability two points of the strength duration curve may be approximated. This allows periodic testing of electrode function and estimation of the safety margin for cardiac pacing. Because of the shape of the strength-duration curve an adequate safety margin should be attained if the pacemaker pulse duration is adjusted to two to three times the pulse duration threshold in the range of thresholds between 0.1 and 0.5 milliseconds and three to four times threshold in the range of thresholds from 0.5 to 2.0 milliseconds.

The safety margin for sensing may also be determined by making the pacemaker progressively less sensitive until sensing is lost. By increasing sensitivity to the maximum the possibility of oversensing or false inhibition may be explored. Programming to the triggered mode during maximum and minimum adjustment will identify the exact point in the QRS complex of the surface ECG where sensing occurs. The pacing rate may be decreased to allow evaluation of the underlying rhythm and the morphology of the normal QRS complex.

Through the use of telemetry other information about the pacemaker system can be obtained such as the current program settings, battery impedance, current drain, hermeticity (i.e., the airtightness of the device), battery voltage, and electrode impedance.

Clinical Experience with Programmability

Preliminary analysis of our experience with multiprogrammable pacemakers at Stanford suggests that programmability plays an important role in extending pacing system longevity by reducing the need for operative revision to correct certain pacing system malfunctions (Table 7-2). Sixty-two consecutive patients receiving single-chamber multiprogrammable (more than four variables) pacemakers were followed for 6 months after implantation. Initially, these pacemakers were only implanted in patients who were thought to be at high risk for pacing system malfunction and in those patients having less than optimal electrode function at the time of generator replacement.

Ninety-seven percent of the pacemakers studied were attached to ventricular electrodes, 87% to unipolar electrodes, and 77% to transvenous

Table 7-2 Clinical experience with multiprogrammable pacemakers

Population characteristics	Results
Number of patients	62
Mean follow-up	6.2 months
Number of patients with some dysfunction detected	16
Number of patients corrected with programmability	14
Number of patients requiring electrode replacement	1
Number of patients requiring pacemaker replacement	1

electrodes. Sixty-six percent of the patients were male. AV block was the most common indication for pacing in our series, accounting for 77% of patients. Twenty percent of patients received pacemakers for sinus node dysfunction, and 3% of individuals received them for the overdrive of ventricular arrhythmias. The greater than usual fraction of cases treated for heart block and with epicardial electrodes is a reflection of Stanford Medical Center's large cardiovascular surgery case load.

In our study programmability was used frequently to adjust the pacemaker to values other than those which would have been available had a nonprogrammable unit been implanted. Forty-eight percent of patients were paced at rates ⩽65 or ⩾80 pulses/min. Twenty-seven percent of patients were adjusted to a pulse duration greater than 0.7 milliseconds. Twenty-one percent of individuals were adjusted to sensitivities other than nominal, and 6% of patients were paced in modes other than inhibited.

Sixteen patients had significant problems that might have led to surgical revision if programmability had not been available. Two patients with unipolar pacemakers developed pectoral muscle stimulation following implantation. In both patients this was relieved by amplitude programmability. False inhibition by skeletal muscle myopotentials was documented in three patients and corrected by programming to the R triggered mode. During the course of follow-up three patients developed pulse duration thresholds greater than 0.5 milliseconds. In two patients this was adequately compensated for by increasing pulse duration with time thresholds decreased. In one patient, however, thresholds continued to increase and electrode revision was eventually required. An increased threshold for sensing was accommodated in three patients by programming to a more sensitive setting. T wave sensing was corrected in two patients by adjustment of the refractory period. One generator required explantation and replacement because of a random component failure during the period of follow-up.

Therefore, of the 62 patients originally implanted, 59 continue in follow-up without intervention. One patient has died without pacemaker dysfunction, one patient's generator required replacement, and one patient had progressive electrode dysfunction that eventually could not be compensated for by programmability, and the electrode was replaced. Based on these data we feel that multiprogrammable pacemakers are effective and reliable, allowing pacemaker function to be closely tailored to individual patient needs. In addition, operative revision is prevented in a significant fraction of patients with pacing system malfunction, thereby extending the longevity of the pacing system and decreasing the lifetime cost of pacing in these patients. On the basis of this study we presently use programmable pacemakers in almost all of our patients.

THE HEMODYNAMICS OF PACING AND THE IMPORTANCE OF THE AV SEQUENCE

Exercise Hemodynamics

The ability to alter cardiac output with exercise is a result of nearly equal contributions from an increase in heart rate and augmentation of stroke volume in the normal subject who is exercising in an upright position. In the supine subject during mild exercise increased output results almost entirely from heart rate augmentation with only a 10%-20% increase in stroke volume even during fairly vigorous activity. The augmentation in stroke volume occurs as a result of increased venous return. The atria serve as a conduit for this venous return, and by contracting in late diastole provide increased ventricular filling and increased diastolic pressure and volume just prior to ventricular systole. This allows ventricular contraction to begin at a point on the pressure-volume curve that is advantageous to increased output according to the Starling hypothesis but at a level much higher than mean diastolic pressure, thereby allowing atrial, systemic, and pulmonary venous pressures to remain low. The loss of atrial contribution in the normal patient is rapidly compensated for by an increase in mean pulmonary arterial and venous pressure. This is usually inconsequential in a normal patient but may be critical in a patient whose pulmonary venous pressure is already elevated. The contribution of the atria is also greater at faster heart rates where diastole is shortened and less time is available for passive ventricular filling.

Pacing in Heart Failure

In patients with heart failure the ability to maintain efficient ventricular contraction and increase stroke output in response to increased venous return may be significantly impaired. These patients are, therefore, dependent on increased heart rate to augment cardiac output during exercise. The effect of various pacing modes on exercise cardiac function in patients with impaired left ventricles is controversial. Benchimol and colleagues (1965) reported the exercise hemodynamics of a small group of patients with compensated heart failure. Only moderate differences in cardiac index were seen between fixed-rate atrial and ventricular pacing. More recently, another study (Greenberg, et al., 1979) noted little atrial contribution to ventricular filling in patients with pulmonary capillary wedge pressures greater than 20 mm/Hg. Other studies have shown significantly improved resting hemodynamics during atrial pacing, as opposed to ventricular pacing (Samet, et al., 1966; Leinbach, et al., 1969; Sutton, et al., 1980).

The patient with persistent bradycardia of any etiology, with or without left ventricular dysfunction, is at a serious hemodynamic disadvantage during exercise. The restoration of ventricular contraction to rates of 70 beats/min neither fully restores normal exercise-related heart rate augmentation of cardiac output nor provides AV synchrony. Therefore, fixed-rate ventricular pacing rarely restores exercise cardiac function to normal in any patient.

Despite growing interest the importance of atrial synchrony versus heart rate augmentation on exercise cardiac output in the setting of AV block and left ventricular dysfunction remains poorly understood. Assessing patients prior to pacemaker implant to determine the most appropriate type of pacemaker is also problematic. The differences in cardiac response to supine and upright exercise and multiple long-term compensatory mechanisms make it difficult to predict a response with data obtained from a single laboratory assessment. The availability of dual-chamber multiprogrammable pacemakers and noninvasive techniques for assessing left ventricular function may allow these determinations to be made with greater ease in the future (Kruse, et al., 1982; Parsonnet, 1982).

The patient with so-called pacemaker syndrome presents a special case. These patients generally do not manifest serious left ventricular impairment but rather develop significant acute symptoms as they change from normal to ventricular paced rhythm. This condition is seen most frequently in those patients having retrograde atrial activation with atrial contraction occurring during ventricular systole. Ogawa and colleagues (1978) demonstrated the severe hemodynamic consequences of V-A pacing. These patients may be effectively treated by any method that maintains the normal AV sequence.

At present, dual-chamber pacing using the most appropriate modality (Table 7-3) is probably indicated in patients with left ventricular dysfunction and a functional atrium, especially those patients with decreased left ventricular compliance such as idiopathic hypertrophic subaortic stenosis.

Table 7-3 Modes of cardiac pacing

Mode*	Atrial functions	Action of A sensing on V pacing	Action of V sensing on A pacing	Ventricular functions
AOO	P	—	—	—
AAI	P, S/I	—	—	—
AAT	P, S/T	—	—	—
VOO	—	—	—	P
VVI	—	—	—	P, S/I
VVT	—	—	—	P, S/T
VAT	S	T	—	P
VDD	S	T	—	P, S/I
DVI	P	—	I	P, S/I
DDD	P, S/I	T	I	P, S/I

*The three-letter code established by the Intersociety Commission for Heart Disease Resources (Parsonnet, et al., 1974) designates the first letter for the chamber(s) paced, the second letter for the chamber(s) sensed, and the third letter for the mode of function. The original code has been expanded to five letters to designate the presence of programmability and tachycardia therapy features (Parsonnet, et al., 1981).

Abbreviations: A = atrial; V = ventricular; O = no effect; D = dual; P = pacing; S = sensing; I = inhibited; T = triggered; S/I = sensing inhibits pacing within the chamber in which sensing has occurred; S/T = sensing triggers a pacing impulse within the chamber in which sensing has occurred.

Pacing Systems for Sequential Pacing

Atrial pacing The simplest technique for maintaining a proper AV sequence is atrial pacing (AAI). This, however, is only useful in those bradycardias of atrial origin that are not accompanied by AV conduction impairment.

Atrial synchronous ventricular pacing Atrial synchronous ventricular pacing (VAT, VDD) is capable of providing both a response to changes in sinus node discharge rate and appropriate AV synchrony in the face of AV block in patients with normal sinus node function. This is accomplished by sensing spontaneous atrial activity and triggering a ventricular impulse after an appropriate delay. The addition of programmability to successive versions of this basic design has provided a pacing system that provides an almost normal situation for those patients with normal SA node function and AV block (Kruse, et al., 1982).

AV sequential pacemaker The present design of the AV sequential pacemaker (DVI) provides for atrial pacing and ventricular pacing and sensing. This system maintains an appropriate AV pacing sequence at a fixed rate unless it is inhibited by a more rapid ventricular rate. However, these pacemakers do not provide paced ventricular rates in synchrony with atrial rates above the basic programmed setting. Thus, this pacing system is most capable of providing AV sequential pacing in patients with atrial bradycardia and AV block. It does not provide for synchronous rate augmentation in the face of exercise or other physiologic stimuli (Leinbach, et al., 1969).

Universal pacemaker Pacemakers are now available with a combination of the atrial synchronous and AV sequential features (DDD) to provide proper AV sequence and appropriate rate augmentation during both atrial bradycardia and normal atrial function. In addition, a pacemaker system has been described that is capable of providing rate augmentation during exercise in patients with no intrinsic atrial function (Cammilli, et al., 1978).

PACEMAKERS IN THE MANAGEMENT OF TACHYARRHYTHMIAS

Techniques

Cardiac pacing may be applied in selected patients for the prevention or termination of a variety of cardiac arrhythmias (see Chapters 2, 9, and 10). Several techniques have been described that utilize atrial, ventricular, and AV sequential pacing. Pacing at normal rates may prevent those tachycardias initiated only during bradycardia, while more rapid (overdrive) pacing may suppress premature beats that give rise to sustained tachyarrhythmias. Cardiac pacing may also be used to induce more acceptable arrhythmias in certain patients. The induction of atrial fibrillation in patients with atrial flutter that is difficult to manage may result in slower ventricular rates. Patients with paroxysmal atrial tachycardias that are unresponsive to drug therapy may be treated by permanent control of the atrial rhythm in very rapid atrial pacing combined with the development of appropriate amounts of AV block by pharmacologic means.

Since the first report by Haft and colleagues (1967), a number of approaches designed to terminate arrhythmias using pacing techniques have been described. These include single random extrastimuli (Ryan, et al., 1968), simultaneous AV sequential pacing (Spurrell and Sowton, 1976), dual-demand pacing (Curry, et al., 1979), orthorhythmic pacing (Zacouto and Guize, 1976), programmed scanning (Critelli, et al., 1979), and both patient-activated (Kahn, et al., 1976) and automatic bursts of rapid pacing (Griffin and Mason, 1980). In a comparison of several of these techniques Fisher and colleagues (1978) demonstrated the more frequent effectiveness of bursts of rapid atrial or ventricular stimulation (see the section on the automatic, programmable tachycardia-terminating pacemaker in this chapter) performed at rates usually 30% or greater than the rate of the tachyarrhythmia and usually lasting less than 10 seconds. The application of these techniques in the management of arrhythmias in the hospitalized patient has been recently reviewed (Cooper, et al., 1978).

Patient-Activated RF Pacemakers

Cardiac pacing is effective in the long-term management of recurrent arrhythmias as well (Fisher, et al., 1982). Patient-activated implantable devices capable of delivering bursts of rapid stimuli have been available for several years, and their efficacy in selected patients for the chronic therapy of supraventricular (Kahn, et al., 1976; Peters, et al., 1978; Waxman, et al., 1978; Todo, et al., 1979) and ventricular (Wyndham, et al., 1977; Hartzler, 1979; Kim, et al., 1979; Ruskin, et al., 1980) tachyarrhythmias (see Figure 10-6). These pacemakers consist of an implanted inductive coil that is powered transcutaneously by a radiofrequency transmitter controlled by either the patient or the physician. The desired pacing rate is adjustable, and the duration of rapid pacing is determined by pressing and releasing a button on the transmitter case. These units are powered by a 9-volt battery and are capable of delivering a 2-millisecond pulse of more than 7-8 volts if positioning is optimal. More recently, an improved transmitter allowing digital control of the pulse duration and pacing duration has been manufactured and is available by special order.*

Although effective in selected patients, patient-activated systems do have several shortcomings:

1. They require the patient to perceive the presence and absence of tachyarrhythmia accurately.
2. They require that the patient have constant access to a transmitter in the event that tachycardia should occur.
3. They are not effective in patients who are rapidly disabled by the tachyarrhythmia.
4. They leave significant symptoms in patients with frequently recurring symptomatic tachycardia as a result of the time required to perceive the arrhythmia and apply the transmitter.
5. They do not provide for backup pacing in the event of postpacing pauses or sinus bradycardia.

---

*Medtronic Incorporated, Minneapolis, Minnesota.

The Automatic, Programmable Tachycardia-Terminating Pacemaker

Although available for a number of years, custom-built automatically activated burst pacemakers have not achieved widespread use (d'Alnoncourt and Luderitz, 1979; Fisher, et al., 1979; Kim, et al., 1979). They possess several advantages over patient-activated devices. The burst pattern is consistent in terms of energy output and duration. In addition, they provide for automatic recognition and tachycardia-terminating response, freeing the patient from the problems of keeping a transmitter available and applying it after the onset of symptoms. However, a significant delay is necessary after the decision for pacing therapy is made because the device has to be adjusted and assembled before it can be furnished to the physician who is to implant it. More importantly, this type of unit does not allow any flexibility in subsequent pacemaker performance because it is not programmable.

Recently, we have used an automatic, multiprogrammable tachycardia-terminating pacemaker in patients with reentrant supraventricular and ventricular arrhythmias (Griffin and Mason, 1980; Griffin, et al., 1980; Griffin, et al., 1981). This pacemaker, the Cybertach-60*, is a bipolar lithium-powered pulse generator that weighs 82 g. It is extensively programmable and fully automatic. It responds with a burst of stimuli of uniform rate (range of 180-1440 beats/min) and duration (range of 0.33-5.3 seconds) after sensing eight consecutive RR intervals shorter than the programmed criteria for the definition of tachycardia (Figure 7-3). For a tachycardia of 150 beats/min less than 6 seconds are usually required for sensing and termination. The tachycardia-terminating response may be inhibited noninvasively. Other programmable variables include two basic pacing rates, 15 pulse durations, and seven input sensitivity levels. The automatic tachycardia-terminating features are also programmable. Twenty-eight combinations of burst rate and duration are available, ranging from 180-270 pulses/min for 1.3-5.4 seconds. The presence of an arrhythmia is determined by rate, and the criteria are programmable with a choice of two rates. Input signals with a frequency greater than 350 beats/min are defined as noise, no tachycardia-terminating response is delivered, and asynchronous pacing is initiated. Application of a magnet converts the device to an asynchronous pacemaker without the tachycardia-terminating response.

Programmability is important in maintaining proper pacemaker function in patients implanted with the Cybertach-60. Frequently, the burst rate most effective for termination changed after the patient was ambulatory and fully recovered from the effects of hospitalization and previous drug therapy. Maintaining optimal pacing and sensing also necessitated adjustment of pulse duration and sensitivity level. The

---

*Intermedics, Inc., Freeport, Texas.

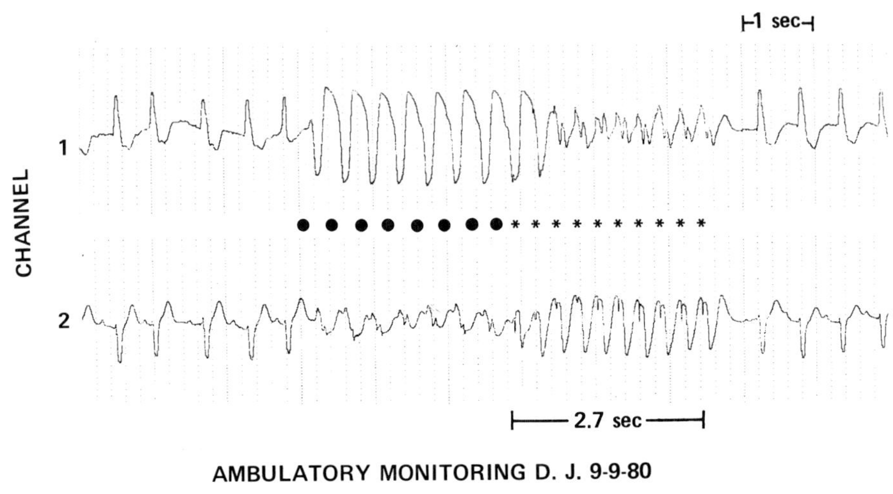

Figure 7-3 Function of the automatic tachycardia-terminating pacemaker. Ten seconds of a two-channel ambulatory ECG recording are displayed. The pacemaker begins to count short R-R intervals (●) beginning with the first wide-complex beat. Coincident with the end of the eighth interval, rapid pacing is initiated (∗) and the ventricular tachycardia is terminated.

pacemaker can record the occurrence of tachyarrhythmias, store this information, and telemeter it upon command to the evaluating physician.

Every patient requires extensive electrophysiologic study prior to implantation. In patients with supraventricular tachycardia particular emphasis is placed on the detection of extranodal pathways. Patients with rapidly conducting antegrade pathways are not considered good candidates for pacing therapy because of the following potential hazards:

1. The induction of atrial fibrillation results in a rapid AV conduction.
2. One-to-one AV conduction of the terminating burst can occur.

The criteria for the selection of patients with ventricular tachycardia for pacing therapy must of necessity be even more strict than for patients with supraventricular arrhythmias. The principal adverse effect of attempted pacing termination is the acceleration of the arrhythmia to more rapid tachycardia and/or fibrillation. For this reason pacing termination of ventricular arrhythmias, particularly with automatic devices, is indicated only when no other effective therapy is available.

Recently, Mirowski and colleagues (1980 and 1981) published their initial results regarding the management of patients with recurrent ventricular tachycardia and fibrillation utilizing an implantable cardiac defibrillator system. Although it is too early to define its role in the management of patients with refractory ventricular arrhythmias, this system would appear to be promising, especially in those patients with primary ventricular fibrillation (see Chapter 10) or with sustained ventricular tachycardia that is resistant to drug therapy.

REFERENCES

Benchimol, A.; Ellis, J. G.; and Diamond, E. G. 1965. Hemodynamic consequences of atrial and ventricular pacing in patients with normal and abnormal hearts. *Am. J. Med.* 39:911-922.

Bilitch, M. 1980. Performance of cardiac pacemaker pulse generators. *PACE* 3:746-751.

Cammilli, L.; Alcidi, L.; Papeschi, G., et al. 1978. Preliminary experience with the pH-triggered pacemaker. *PACE* 1:448-457.

Curry, P. J. L.; Rowland, E.; and Krikler, D. M. 1979. Dual-demand pacing for refractory atrioventricular reentry tachycardia. *PACE* 2:137-151.

Cooper, T. B.; MacLean, W. A. H.; and Waldo, A. L. 1978. Overdrive pacing for supraventricular tachycardia: a review of theoretical implications and therapeutic techniques. *PACE* 1:196-221.

Critelli, G.; Grassi, G.; Chiariello, M., et al. 1979. Automatic "scanning" by radiofrequency in the long-term electrical treatment of arrhythmias. *PACE* 2:289-296.

d'Alnoncourt, C. N.; and Luderitz, B. 1979. Therapie tachykarder Rhythmusstorungen mit implantierten Schrittmachern. *Dtsch. med. Wschr.* 104:1009-1014.

Elmquist, R.; and Senning, A. 1959. An implantable pacemaker for the heart. (Proceedings of the Second International Conference on Medical Electronics, Paris, June 1959.) *Medical Electronics.* London: Iliffe. p. 253.

Fisher, J. D.; Kim, S. G.; Furman, S., et al. 1982. Role of implantable pacemakers in control of recurrent ventricular tachycardia. *Am. J. Cardiol.* 49:194-206.

Fisher, J. D.; Furman, S.; and Duffin, E. G. 1979. Automatic implanted rapid burst pacer for refractory ventricular tachycardia (abstract). *Clin. Res.* 27:164A.

Fisher, J. D.; Mehra, R.; and Furman, S. 1978. Termination of ventricular tachycardia with bursts of rapid ventricular pacing. *Am. J. Cardiol.* 41:94-102.

Greatbatch, W.; Lee, J. H.; Mathias, W., et al. 1971. The solid-state lithium battery: a new improved chemical power source for implantable cardiac pacemakers. *I.E.E.E.* 18:317-324.

Greenberg, B.; Chatterjee, K.; Parmley, W. W., et al. 1979. The influence of left ventricular filling pressure on atrial contribution to cardiac output. *Am. Heart J.* 98:742-751.

Griffin, J. C.; and Mason, J. W. 1980. Clinical use of an implantable automatic tachycardia-terminating pacemaker (abstract). *Clin. Res.* 28:177A.

Griffin, J. C.; Mason, J. W.; and Calfee, R. V. 1980. Clinical use of an implantable automatic tachycardia-terminating pacemaker. *Am. Heart J.* 100:1093-1096.

Griffin, J. C.; Mason, J. W.; Ross, D. L., et al. 1981. The treatment of ventricular tachycardia using an automatic tachycardia-terminating pacemaker. *PACE* 4:582-588.

Haft, J. I.; Kosowsky, B. D.; Lau, S. L., et al. 1967. Termination of atrial flutter by rapid electrical pacing of the atrium. *Am. J. Cardiol.* 20:239-244.

Hartzler, G. O. 1979. Treatment of recurrent ventricular tachycardia by patient-activated radiofrequency ventricular stimulation. *Mayo Clin. Proc.* 54:75-82.

Hauser, R. G.; and Giuffre, V. W. 1979. Clinical assessment of cardiac pacemaker performance. *J.C.E. Cardiol.* 14(1):19-35.

Hurzeler, P.; Morse, D.; Leach, C., et al. 1980. Longevity comparisons among lithium anode power cells for cardiac pacemakers. *PACE* 3:555-561.

Kahn, A.; Morris, J. J.; and Citron, P. 1976. Patient-initiated rapid atrial pacing to manage supraventricular tachycardia. *Am. J. Cardiol.* 38:200-204.

Kim, S. G.; Fisher, J. D.; Furman, S., et al. 1979. Implantable ventricular burst pacemakers for termination of ventricular tachycardia. In *Proceedings of the seventh world symposium on cardiac pacing.* Claude Meere, ed. Montreal: PACE SYMPOSIA, pp. 6-12.

Kruse, I.; Arnman, K.; Couradson, T.-B., et al. 1982. A comparison of the acute and long-term hemodynamic effects of ventricular inhibited and atrial synchronous ventricular inhibited pacing. *Circulation* 65:846-855.

Leinbach, R. C.; Chamberlain, D. A.; Kastor, J. A., et al. 1969. A comparison of the hemodynamic effects of ventricular and sequential AV pacing in patients with heart block. *Am. Heart J.* 78:502-508.

Mirowski, M.; Reid, P. R.; Mower, M. M., et al. 1980. Termination of malignant ventricular arrhythmias with an implanted automatic defibrillator in human beings. *N. Engl. J. Med.* 303:322-324.

Mirowski, M.; Reid, P. R.; Watkins, L., et al. 1981. Clinical treatment of life-threatening ventricular tachyarrhythmias with the automatic implantable defibrillator. *Am. Heart J.* 102:265-270.

Ogawa, S.; Dreifus, L. S.; Shenoy, P. N., et al. 1978. Hemodynamic consequences of atrioventricular and ventriculoatrial pacing. *PACE* 1:8-15.

Parsonnet, V.; Furman, S.; Smyth, N. P. D. 1974. Implantable cardiac pacemakers: status report and resource guideline. Pacemaker Study Group (ICHD). *Circulation* 50:A-21.

Parsonnet, V. 1977. Cardiac pacing and pacemakers: VII. Power sources for implantable pacemakers, Parts I and II. *Am. Heart J.* 94:517-528 and 658-664.

Parsonnet, V. 1979. Survey of pacemaker practices in the United States—1978. In *Proceedings of the seventh world symposium on cardiac pacing.* Claude Meere, ed. Montreal: PACE SYMPOSIA. pp. 41-43.

Parsonnet, V. 1982. The proliferation of cardiac pacing: medical, technical, and socioeconomic dilemmas. *Circulation* 65:841-845.

Parsonnet, V.; Furman, S.; and Smyth, N. P. D. 1981. A revised code for pacemaker identification. *PACE* 4:400-403.

Peters, R. W.; Shafton, E.; Frank, S., et al. 1978. Radiofrequency-triggered pacemakers: use and limitations. *Ann. Intern. Med.* 88:17.

Ruskin, J. N.; Garan, H.; Poulin, F., et al. 1980. Permanent radiofrequency ventricular pacing for management of drug-resistant ventricular tachycardia. *Am. J. Cardiol.* 46:317-321.

Ryan, G. F.; Easley, R. M.; Zaroff, L. I., et al. 1968. Paradoxical use of a demand pacemaker in the treatment of supraventricular tachycardia due to the Wolff-Parkinson-White syndrome. *Circulation* 38:1037.

Samet, P.; Castillo, C.; and Bernstein, W. H. 1966. Hemodynamic sequela of atrial, ventricular, and sequential atrioventricular pacing. *Am. Heart J.* 72:725.

Spurrell, R. A. J.; and Sowton, E. 1976. Pacing techniques in the management of supraventricular tachycardias. *J. Electrocardiol.* 9(1):89-96.

Sutton, R.; Perrins, J.; and Citron, P. 1980. Physiological cardiac pacing. *PACE* 3:207-219.

Todo, K.; Kaneko, S.; Fujiwara, T., et al. 1979. Patient-controlled rapid atrial pacing in the long-term management of recurrent supraventricular tachycardias. In *Proceedings of the seventh world symposium on cardiac pacing.* Claude Meere, ed. Montreal: PACE SYMPOSIA. pp. 9-16.

Tyers, F. G. O.; and Brownlee, R. R. 1978. Current status of pacemaker power sources. *Ann. Thorac. Surg.* 25:571-587.

Waxman, M. B.; Wald, R. W.; Bonnet, J. F., et al. 1978. Self-conversion of supraventricular tachycardia by rapid atrial pacing. *PACE* 1:35.

Welti, J. J. 1980. STIMAREC reports. Paris: Hôpital Fernand-Widal.

Wyndham, C.; Meeran, M.; Denes, P., et al. 1977. New uses for the externally controlled radiofrequency pacemaker (abstract). *Am. J. Cardiol.* 39:306.

Zacouto, F. I.; and Guize, L. J. 1976. *Fundamentals of orthorhythmic pacing in cardiac pacing.* B. Luderitz, ed. Berlin: Springer-Verlag. pp. 212-218.

8 Multifocal Atrial Tachycardia, Atrial Flutter, and Atrial Fibrillation

Jeffrey L. Anderson, M.D.

Associate Professor of Internal Medicine (Cardiology)
University of Utah College of Medicine
Salt Lake City, Utah

This chapter deals with the irregular atrial tachyarrhythmias, which include atrial flutter, atrial fibrillation, and multifocal atrial tachycardia. These arrhythmias are among those most commonly seen in clinical practice. Because the clinical significance of and therapeutic approaches to these conditions vary widely, individual evaluation and clinical judgment are required. Thus, the clinician should have a thorough understanding of these arrhythmias.

MULTIFOCAL ATRIAL TACHYCARDIA

Multifocal atrial tachycardia (MAT) is a chaotic supraventricular tachyarrhythmia whose clinical and electrocardiographic features have been evident since the late 1960s. As familiarity with MAT has increased, so also has the medical community's ability to recognize it. The distinct nature of MAT's clinical presentation, the ease with which it is confused with atrial fibrillation or flutter, and the unique therapeutic implications it raises are points worth careful consideration (Shine, et al., 1968; Phillips, et al., 1969; Lipson and Naimi, 1970; Chung, 1971; Berlinerblau and Feder, 1972; D'Cruz, et al., 1974; Clark, 1977).

Diagnosis

MAT appears in 0.5-2.5/1000 ECGs performed in large series (Shine, et al., 1968; Phillips, et al., 1969; Lipson and Naimi, 1970; Chung, 1971; Berlinerblau and Feder, 1972; Clark, 1977; see Figure 8-1). The diagnosis of MAT depends on the presence of the following:

1. Well-organized, discrete P waves of varying morphology from at least three foci. There is no evidence of a dominant pacemaker (sinus or other).
2. Irregular variation in PP intervals, with an isoelectric baseline. Phasic respiratory variation in P-wave morphology should be excluded. The PR and RR intervals also vary.

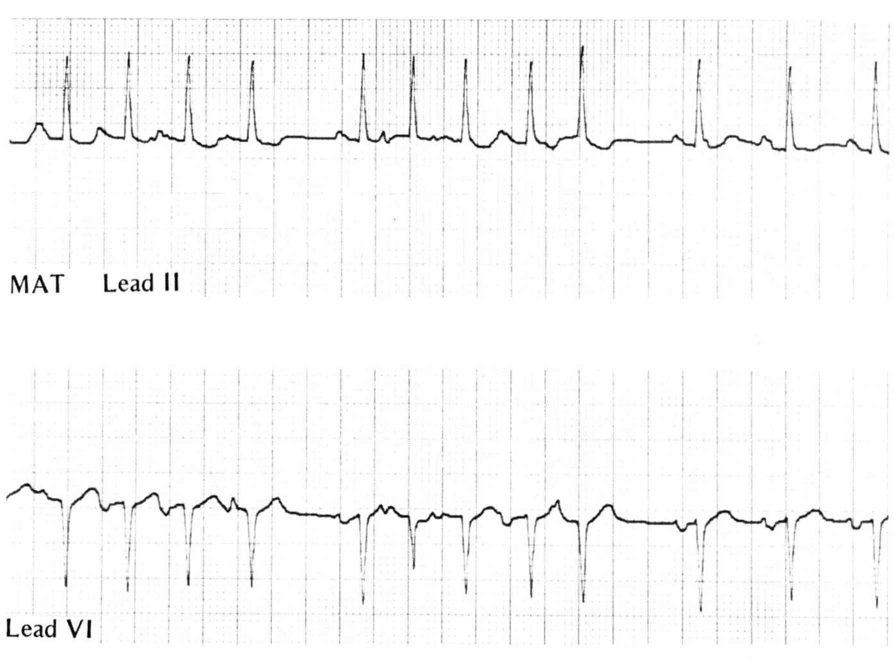

Figure 8-1 Rhythm strip demonstrating multifocal atrial tachycardia. Leads II and V_1 are shown.

3. Atrial rate usually greater than 100 beats/min and less than 250 beats/min. Occasionally, a rhythm with a similar mechanism occurs, but a rate of less than 100 beats/min is seen. In this case the term multifocal atrial rhythm is used.

The morphology of ectopic P waves in this rhythm may be extremely varied. Frequently, peaked and tented forms are present, especially in patients with severe underlying pulmonary disease.

The ventricular rate in untreated MAT is commonly 100-150 beats/min. One to one AV conduction usually predominates, but nonconducted ectopic P waves are common, especially at higher atrial rates. When the RP interval is less than the QT interval, nonconduction is physiologic. When the RP interval is greater, nonconduction signifies AV block (Shine, et al., 1968). As is the case with atrial fibrillation, RR intervals are irregularly irregular and are occasionally as slow as 50-60 beats/min or faster than 150 beats/min. The QRS interval is narrow unless an underlying intraventricular conduction delay is present. Aberrant conduction may accompany short RR cycles. Premature ventricular complexes are frequently seen in association with MAT and must be distinguished from supraventricular complexes with aberrancy.

Onset-Termination

Sinus rhythm with premature atrial complexes, usually multifocal, is the most common rhythm preceding and succeeding MAT (Shine, et al., 1968; Berlinerblau and Feder, 1972). Multifocal or wandering atrial pacemaker is also a relatively common preexisting and terminating rhythm (Shine, et al., 1968; Phillips, et al., 1969; Lipson and Naimi, 1970; Berlinerblau and Feder, 1972). Atrial fibrillation and flutter may precede MAT. Digitalization may result in conversion of atrial fibrillation to MAT (Shine, et al., 1968). MAT may end in atrial fibrillation, serving as a transition rhythm between sinus rhythm with premature atrial complexes and atrial fibrillation (Lipson and Naimi, 1970). Incremental digitalis administration may transform MAT into a regularized paroxysmal atrial tachycardia with block or a junctional rhythm, probably as a result of toxicity (Shine, et al., 1968).

Differential Diagnosis

MAT masquerades as a number of rhythms, especially atrial fibrillation. The following is a list of the differential points (Table 8-1):

1. *Atrial fibrillation:* Differentiation must be made on the basis of ECG recordings. Atrial flutter-fibrillation causes the most diagnostic problems. Here, the atrial rate is greater than 350 beats/min, P waves are not discrete, and the baseline is not isoelectric. The ventricular response is usually less than 1:1.
2. *Atrial flutter:* The greatest difficulty occurs when an irregular AV block is present. The atrial mechanism is differentiated by its characteristic "sawtooth" morphology, an atrial rate of 250-350 beats/min, and a baseline that is not isoelectric. The ventricular response is usually less than 1:1.
3. *Sinus rhythm with multifocal premature atrial complexes:* A dominant sinus rhythm with basically regular PP intervals can be identified.
4. *Atrial tachycardia with block:* The P-wave morphology is unvarying, although it differs from sinus P-wave morphology. The PP interval is basically regular, although some ventriculophasic variation may be present.
5. *Wandering atrial pacemaker:* At rates less than 100 beats/min this condition may be indistinguishable from multifocal atrial rhythm. Changes in P-wave morphology and PP intervals are said to evolve more regularly or gradually.

Table 8-1 Differential diagnosis of multifocal atrial tachycardia (MAT)

Rhythm	Similarities to MAT	Differentiating characteristics
MAT	—	Discrete P waves ⩾3 forms. Irregular PP interval. Rate usually 100-250 beats/min
Atrial fibrillation	Ventricular response is irregularly irregular. Confusion if discrete F wave in atrial flutter-fibrillation	A rate ⩾350 beats/min. P (F) waves not discrete. Baseline not isoelectric. Ventricular response <1:1
Atrial flutter	Chaotic ventricular response if irregular AV block	Sawtooth F waves. Baseline not isoelectric. Ventricular response <1:1
Sinus rhythm (or tachycardia) with multifocal premature atrial complexes	Chaotic rhythm, multifocal P waves	Dominant P waves present. Regular underlying PP interval
Atrial tachycardia with block	Irregular AV block → irregular pulse, discrete P waves	Constant P-wave morphology. Ventricular response <1:1
Wandering atrial pacemaker	Multifocal P waves	Rate <100 beats/min. Gradually evolving P waves, PP interval

6. *Slow, benign (ectopic) paroxysmal atrial tachycardia:* The duration is characteristically brief (usually 3-20 beats). The P waves of the entire episode tend to be similar. Regularization of PP and RR intervals occurs after warm-up beats. Some variation persists, however. This condition is seen in a somewhat younger, less symptomatic population (Stemple, 1977).

7. *Sinus arrhythmia:* The PP interval variation is usually phasic with respiration (although not necessarily). P-wave morphology is constant or shows mild phasic variation. The atrial rate is slow, less than 100 beats/min.

8. *Ventricular tachycardia:* Ventricular tachycardia is occasionally mistakenly diagnosed when MAT is associated with a rapid ventricular response and aberrant conduction. In this case irregular ventricular tachycardia or flutter with a suggestion of capture beats may be simulated. MAT is differentiated by ectopic P waves preceding the bizarre QRS complexes.

Electrical Mechanism

The electrophysiologic mechanisms of MAT still have not been adequately described (Berlinerblau and Feder, 1972; D'Cruz, et al., 1974). Electrocardiographically, the arrhythmia suggests multiple, competing ectopic foci, as its name implies. MAT may be an accentuated and accelerated form of wandering atrial pacemaker with premature atrial complexes (Berlinerblau and Feder, 1972). On the other hand, D'Cruz and colleagues (1974) noted atrial refractoriness to pacing in MAT and argued for a multiple reentrant mechanism. In this model the reentrant circuits vary in duration, as well as anatomic course, from beat to beat, depending on the degree of local impariment of conduction in the atria. Similarity between the mechanisms of MAT and atrial fibrillation has been suggested by their frequent association (Lipson and Naimi, 1970). In one series 8 out of 32 cases of MAT occurred during digitalis therapy for atrial fibrillation (Shine, et al., 1968). Two additional patients developed fibrillation or flutter during maintenance digitalis therapy for MAT. In another study atrial fibrillation or flutter preceded MAT in seven out of 31 cases and followed MAT in 5 out of 31 instances (Phillips, et al., 1969). In a third series MAT progressed to atrial flutter or fibrillation in 17 out of 31 patients (55%) (Lipson and Naimi, 1970). Sinus tachycardia (61%) and premature atrial complexes (64%) commonly preceded MAT in this study. In the fourth study atrial fibrillation or flutter preceded or followed MAT in nine out of 31 cases (Berlinerblau and Feder, 1972). Lipson and Naimi (1970) demonstrated cases of transitions back and forth between atrial fibrillation and MAT and suggested a similar pathogenetic mechanism.

Etiologic Factors

The following is a list of the etiologic factors for MAT:

A. *Associated underlying diseases*
   1. Severe pulmonary disease (in ⩾50% of patients), chronic or acute
      a. Frequently with cor pulmonale
      b. Acute pulmonary embolus (in ≈10% of patients)
   2. Hypertensive or coronary heart disease (in ⩾50% of patients)
   3. Complicated postoperative course
   4. Severe systemic illness

B. *Associated metabolic abnormalities*
   1. Blood gas abnormality (i.e., hypoxia, hypercarbia, or acidosis)
   2. Electrolyte abnormality (i.e., hyponatremia, hypokalemia, hypocalcemia)
   3. Fever, infections (i.e., bronchitis)
   4. Anemia
   5. Uremia

C. *Associated drugs*
   1. Excessive bronchodilators (theophylline, catecholamines)
   2. Digitalis (avoid intoxication, although it is not usually a cause)

Associated cardiopulmonary disease Although exceptions occur, MAT is found primarily in elderly patients with cardiopulmonary disease or acute systemic illness. The average age of a patient who develops MAT is about 70 years (Shine, et al., 1968; Phillips, et al., 1969; Lipson and Naimi, 1970; Chung, 1971; Berlinerblau and Feder, 1972; Clark, 1977). Severe cardiopulmonary disease has been described in 35%-90% of patients. The majority of these patients also have cor pulmonale. Evidence for associated coronary artery disease or hypertensive heart disease is also very common (50%-90% prevalence). MAT is commonly found in patients in four clinical settings: (1) severe chronic or acute pulmonary disease; (2) complicated postoperative period; (3) severe congestive heart failure; and (4) miscellaneous severe systemic illness (Shine, et al., 1968).

Specific associated or initiating factors No specific metabolic factors are common to all patients developing MAT but one or more of the following are frequently present: fever, infections (i.e., bronchitis), abnormalities of blood gases (hypoxia, hypercarbia, pH abnormalities), electrolyte abnormalities (hypokalemia, hyponatremia, hypocalcemia), anemia, and uremia. Thyroid abnormalities have not been well defined (Phillips, et al., 1969). An unusually high incidence of glucose intolerance was found in one study (Phillips, et al., 1969) but has also been attributed to physiologic aging (Berlinerblau and Feder, 1972). Acute pulmonary embolism may occur in up to 12% of patients (Phillips, et al., 1969; Chung, 1971) and is an important initiating factor to recognize.

Digitalis intoxication does not appear to be a common initiating mechanism, although signs of digitalis intoxication may be present in some patients when MAT is diagnosed (Shine, et al., 1968; Phillips, et al., 1969; Lipson and Naimi, 1970; Chung, 1971; Berlinerblau and Feder, 1972). Bronchodilator drugs are frequently used in patients developing MAT and may contribute to the initiation or production of rapid heart rates (Shine, et al., 1968). In rare cases multifocal atrial tachycardia/rhythm may be seen in younger patients who lack evident cardiac disease or initiating factors (D'Cruz, et al., 1974). In these patients, the atrial rate is usually slower, and the rhythm may be chronic.

MAT commonly signifies diffuse atrial pathology, especially right atrial disease. Several researchers have suggested that atrial ischemia, fibrosis, distention, stress, and sinus node damage are important predisposing factors. Chronic pulmonary disease with pulmonary hypertension and coronary artery disease would sustain these processes. Precise pathophysiologic correlations have not as yet been made, however.

Thyrotoxicosis, myocarditis, iron deficiency anemia, cancer of the lung, recent myocardial infarction, recent cerebral vascular accidents, or systemic lupus erythematosus have been associated with MAT in rare instances.

Clinical Findings

Dyspnea and palpitation are the predominant clinical symptoms of MAT. The irregularly irregular pulse (100 beats/min in two-thirds of patients) must be distinguished from atrial fibrillation by ECG recordings.

Hemodynamic Consequences

No documentation exists of the hemodynamic changes accompanying acute transitions between MAT and sinus rhythm. Tachycardia, irregular atrial and ventricular filling, and variable effectiveness of the atrial mechanism must contribute adversely to cardiac hemodynamics. Rapid heart rates are particularly poorly tolerated in ill and elderly patients, who are also most commonly affected by MAT. The atrial rate is generally slower in MAT than in atrial fibrillation or flutter; extremely rapid ventricular responses resulting in immediate hemodynamic deterioration are infrequent. Hemodynamic deterioration in patients with MAT is usually more dependent on severity of the underlying cardiopulmonary disease.

Prognosis

The mortality rate for patients developing MAT is 30%-50%. However, despite the high associated mortality the rhythm disturbance per se appears to carry a benign prognosis. In Lipson's study no deaths could be attributed directly to MAT (Lipson and Naimi, 1970).

The duration of MAT varies from seconds to years. In one-third of patients the MAT may terminate within 1-3 days, most of the rest of the MATs have ended by 1-2 weeks, and in a few patients the MAT rhythm may persist for years (Shine, et al., 1968; Phillips, et al., 1969; Lipson and Naimi, 1970; Berlinerblau and Feder, 1972; D'Cruz, et al., 1974).

Treatment

Therapy for MAT is directed primarily at the underlying disease and secondarily at the rhythm itself. Improved oxygenation, control of infection, correction of specific metabolic abnormalities or anemia, and optimization (reduction whenever possible) of bronchodilator dosage should constitute the principal therapeutic approach.

The role of digitalis requires careful consideration. Most studies report an inconsistent relationship of digitalis to MAT. If digitalis intoxication is suspected, the drug should be omitted; otherwise, maintenance digitalization may be continued. Careful digitalization may be undertaken in patients not already receiving the drug. The majority of patients will show little response in atrial rate after the addition of digitalis (Shine, et al., 1968; Phillips, et al., 1969; Lipson and Naimi, 1970; Berlinerblau and Feder, 1972). Some decrease in ventricular rate or conversion to sinus rhythm occurs in about one-third of digitalized patients, but a causal relationship is often difficult to prove; discontinuation of digitalis has also been associated with the termination of MAT in a few cases. Treatment of concurrent heart failure and prophylaxis against atrial fibrillation may provide the rationale for cautious digitalization in certain patients with MAT.

In contrast to maintenance digitalis, incremental dosing in MAT, usually given for rate control when MAT is mistakenly diagnosed as atrial fibrillation, may produce high-grade AV block, regularized atrial tachycardia with block, nodal rhythm, or ventricular irritability (Shine, et al., 1968). Digitalis intoxication may, therefore, be precipitated if it is not already present (see Chapter 13).

Cardioversion is usually unsuccessful or only temporarily successful and may be dangerous, especially in patients who are receiving digitalis (Chung, 1971; Berlinerblau and Feder, 1972). Success with rapid atrial pacing has not been reported, and atrial capture may be difficult in MAT (D'Cruz, et al., 1974) (see Chapter 13).

Beta-adrenergic blocking drugs may offer potential for therapeutic success in MAT (Wang, et al., 1977) but are frequently contraindicated and have not been used extensively. Propranolol is contraindicated when heart failure and bronchospastic pulmonary disease are present, which means the majority of patients with MAT. Newer, more cardioselective beta blocking agents (e.g., acebutolol, atenolol, metoprolol) given in low doses may be adequately tolerated by selected patients and have been successful in terminating or slowing MAT in several cases (Williams, 1979). More experience will be required to firmly establish the role of beta blocking agents.

The calcium entry blocker verapamil deserves therapeutic trial in MAT because of its better tolerance than beta blockers in patients with pulmonary disease and its known effects on sinus and AV nodal conduction (Ellrodt, et al., 1980). However, adequate clinical studies are not yet available.

Other antiarrhythmic agents have been generally ineffective or only poorly effective (Shine, et al., 1968; Berlinerblau and Feder, 1972). In occasional patients quinidine or procainamide have been useful with or without propranolol, but MAT does not respond to lidocaine, phenytoin, and usually not to procainamide or quinidine. The adverse interaction of quinidine with digitalis should also be considered (see Chapter 13).

ATRIAL FLUTTER

In its classic form atrial flutter can be identified readily by its characteristically regular, sawtooth appearance on the ECG (Katz and Pick, 1956; Chung, 1977; Marriott and Myerburg, 1978). It is less common than its sister rhythm, atrial fibrillation, with a prevalence ratio estimated at between 1:10 and 1:20. The clinical significance and therapeutic response of atrial flutter are relatively distinct from those of atrial fibrillation and supraventricular tachycardia and deserve separate consideration.

Diagnosis

Atrial activity in uncomplicated atrial flutter is characteristically regular with a rate of 250-350 beats/min (Katz and Pick, 1956; Chung, 1977; Marriott and Myerburg, 1978). Atrial flutter waves are usually more prominent in inferior leads and V_1, where a sawtooth pattern is characteristically present (Figure 8-2). An atrial rate of 200-250 beats/min (occasionally less) may also be seen with atrial flutter. At times the differential diagnosis between atrial flutter and atrial (supraventricular) tachycardia is difficult to make. In addition to atrial rate and morphology, the presence or absence of AV block and response to vagal stimulation may be useful in distinguishing between the two arrhythmias. Categorical separation, however, is not always possible (Marriott and Myerburg, 1978). Rates of 200 beats/min or less are commonly associated with quinidine (or procainamide or disopyramide) therapy. Conversely, carotid sinus massage or digitalis may enhance the atrial flutter rate. Transitional rhythms between atrial flutter and atrial fibrillation are also seen clinically. The term atrial impure flutter has been applied to flutter with faster atrial rates (350-400 beats/min) (Chung, 1977). Similarly, Wells and colleagues (1979) separated atrial flutter arising after open heart surgery into types I (classical) and II (uncommon). In both types the atrial flutter waves are regular and uniform, but in type II the rates are faster (340-430 beats/min) and the response to rapid atrial pacing is unreliable. The term atrial flutter-fibrillation describes faster atrial rhythms (>350 beats/min) with slight variations in atrial cycle length and morphology. Atrial mechanisms with rates of about 400-450 beats/min and with more obvious variations of configuration and cycle length are referred to as coarse atrial fibrillation.

Intracardiac recordings from patients with atrial flutter-fibrillation and coarse atrial fibrillation suggest a spectrum of rhythms. One study found biatrial coarse fibrillation in 50% of these patients, but periods of dissimilar rhythms were found in the other 50% of patients (Schaal and Leier, 1978). These other rhythms included flutter in one atrium (right or left) and contralateral (dissociated) fibrillation, atrial tachycardia, distinct flutter, or quiescence. Simultaneous unilateral flutter with fast flutter, fragmented flutter, or fibrillation was also seen. Sinus rhythm

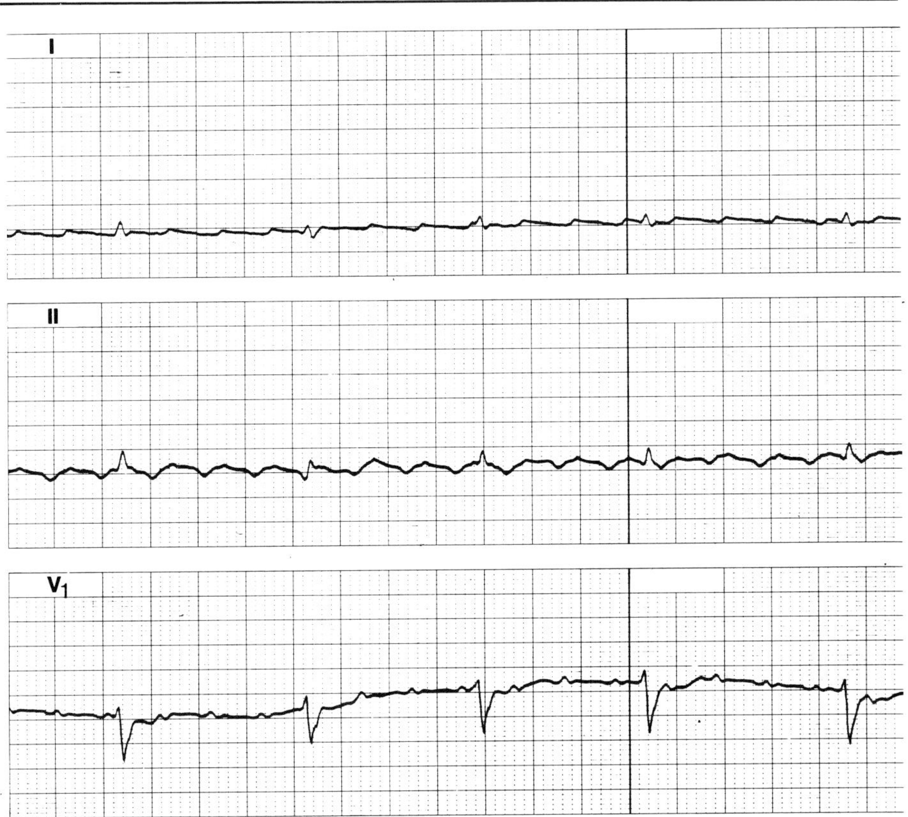

Figure 8-2 Rhythm strip demonstrating atrial flutter. Characteristic sawtooth atrial morphology can be seen in lead II. The ventricular response is slightly irregular.

with atrial dissociation and unilateral atrial flutter is possible but is extremely rare (Chung, 1977).

It is evident that an overlapping spectrum of rhythms exists between atrial tachycardia, with or without block, and atrial fibrillation, and that classifications of atrial tachyarrhythmias within this continuous spectrum based on electrocardiographic criteria are at times difficult or arbitrary.

Electrocardiographic Features

The flutter wave The flutter wave (F wave) in V_1 consists of two components that are oppositely directed. The initial (positive) deflection of atrial depolarization (P wave) is followed by a negative deflection of atrial repolarization (T wave).

The atrial mechanism may occasionally be well defined in only one or two leads. It is best seen most commonly in an inferior lead or lead V_1. When the atrial mechanism is poorly defined in all leads, the diagnosis may be aided by transsternal (Lewis) leads, by echocardiographic analysis of mitral valve motion (Fujiia, et al., 1978; Greenberg, et al., 1979), or by a readily used electrode pill (Jenkins, et al., 1979) or other esophageal electrode.

Atrial flutter with F waves that simulate P waves of atrial (supraventricular) tachycardia in all leads, but at a rate of 250 beats/min or more, may be seen occasionally. Untreated atrial flutter with 2:1 AV block may masquerade as atrial, junctional, or sinus tachycardia. Alternate flutter waves are camouflaged by superimposed portions of the QRS, ST, or T waves.

Ventricular response The ventricular rate in atrial flutter depends both on the atrial rate and the state of AV nodal conduction. Untreated atrial flutter presents most often with 2:1 AV conduction and a ventricular response of 140-175 beats/min. Fortunately, the physiologic refractory period in normal AV junctional tissue prevents a 1:1 AV response, with rare exceptions (Patton and Helfant, 1969; Kennelly and Lane, 1978). Hemodynamic compromise is thereby avoided. Digitalization, vagal stimulation, or preexisting AV conduction delay result in increased AV conduction ratios, most commonly 4:1 and occasionally 6:1. Odd AV ratios (3:1, 5:1) are relatively rare. A pattern of alternating 2:1 and 4:1 AV responses occurs often and may simulate bigeminy. Atrial flutter associated with Wenckebach AV block may result in a "regularly irregular" ventricular response. Varying AV block causes an irregularly irregular ventricular response, which simulates atrial fibrillation. Quinidine (or procainamide or disopyramide) therapy may slow the atrial rate, facilitate AV conduction, and increase ventricular conduction.

The common occurrence of even AV ratios (2:1, 4:1) has been explained by postulating two regions (upper and lower) of AV junctional block (Besoain-Santander, et al., 1950; see Figure 8-3). Varying penetration of impulses into AV junctional tissue without transmission to the ventricles (concealed conduction) may explain the spectrum of AV transmission that can be observed clinically (Katz and Pick, 1956). AV conduction in transitional rhythms (i.e., flutter-fibrillation) is characteristically irregular.

Independent, regular ventricular activity in atrial flutter may indicate complete heart block with a subsidiary escape rhythm or AV dissociation with ventricular tachycardia.

The QRS complex is usually normal in atrial flutter. Aberrancy, when present, suggests His-Purkinje or intraventricular conduction delay that may be fixed or rate-related or caused by ventricular preexcitation (Wolff-Parkinson-White syndrome).

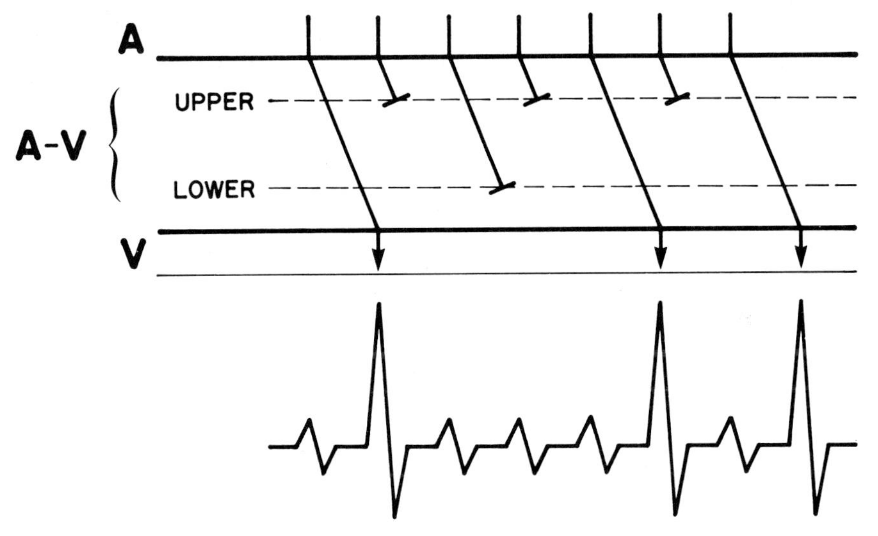

Figure 8-3 Schematic diagram explaining alternating 4:1 and 2:1 AV block in atrial flutter by postulating two regions (upper and lower) of alternating AV junctional block.

Onset-termination Atrial flutter is frequently initiated by a critically timed atrial premature complex. Flutter may terminate spontaneously with resumption of sinus rhythm or an escape junctional rhythm, which is usually transient. Transitions back and forth between atrial fibrillation (or occasionally tachycardia) and atrial flutter may be observed spontaneously or during therapeutic maneuvers (Katz and Pick, 1956). Atrial flutter may also be initiated by a ventricular premature complex with retrograde conduction to the atrium. It is clear from intracardiac electrophysiologic studies that atrial flutter can be induced in susceptible patients by one or two very early premature atrial complexes, timed just beyond the atrial refractory zone (Watson and Josephson, 1980). Bursts of very rapid atrial pacing (150-350 beats/min) are another effective method for inducing flutter in these patients. Recent clinical observations suggest that a range of coupling intervals characterizes the initiating atrial premature beats, including relatively long, as well as short, intervals (Cooper, et al., 1979b).

Clinical Findings

Atrial flutter may go unnoticed, may cause palpitations, or may be associated with significant hemodynamic compromise and hypotension.

The ventricular response rate and cardiac state determine the patient's tolerance to atrial flutter. On examination the patient's pulse may be either regular or irregular. The irregularity may be bigeminal, cyclically (regularly) irregular, or irregularly irregular. Commonly, a regular tachycardia of 150-160 beats/min is initially present and indistinguishable from that of other forms of supraventricular tachycardia. Inspecting the patient's neck veins may be very helpful in making a diagnosis. The presence of rapid (250-350 beats/min) and regular undulatory waves in the jugular system suggests atrial flutter. If carotid sinus massage produces abrupt halving of the ventricular rate (to 75-80 beats/min), atrial flutter should be suspected and can be confirmed by ECG recordings. The intensity of the heart sounds may vary. Greenburg and colleagues (1979) used ECG recordings to show that the intensity of S_1 relates inversely to the degree of mitral valve closure at the onset of systole. Atrial sounds can occasionally be heard and recorded in atrial flutter (Neporent, 1964). The signs and symptoms of underlying heart disease are frequently present. In addition, pulsus alternans may occasionally be found, usually with 2:1 AV conduction. If the ventricular rate is quite irregular, a pulse deficit is often present. Sudden heart failure and/or hypotension may be manifestations of acute atrial flutter in compromised patients.

Differential Diagnosis

Analysis of the atrial flutter wave on the ECG usually differentiates flutter from allied rhythms. Carotid sinus massage may frequently aid in the identification by slowing AV conduction, usually from 2:1 to 4:1, revealing the underlying flutter mechanism. Atrial flutter with 2:1 AV conduction must be differentiated from atrial, AV junctional, and sinus tachycardia, and, when associated with ventricular aberrancy, from ventricular tachycardia (Wellens, et al., 1978b). Atrial flutter with an irregularly irregular ventricular response must be differentiated from atrial fibrillation and MAT.

Artifacts may simulate atrial flutter. Tracings from patients with regularly occurring muscle tremors, such as those caused by Parkinson's disease, and diaphragmatic flutter may produce a false flutter wave on the ECG, especially in the limb leads. Close inspection of all leads will show the underlying atrial mechanism to be sinus in these cases.

Mechanism

The mechanisms of atrial flutter and fibrillation have been the subject of controversy since the 1950s (Hecht, 1953; Katz and Pick, 1953). The two major competing theories, those of automaticity and reentry, continue to evolve, and both theories may apply. Several studies suggest that the mechanisms of atrial flutter and fibrillation are similar (Hecht, 1953; Katz and Pick, 1953; Schaal and Leier, 1978; Wells, et al., 1979).

The theory of macro-reentry circuits (circus movement) was initially championed by Lewis (Lewis, 1918). The automatic focus theory was given impetus by studies, such as those of Scherf, concluding that local atrial application of aconitine could induce atrial fibrillation (Scherf, 1947). Pick, Katz, and Hecht integrated previous observations into a theory of multiple atrial reentry (Hecht, 1953; Katz and Pick, 1953). In fibrillation the pathways might be less organized and more microscopic than in flutter. Perpetuation of atrial flutter and fibrillation could depend on prolongation of the refractory period and an unequal recovery of excitability. Another research team (Moe and Abildskov, 1959) gathered additional experimental evidence to prove that atrial fibrillation is a self-sustained arrhythmia independent of focal discharge. Pastelin and colleagues (1978) showed experimentally that circus movement using the specialized atrial conduction pathways might occur and could explain features of atrial flutter. Recent clinical (four patients) and experimental studies of the effects of atrial extrastimulation and rapid pacing on the atrial flutter cycle have also been interpreted as favoring macro-reentry as the mechanism of atrial flutter (Inone, et al., 1981).

Several recent studies suggest localized reentry, thus supporting both a focal origin and a reentrant mechanism. In atrial flutter electronic pacing can occasionally capture portions of the atrium without interrupting the underlying rhythm, which remains after termination of pacing; this argues against macro-reentry (Waldo, et al., 1977; Friedman, et al., 1982). Vectoral ECG analysis assigns the origin of the typical flutter wave to the left posterior atrium with subsequent cephalad conduction (Mirowski and Alkan, 1967; Waldo, et al., 1977). Rapid coronary sinus pacing simulates atrial flutter on ECG recordings (Rosen, et al., 1969). Atrial endocardial mapping similarly places the onset of the atrial wave at the lower right atrium or the proximal coronary sinus (Watson and Josephson, 1980). Further evidence of focalization is presented by clinical examples of atrial flutter with exit block (Homcy, et al., 1979). Dual echocardiography of the mitral and tricuspid valves demonstrates reversal of the normal contraction sequence in atrial flutter, with left atrial preceding right atrial contraction (Fujiia, et al., 1978). The feasibility of sustained micro-reentrant circuits in mammalian atria has now been demonstrated experimentally by the elegant studies of Allessie and colleagues (1976). Clinical evidence for focal reentry at electrophysiologic study has been presented recently (Friedman, et al., 1982).

The phenomenon of triggered automaticity has also added new interest and uncertainty to this picture (Cranefield, 1977). Sustained ectopic activity in fibers within the coronary sinus and mitral valve apparatus can be induced experimentally by premature atrial complexes or rapid atrial stimulation (Cranefield, 1977; Wit and Cranefield, 1977). Thus, the initiation and termination of atrial tachyarrhythmias by pacing techniques may not always signify underlying reentry, but may alternatively represent triggered activity in fibers with rate-sensitive after-depolarizations (see Chapter 1). The bulk of electrophysiologic and pharmacologic evidence, nonetheless, supports reentry as the usual mechanism (Watson and Josephson, 1980; Friedman, et al., 1982).

Etiologic Considerations

Underlying heart disease Both acute and chronic atrial flutter are usually manifestations of underlying organic heart disease of many causes. Atrial flutter is rare in apparently healthy patients and usually appears in paroxysmal form in these cases. Atrial flutter was found in only one of 67,000 ECGs of asymptomatic United States Air Force personnel (Fosmoe, et al., 1960). It is seen more commonly in infancy than atrial fibrillation (Langendorf and Pick, 1966). Atrial flutter is usually a manifestation of coronary artery disease, hypertensive heart disease, or rheumatic heart disease (mitral valve stenosis). Atrial flutter complicates 2%-5% of cases of acute myocardial infarction, being less frequent than atrial fibrillation or supraventricular tachycardia (Liberthson, et al., 1976; Marriott and Myerburg, 1978). Less common cardiac etiologies include nonrheumatic mitral valve disease (i.e., mitral valve prolapse), pericarditis, myocarditis, cardiomyopathy, Wolff-Parkinson-White syndrome, thyrotoxicosis, and chronic obstructive pulmonary disease.

Specific initiating factors Atrial flutter is an unusual manifestation of digitalis intoxication (Agarwal, et al., 1972). Hemodynamic factors, such as exercise, may initiate atrial flutter in predisposed patients. Positional paroxysmal atrial flutter has been reported (Desser, et al., 1979). Electrolyte abnormalities, such as hypokalemia, may be implicated, particularly in patients who are receiving diuretics. Atrial flutter may occur in association with a viral syndrome, suggesting pericardial or myocardial involvement. Perioperative hormonal, electrolyte, or hemodynamic aberration may result in atrial flutter. Quinidine and other membrane-active drugs may occasionally convert atrial fibrillation into atrial flutter.

Hemodynamic Consequences

The hemodynamic consequences of atrial flutter vary greatly, depending primarily on the ventricular rate, underlying myocardial functional state, and duration of the rhythm disturbance. With 1:1 AV conduction hemodynamic impairment is almost always observed because of the rapid ventricular rate. More commonly, 2:1 AV conduction presents initiating symptoms of congestive heart failure in one-third to one-half of patients with underlying heart disease. Angina pectoris may develop as a consequence of reduced cardiac output and, hence, coronary flow. Acute hypotension may ensue, associated with lightheadedness, dizziness, confusion, or syncope. These manifestations are more likely to occur in elderly patients and in individuals with advanced underlying heart disease.

Little hemodynamic information is available to assess cardiac performance before and directly after conversion of atrial flutter to sinus rhythm (Lequime, 1942; Harvey, et al., 1955; McIntosh, et al., 1964). Harvey and colleagues (1955) noted depressed cardiac output in 11 of 12 patients who had atrial flutter and compensated hearts. Cardiac output increased by 25%-50% in the five patients in whom atrial flutter was converted to sinus rhythm by quinidine administration. Similarly, Lequime (1942) found that cardiac output increased by 40% in two patients who were converted from 2:1 atrial flutter. McIntosh and colleagues (1964) reported that the normal increase in cardiac output during exercise was also blunted during atrial flutter.

Clinical Significance

The clinical significance of atrial flutter may be reduced to hemodynamic, etiologic, prognostic, and therapeutic considerations. Atrial flutter associated with acute hemodynamic compromise obviously demands immediate therapeutic intervention. Newly appearing atrial flutter may lead to the diagnosis of otherwise occult heart disease or focus the clinician's attention on the cardiac consequences of systemic disease.

Prognosis

A prognostic evaluation of atrial flutter includes prognosis of the rhythm disturbance itself and prognosis of the underlying heart disease. The increasing duration of atrial flutter, increasing patient age, the presence of significant heart disease, and rapid ("impure") atrial flutter suggest a poor prognosis for conversion to and maintenance of sinus rhythm. The prognosis is better when specific initiating factors can be uncovered, such as the early postoperative period, electrolyte or acid-base imbalance, acute pulmonary abnormalities, thyroid disease, or hormonal imbalance. Atrial flutter in myocardial infarction and heart failure is associated with a high mortality rate that is more directly related to myocardial failure than the rhythm disturbance per se (Liberthson, et al., 1976).

Treatment

The therapeutic approach to atrial flutter will depend on the clinical setting. Drug therapy is similar to that for atrial fibrillation, but the responses may differ. Cardioversion is almost universally effective, frequently at low energy levels (Selzer, et al., 1966; Lown, 1967a; Resnekov and McDonald, 1968). Rapid atrial pacing has emerged as a useful alternative method of converting atrial flutter to sinus rhythm but is usually ineffective for treating atrial fibrillation or flutter-fibrillation (Waldo, et al., 1977).

Drug therapy Atrial flutter with a rapid ventricular rate (usually 2:1 AV conduction) requires treatment. When drug therapy is appropriate, a digitalis glycoside (i.e., digoxin) is often the agent of first choice (Smith and Haber, 1963). Digitalis slows AV nodal conduction and frequently converts 2:1 AV block to 4:1. Conversion to sinus rhythm may also ensue. Digitalis also decreases atrial vulnerability to flutter by narrowing the vulnerable zone for the initiation of flutter by a premature beat (Engel and Gonzalez, 1978). Larger doses of digoxin are often required to obtain rate control in atrial flutter than in atrial fibrillation.

Intravenous or oral therapy with propranolol is an alternative initial drug approach (Harrison, et al., 1965; Wolfson, et al., 1967; Frieden, et al., 1968; Lemberg, et al., 1970; Singh and Jewitt, 1974). Ventricular response slows reliably (AV block increases) when atrial flutter is treated with incremental intravenous propranolol (Harrison, et al., 1965). Conversion to sinus rhythm occurs occasionally to frequently, depending on the chronicity of the flutter and the type of heart disease (Wolfson, et al., 1967; Lemberg, et al., 1970). Several other beta-adrenoreceptor blocking drugs have recently been approved in the United States (see Chapter 3). Metoprolol, nadolol, atenolol, and pindolol are now approved for treatment of hypertension, and timolol has been approved for prevention of sudden death in post-myocardial infarction patients. At least several of these newer agents appear to possess antiarrhythmic properties similar to propranolol (Singh and Jewitt, 1974; Winchester, et al., 1978; Frishman, 1979; Williams, 1979). Cardioselective agents may offer an advantage over propranolol in patients with bronchospastic pulmonary disease. The addition of beta blocking drugs to digitalis therapy allows for easier rate control and avoids the potential adverse reactions of high digitalis doses (Frieden, et al., 1968; Singh and Jewitt, 1974). Although rate control has become a major therapeutic indication for beta blockers, many patients with atrial flutter unfortunately have significant left ventricular dysfunction, which may preclude the use of beta blocking drugs.

Verapamil, a membrane antagonist of calcium-carrying ionic currents, is a highly effective drug for slowing the ventricular rate in atrial flutter and sometimes allows conversion to normal sinus rhythm (Schamroth, et al., 1972; Heng, et al., 1975; Hagemeijer, 1978; Singh, et al., 1978; Ellrodt, et al., 1980; Klein and Kaplinsky, 1982). Whether it is useful in maintaining sinus rhythm after conversion is unknown (Singh, et al., 1978). This drug is generally well tolerated intravenously but is a vasodilating agent and can cause a clinically significant fall in blood pressure in some patients. Verapamil is also a sinus node depressant and should not be used in individuals with the brady-tachy syndrome.

Quinidine, procainamide, and disopyramide may all lead to pharmacologic conversion of atrial flutter to normal sinus rhythm (Anderson, et al., 1978; Luoma, et al., 1978). However, electrical conversion is preferred to high-dose loading regimens for this purpose because of the frequent side-effects of the latter treatment modality (Hurst and Myerburg, 1968). When these drugs are administered in standard dosages for 1-2 days prior to electroversion, they may still occasionally restore sinus rhythm, which avoids electroversion (Marriott and Myerburg, 1978). These drugs are usually given only after digitalization to avoid the possibility of a parodoxical increase in ventricular rate caused by facilitated AV conduction (Hoffman, et al., 1975). Antiarrhythmic therapy is frequently given after cardioversion in an attempt to maintain sinus rhythm, as is discussed in the section on atrial fibrillation. Quinidine, disopyramide, and quinidine plus propranolol are frequent choices for maintenance therapy (Fors, et al., 1971; Sodermark, et al., 1975; Anderson, et al., 1978) if a recurrence is likely. Digitalis or propranolol alone may be tried initially for the prevention of paroxysmal atrial flutter, but these drugs are probably less effective.

Electrical cardioversion Electrical cardioversion is over 95% effective in restoring sinus rhythm in patients with atrial flutter if the sinus mechanism is intact (Selzer, et al., 1966; Lown, 1967a; Resnekov and McDonald, 1968). Flutter can often be converted to sinus rhythm with low energy settings in the range of 5-50 joules. Both to avoid the need for repeated cardioversion and to lower the risk of conversion to atrial fibrillation (Guiney and Lown, 1972), a minimum of 50 joules may be chosen initially (Marriott and Myerburg, 1978) unless the patient has been given significant amounts of digitalis, in which case the lower energies should be used in the beginning.

Rapid atrial pacing Rapid atrial pacing, when readily available, is an alternative to electrocardioversion for the acute management of atrial flutter (Pittman, et al., 1973; Orlando, et al., 1977; Waldo, et al., 1977; Das, et al., 1978; Wellens, et al., 1978a). This therapeutic modality is preferred if digitalis intoxication is suspected (Das, et al., 1978), in the postoperative cardiac patient who has atrial leads in place (Pittman, et al., 1973; Wells, et al., 1979), in patients with severe pulmonary disease (Orlando, et al., 1977), and when anesthesia or sedation cannot be given. Technically, the transvenous pacing catheter is guided fluoroscopically against the right atrial wall. Pacing is then initiated at 10%-20% above the intrinsic atrial rate for 3-60 seconds. The rates are progressively increased as needed to as high as 600-1500 beats/min. The current may also be increased if success is not achieved (to 5-15 milliamperes). After the atrium is captured by the pacemaker for several seconds at each setting pacing is abruptly discontinued. This maneuver may result in the return to normal sinus rhythm. Return to atrial flutter implies a failure to capture the entire atrium, and a higher rate is selected for the next trial. The underlying atrial flutter rate may accelerate, suggesting entrainment of the atrium to the paced rate (Waldo, et al., 1977; Watson and Josephson, 1980). Rapid (type II) flutter is not reliably converted by rapid atrial pacing (Wellens, et al., 1978a; Wells, et al., 1979). Rapid atrial pacing allows an overall 80%-90% conversion rate of atrial flutter to sinus rhythm. However, in about one-third of cases transient atrial fibrillation may be initiated with subsequent spontaneous conversion to sinus rhythm.

Individualization of therapy *Emergent therapy* Patients with substantial hemodynamic compromise as a result of a rapid ventricular rate should be treated immediately with cardioversion.

Urgent therapy Atrial flutter with initial hemodynamic compensation but with rapid ventricular rate requires immediate attention. If immediate conversion is desired, electroversion or rapid atrial pacing is employed. If rate control is an acceptable goal, drug therapy is used.

Elective therapy In occasional cases atrial flutter will present with moderate ventricular response and no hemodynamic compromise. No therapy may be required, or electrical or drug conversion may be attempted. The therapeutic decision will depend on the underlying heart disease and the prognosis for return to sinus rhythm. Excessive slowing of the ventricular rate in response to digitalis may indicate underlying AV nodal disease. A demand pacemaker is usually required prior to prophylactic antiarrhythmic therapy in atrial flutter associated with the bradycardia-tachycardia variant of the sick sinus syndrome.

Atrial flutter in preexcitation syndromes Recurrent atrial flutter in the Wolff-Parkinson-White syndrome with dangerously rapid (1:1) conduction to the ventricles requires emergent therapy, usually with electrical cardioversion. If time permits the use of drug therapy, intravenous procainamide and/or lidocaine may block conduction in the accessory pathway effectively. A similar result may occur with quinidine therapy. Selection of an effective drug regimen for the Wolff-Parkinson-White syndrome with associated supraventricular tachyarrhythmias may be aided by electrophysiologic studies (Denes, et al., 1979; see Chapters 2 and 9). Epicardial mapping and surgical division of the anomalous bypass tract may be necessary as definitive therapy in selected cases (Denes, et al., 1979; see Chapter 11). Cryoablation, surgical interruption, or catheter ablation of the AV node with permanent ventricular or AV sequential pacing are approaches to controlling the ventricular response in atrial flutter and fibrillation when the ventricular response cannot be slowed by other therapy (Sealy, et al., 1977).

ATRIAL FIBRILLATION

Atrial fibrillation is the most common sustained rhythm, other than a sinus mechanism, noted in clinical practice (Katz and Pick, 1956; Kannel, et al., 1982). Mechanisms, associated cardiac disease, and therapy compare closely to those of atrial flutter, although some differences exist. Prognosis, significance, and therapeutic approaches vary depending on the clinical setting and require individual judgment.

Diagnosis

Irregularity of cardiac impulse on physical examination and of QRS complexes on the ECG usually first draw attention to the possibility of atrial fibrillation. Inspection of the ECG shows that P-wave activity has been replaced by irregular, oscillating atrial fibrillatory waves (Figure 8-4).

Atrial morphology and rate The atrial fibrillatory (F) wave is characterized by varying morphology, amplitude, and cycle length, and has a rate of 400-650 beats/min. ECG leads II and V_1 often show the most prominent fibrillatory activity. The amplitude is generally less than that of the flutter waves, but the spectrum ranges from coarse, flutterlike waves (usually at slower rates) to waves so fine that atrial activity cannot be discerned on the ECG. In the latter case a presumptive diagnosis of atrial fibrillation is frequently made when the ventricular rhythm is grossly irregular. Confusing baseline artifacts associated with somewhat irregular ventricular rates may lead occasionally to a false diagnosis of atrial fibrillation. Transsternal, esophageal, or intra-atrial leads may be required to establish the diagnosis (Bellet, 1971; Fowler, 1977; Chung, 1977). Echocardiographic analysis of diastolic mitral valve motion may help assess atrial rhythm. Dissociation of atrial rhythms between or within the atria is rarely diagnosed by scalar ECG but may be seen more often on intracardiac studies (Schaal and Leier, 1978). In this instance atrial fibrillation controls only a portion of the atria, and another rhythm (i.e., atrial flutter, tachycardia, and sinus rhythm) controls the residual atria.

Ventricular response The ventricular response to atrial fibrillation is typically irregularly irregular (Bellet, 1971). In untreated atrial fibrillation the ventricular rate is usually rapid (120-180 beats/min). Slower rates occur when preexisting AV conduction delay is present. Initially rapid ventricular rates of 180-220 beats/min are seen occasionally, especially in children. Ventricular transmission of rates above 220 beats/min is

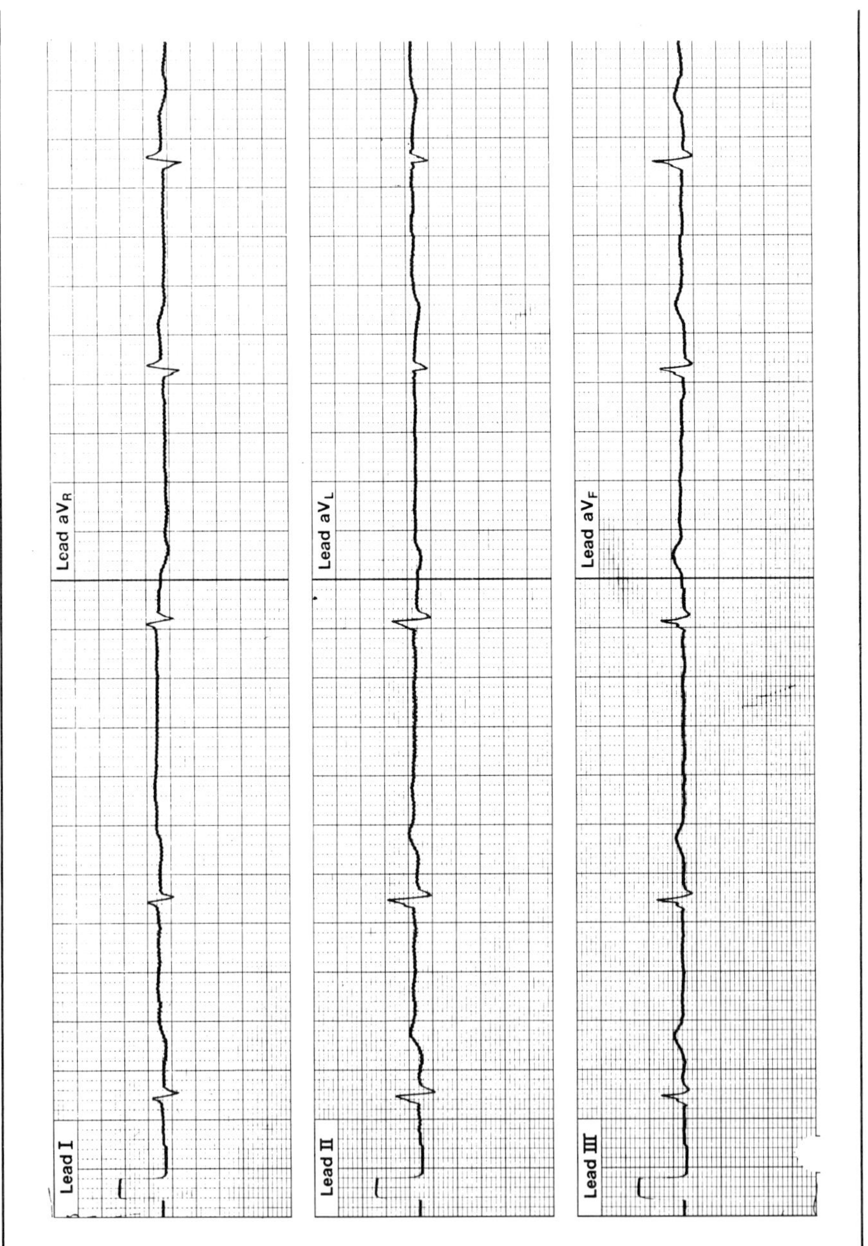

Figure 8-4 Coarse atrial fibrillation recorded in limb leads and precordial leads. The atrial mechanism is only apparent in right precordial leads (especially V_1).

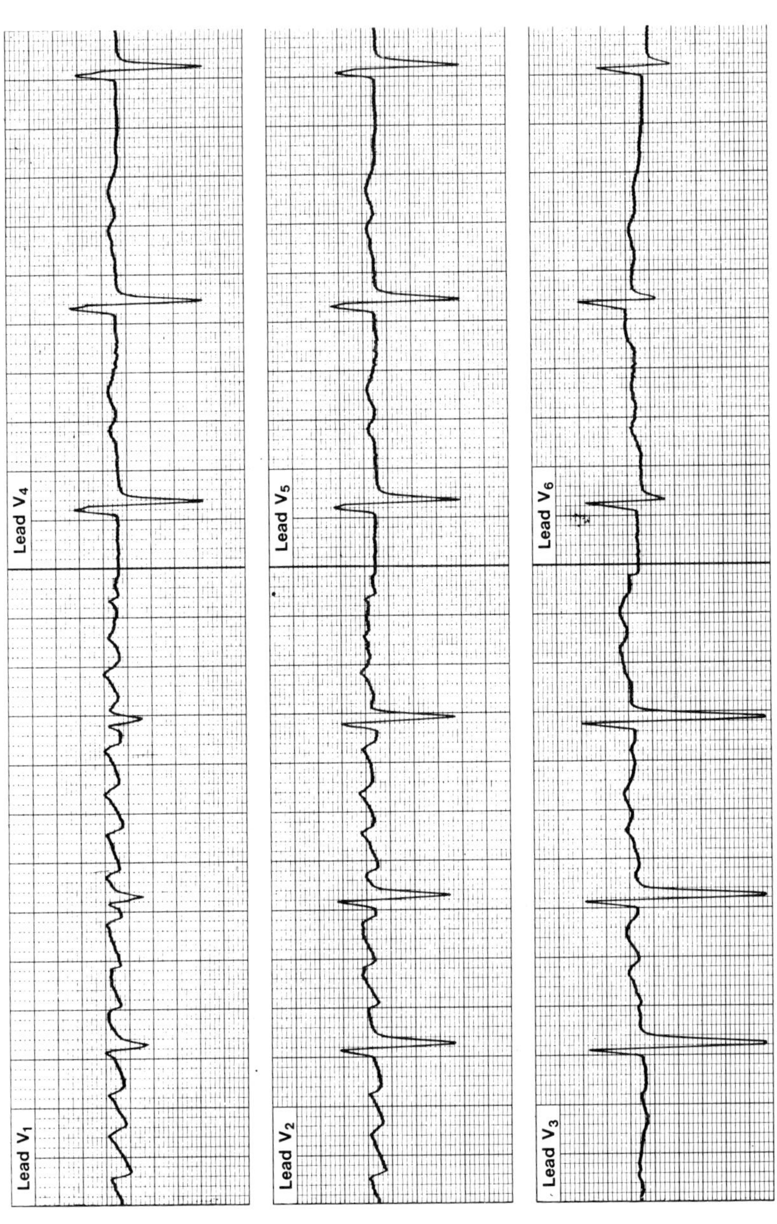
Lead V_1
Lead V_4
Lead V_2
Lead V_5
Lead V_3
Lead V_6

normally limited by the physiologic refractoriness of AV junctional tissue but may be seen in preexcitation syndromes.

An irregular ventricular response is attributed to irregularly irregular atrial fibrillatory activity and concealed conduction in the AV junction (Langendorf, et al., 1965; Cohen, et al., 1970). Approximately every third to sixth atrial impulse arriving at the AV junction passes through to the ventricles. Other atrial impulses penetrate into the AV junction but are blocked at different levels, depending on local refractoriness.

Conduction of each impulse sets conditions for the subsequent impulse. The net response is a grossly irregular rhythm. In the intracardiac electrogram atrial activity is chaotic, and each ventricular complex is preceded at a fixed, appropriate interval by a His bundle deflection (Lister, et al., 1976).

Atrial fibrillation occurring in otherwise normal individuals may be subject to a high degree of physiologic junctional delay, resulting in relatively slow rates. Ventricular rates of 60-100 beats/min, when seen in untreated elderly patients, usually signify intrinsic AV junctional disease. A high degree of AV disease should be suspected when the untreated ventricular rate is slower than 60 beats/min.

In atrial fibrillation with a regular ventricular response AV dissociation may be seen with heart block or AV junctional tachycardia. The patient is usually elderly, or digitalis toxicity is present. In these cases the ventricular response is regular, and the rate is determined by the subsidiary junctional, ventricular, or electronic pacemaker.

QRS configuration in atrial fibrillation The QRS configuration is generally roughly similar to that of normal sinus rhythm. The QRS contour is subject to some variation because of superimposition of fibrillatory waves, respiratory variation, or underlying conduction disturbance. Preexisting right or left bundle branch block, rate-dependent bundle branch block, or aberrant conduction because of the Wolff-Parkinson-White syndrome may be present. Differentiating aberrantly conducted supraventricular from ventricular premature complexes is a challenge (Gouaux and Ashman, 1947; Langendorf, et al., 1955; Marriott and Sandler, 1966; Wellens, et al., 1978b). Commonly, aberrant ventricular conduction occurs when a short cycle, after a relatively long cycle, finds the ventricle partially refractory. The term Ashman phenomenon describes this well-known and frequently observed finding (Gouaux and Ashman, 1947; Marriott and Sandler, 1966). Aberrant conduction frequently shows an RSR pattern resembling right bundle branch block because of the longer refractoriness of the right bundle branch. The initial QRS forces are also similar to those of normal beats. In supraventricular beats that exhibit aberrant conduction the HV interval may be prolonged on the intracardiac electrogram (Lister, et al., 1976). A salvo of aberrantly conducted beats may simulate a run of ventricular tachycardia. Ventricular ectopic beats, on the other hand, tend to be monophasic or biphasic in lead V_1 and to have abnormal initial QRS forces.

Onset-termination Atrial fibrillation may be initiated by a single, critically timed atrial premature complex (Killip and Gault, 1965), may appear in transition from sinus rhythm with premature atrial complexes, atrial flutter, or tachycardia, or occur spontaneously during sinus rhythm. Recent observations suggest that a range of coupling intervals characterize initiating atrial premature beats, including both relatively long and short intervals (Priest, et al., 1979). Atrial fibrillation may present in brief paroxysms or be chronically self-sustaining. A prolonged PR interval or a broad P wave is said to be a predisposing factor for the initiation of atrial fibrillation (Lown, 1967a; Buxton, et al., 1979). Atrial fibrillation may terminate spontaneously or after drug therapy or electroversion, allowing resumption of sinus rhythm. Less commonly, transformation to atrial flutter or tachycardia occurs. AV junctional escape frequently precedes the reestablishment of sinus rhythm. Symptomatic bradycardia, sinus arrest, or syncope may sometimes herald the return of sinus rhythm from atrial fibrillation (Lown, 1967a; Ferrer, 1974). Transient atrial or ventricular standstill may be caused by depression of the sinus and subsidiary pacemakers (postdrive inhibition) or signify intrinsic conduction system disease. The bradycardia-tachycardia (sick sinus) syndrome, often seen in the elderly, may be characterized on ambulatory ECG monitoring by periods of atrial fibrillation, atrial flutter, and tachycardia in transition with sinus bradycardia or first-degree and higher AV block (Ferrer, 1974).

In susceptible individuals atrial fibrillation can be induced in the electrophysiologic laboratory by one or two critically timed atrial premature contractions near the refractory period or by bursts of rapid atrial pacing (Lister, et al., 1976). Unless sufficient atrial enlargement is present, atrial fibrillation will not usually be maintained (Moore, et al., 1962). Rapid atrial pacing, electroversion, and drug therapy frequently convert atrial flutter initially to atrial fibrillation (Guiney and Lown, 1972; Pittman, et al., 1973; Orlando, et al., 1977; Das, et al., 1978; Wellens, et al., 1978a).

Clinical Findings

The onset of atrial fibrillation may either go unnoticed or be associated with palpitations, dyspnea, lightheadedness, or precordial oppression. Ventricular rate and cardiac state determine whether heart failure is present. On examination the pulse is irregularly irregular and a deficit is evident. (The apical rate exceeds the peripheral pulse rate.) Blood pressure may be reduced. The jugular pulse is irregular and has a ventricular form, with no "a" wave. Rales, signs of pleural effusion, peripheral edema, or ascites suggest associated heart failure. The intensity of S_1 is variable, caused mainly by varying mitral valve position at onset of systole (Greenburg, et al., 1979). Atrial sounds may be heard occasionally (Neporent, 1964). Auscultatory and other signs of associated heart disease are often present (Bellet, 1971). The cardiac silhouette is frequently enlarged on chest roentgenogram.

Differential Diagnosis

Atrial fibrillation must be differentiated from sinus rhythm with frequent atrial or ventricular premature beats, MAT, and atrial flutter or atrial tachycardia with varying AV block. Differentiation can be achieved by paying attention to atrial activity. When rapid transmission to the ventricles occurs (rates over 150 beats/min), less variation in cycle length is present; atrial fibrillation may mimic irregular supraventricular or even ventricular tachycardia if aberrant ventricular conduction occurs (Gouaux and Ashman, 1947; Wellens, et al., 1978b). Carotid sinus massage may slow the ventricular rate in atrial fibrillation but not in ventricular or supraventricular tachycardia.

Mechanism

Clinical and experimental observations attest to the similarities of mechanism between atrial fibrillation and flutter. The evolution of the competing theories of reentry and automaticity was presented earlier in the chapter in the section on atrial flutter. The concept of multiple atrial reentry, as developed by Pick, Katz and Hecht, and others, was a major conceptual advance in explaining atrial fibrillation (Hecht, 1953; Katz and Pick, 1953). Prinzmetal (1953) photographed the microscopic atrial contraction pattern in patients with atrial fibrillation at surgery using high-speed cinematography. Moe and Abildskov (1959) showed that atrial fibrillation could be a self-sustained rhythm, independent of focal discharge. Moore and colleagues (1962) emphasized the importance of increased atrial mass to the maintenance of atrial fibrillation (Bellet, 1971; Moore, et al., 1962). The factors predisposing to sustained atrial fibrillatory mechanism may be summarized as a large atrial mass, irregular atrial refractoriness, prolonged atrial conduction, shortened atrial refractoriness, and premature stimulation of the atria (Schamroth, 1971).

In the Wolff-Parkinson-White syndrome the relationship between macro-reentrant tachycardia and atrial fibrillation appears to be complex (Wellens and Durrer, 1974; Campbell, et al., 1977). Amelioration after surgical sectioning points to the participation of the bypass tract (Sealy, et al., 1977). Fragmentation of atrial impulses at short atrial cycles in paroxysmal supraventricular tachycardia in the Wolff-Parkinson-White syndrome may be an important mechanism for initiating atrial fibrillation (Sung, et al., 1977; Wyndham, et al., 1977).

Etiologic Considerations

Underlying heart disease The following is a list of the etiologic factors underlying organic heart disease in atrial fibrillation:

1. Coronary artery disease (atherosclerotic)
   a. Chronic, with or without symptoms
   b. Acute myocardial infarction
2. Hypertensive heart disease
3. Rheumatic (mitral) valvular heart disease
4. Nonrheumatic mitral disease with mitral regurgitation
5. Cardiomyopathy, usually advanced (hypertrophic, dilated, restrictive, toxic, myocarditis, pericarditis)
6. Conduction system disease (sick sinus syndrome, Wolff-Parkinson-White syndrome, familial)
7. Thyrotoxicosis (overt or occult)
8. Congenital heart disease (i.e., atrial septal defect)
9. Constrictive pericarditis
10. Other causes of large atrium or heart failure
11. None (uncommon—"lone" atrial fibrillator)

Atrial fibrillation is most commonly encountered in patients who are over 40 years old in association with ischemic heart disease, hypertensive heart disease, or mitral valve disease (Kannel, et al., 1982). In the general population its prevalence is about four out of 1,000 people (Ostrander, et al., 1965). Atrial fibrillation comprises 9%-12% of ECGs performed in large hospital studies (Katz and Pick, 1956). It is rare in apparently normal individuals but is found more often than atrial flutter. In one study atrial fibrillation was found on the ECGs of five out of 67,000 asymptomatic United States Air Force personnel (Fosmoe, et al., 1960). In another study paroxysmal atrial fibrillation occurred in 125 out of 750,000 healthy airmen (Busby and Davis, 1976). Sustained atrial fibrillation unassociated with manifest heart disease (idiopathic, benign, or lone atrial fibrillation) comprises up to 5% of large clinical series of atrial fibrillation (Evans and Swann, 1954; Bellet, 1971). Atrial fibrillation in a representative hospital population was associated with atherosclerotic cardiovascular disease in 43% of patients, hypertensive heart disease in 14% of patients, rheumatic heart disease in 11% of patients, and other disease in the remaining 32% of patients (Aberg, 1968). About one-third of the patients followed for mitral valve stenosis are in atrial fibrillation (Fowler, 1977). Nonrheumatic mitral valve diseases (i.e., myxomatous degeneration or ischemic disease) are assuming increasing importance.

Acute myocardial infarction may lead to atrial fibrillation in 7%-16% of patients (Julian, et al., 1964; Meltzer and Kitchell, 1966; Jewitt, et al., 1967; Lown, 1967a; DeSanctis, et al., 1972; Liberthson, et al., 1976). About one-third of patients who are followed for cardiomyopathy are in atrial fibrillation (Schamroth, 1971). Dilated, hypertrophic (especially obstructive), infiltrative, and restrictive forms of advanced cardiomyopathy may all be accompanied by atrial fibrillation (Watson, et al., 1977). Atrial fibrillation is clearly associated with chronic constructive pericarditis, occurring in about 25% of patients (Dalton, et al., 1956).

Atrial fibrillation occurs in infancy only rarely and usually signifies congenital heart disease (i.e., atrial septal defect, Ebstein's anomaly, or transposition of the great vessels) (Langendorf and Pick, 1966). The prevalence of atrial fibrillation with atrial septal defects is 10%-15% in patients who are over 45 years old (Campbell, et al., 1957). Chronic cor pulmonale is a relatively uncommon cause of chronic atrial fibrillation but is frequently associated with paroxysmal atrial fibrillation (Corazza and Pastor, 1958; Schamroth, 1971).

Atrial fibrillation is being recognized increasingly as a manifestation of diffuse conduction system disease in elderly patients (sick sinus syndrome) (Kaplan, et al., 1973; Ferrer, 1974). Preexcitation, as in the Wolff-Parkinson-White syndrome, is associated with a predisposition to atrial fibrillation (Wellens and Durrer, 1974).

Lone (idiopathic) atrial fibrillation is perhaps best exemplified in studies of young patients in whom occult coronary artery disease is unlikely. Of 106 cases of atrial fibrillation reported in military personnel, 95% were paroxysmal, 60% occurred just once, and only 5% were chronic (Class, 1957; Lamb and Pollard, 1964; Peter, et al., 1968). Cases of familial atrial fibrillation have been reported, suggesting that heritable factors may be important in some patients (Gould, 1957; Phair, 1963).

Specific initiating factors The following is a list of the precipitating factors for atrial fibrillation:

1. Premature atrial contractions
2. Metabolic imbalance (abnormalities of electrolytes, acid-base, and blood gases, catecholamines, hypoglycemia, fever/sepsis)
3. Surgery (especially cardiac surgery)
4. Neurogenic imbalance [i.e., sudden emotion, violent exertion, nausea/vomiting, trauma, cerebrovascular accidents, or combined sympathetic/parasympathetic (vagal) discharge]
5. Thyrotoxicosis
6. Toxic substances (alcohol, caffeine, cigarettes)
7. Noxious factors (i.e., electrocution, hypothermia, or asphyxia)

The proximate cause of atrial fibrillation is usually premature atrial contractions. Atrial fibrillation may occur postoperatively and be attributed to imbalances in acid-base, blood gases, electrolytes, or catecholamines. Cardiac surgery is a much more common precipitant of atrial fibrillation than noncardiac surgery (Bellet, 1971). Electrolyte disturbance in patients who are taking diuretics (i.e., hypokalemia) may be an initiating factor of atrial fibrillation.

Thyrotoxicosis, often occult, may be found in 5%-10% of patients who present with atrial fibrillation. A recent study reported subtle thyroid abnormalities in 13% of patients with atrial fibrillation (Class, 1957). Atrial fibrillation is present in about 10% of patients who are seen for thyrotoxicosis (Schamroth, 1971). Screening for thyroid abnormalities is, therefore, suggested in patients who present with atrial fibrillation without an obvious cause.

Paroxysmal atrial fibrillation may occur in otherwise normal individuals in association with excessive alcohol or caffeine intake, cigarette use, or sudden emotional excitement. Nausea, vomiting, coughing, severe pain, carotid sinus massage, and combined sympathetic/parasympathetic discharge are other reported precipitants of atrial fibrillation, as are hypoglycemia, hypothermia, asphyxia, systemic infection, or electrocution (Bellet, 1971). Chest and head trauma and subarachnoid hemorrhage may initiate this rhythm on occasion. Atrial fibrillation may also develop in the setting of a viral syndrome, suggesting pericarditis or myocarditis. The therapy of atrial flutter may precipitate fibrillation, as was discussed in the previous section on atrial flutter.

Hemodynamic Consequences

Atrial fibrillation may have little recognizable hemodynamic effect in otherwise normal subjects but may be potentially serious for patients with severe mitral valve disease or heart failure. Adverse hemodynamic consequences may be expected because of loss of atrial systolic "kick," increased resting ventricular rate with decreased diastolic filling, and disproportionate rate acceleration with exercise. The atrial kick acts to rapidly increase end-diastolic ventricular pressure and hence volume, augmenting ventricular contraction and stroke volume (Skinner, et al., 1963; Kosowsky, et al., 1968). Loss of atrial kick decreases volume, which must be recovered by increased mean diastolic pressure. The atrial kick facilitates mitral and tricuspid valve closure by establishing a reverse pressure gradient between the atrium and ventricle. Loss of the atrial kick leads to sluggish valve closure and may allow early systolic valvular insufficiency (Daley, et al., 1965). Braunwald and colleagues (1960) confirmed the applicability of Starling's law relating ventricular filling and contraction to atrial fibrillation.

Excessive ventricular rates are hemodynamically important in mitral valve stenosis where diastolic filling is slowed; rapid rates may substantially decrease cardiac output. A decrease in exertional capacity may result in most patients with atrial fibrillation because of disproportionate acceleration of ventricular rates with exercise (Benchimol, et al., 1965; Kaplan, et al., 1968). Cardioactive drugs, neurocirculatory effects, and underlying disease states also contribute to hemodynamic alterations. Atrial fibrillation in acute myocardial infarction is well tolerated in approximately 20% of patients, causes marginal compromise in almost 60% of patients, and severe hemodynamic deterioration in the remaining 20% of patients (Liberthson, et al., 1976).

Several studies have confirmed the hemodynamic benefit of conversion of atrial fibrillation to sinus rhythm, although the onset and magnitude of benefit have varied (Oram, 1963; Kahn, et al., 1964; Killip and Baer, 1964; Morris, et al., 1964; Reale, 1965; Rodman, et al., 1966; Resnekov, 1967; Ikram, et al., 1968; Shapiro and Klein, 1968; Scott and Patterson, 1969; DeMaria, et al., 1975). DeMaria and colleagues (1975) found increases in the left ventricular end-diastolic dimension, ejection fraction, stroke volume, and estimated cardiac index (+0.3 L/min/m^2) in 35 patients who were studied echocardiographically 1 hour after electroversion to sinus rhythm. The cardiac index rose 0.7 L/min/m^2 in those patients with depressed function (<2.5 L/min/m^2). Killip and Baer (1964) noted a 33% rise in the resting cardiac output after electroversion of atrial fibrillation in nine patients with underlying mitral valve stenosis but no change in four patients with normal hearts. Morris and colleagues (1964) reported a similar rise in the resting cardiac output within 2-3 hours in eight of eleven patients at rest and a 17% rise in the exercise cardiac output in all of five patients. The reestablishment of sinus rhythm after mitral valvuloplasty was associated with an approximately 25% rise in both resting and exercise cardiac outputs by 6-12 hours in the study conducted by Kahn and colleagues (1964). Another study noted a fall in elevated end-diastolic pressures and a variable change in cardiac output in twelve patients at one-half hour (Reale, 1965). Shapiro and Klein (1968) noted a small increase in output, significant only with exercise, in 10 patients at one-half hour. Oram and colleagues (1963) found a significant increment of cardiac output in 10 patients studied 3-16 days after conversion. A lack of immediate improvement was attributed to anesthesia. Similarly, another study showed a gradual increase in the cardiac index (+12%) over 3 hours to 1 week after electroversion of chronic atrial fibrillation (Rodman, et al., 1966). An increase in the cardiac index (+22%) also occurred in 26 patients in whom atrial fibrillation was converted to sinus rhythm with quinidine. Resnekov (1967) found that an increase in the resting cardiac output (+12%) accompanied electroversion of atrial fibrillation in patients with abnormal hearts, and an increase in the exercise cardiac output in patients with both normal and abnormal hearts. MacIntosh, et al., (1964) reviewed these and other earlier studies and evaluated several patients of their own. A 25%-33% rise in the resting and exercise cardiac outputs followed the return to sinus rhythm in about two-thirds of patients who were reviewed. Scott and Patterson (1969) showed that a delayed rise in cardiac output occurred over 3 days after electroversion. Ikram, et al. (1968) presented evidence that delayed improvement may be caused by a delay in the return of atrial mechanical function (Scott and Patterson, 1969). Early atrial electromechanical dissociation was noted echocardiographically in two patients in DeMaria's series (DeMaria, et al., 1975). To summarize, atrial fibrillation compromises the resting cardiac output in abnormal hearts and exercise output in both abnormal and normal hearts. A delay in the full benefit, lasting hours to several days, may follow cardioversion; a delay in the return of atrial mechanical function can be documented in some of these cases.

Prognosis

The severity of underlying heart disease and the duration of atrial fibrillation generally determine the prognosis. The short-term prognosis for establishing sinus rhythm is excellent (80%-95%) with the availability of electrical conversion techniques, provided that the sinus mechanism is intact (Selzer, et al., 1966; Lown, 1967a; Resnekov and McDonald, 1968). The prognosis for maintaining sinus rhythm for at least several months, on the other hand, is relatively poor, even with drug therapy (Hurst, et al., 1964; Selzer, et al., 1966; Lown, 1967a; Resnekov and McDonald, 1968; Szekely, et al., 1970; Takkunen, et al., 1970; Sodermark, et al., 1975). Fifty to one hundred percent of patients (average 70%-75%) will revert to atrial fibrillation within 3-12 months, the majority of patients within 1 day to 1 month. With optimal drug therapy 30%-50% of patients will revert in 3-12 months. Both short-term and long-term success are inversely related to the duration of atrial fibrillation. When atrial fibrillation has been present for 5 or more years, the chances of establishing and, particularly, of maintaining sinus rhythm are very low. The prognosis of atrial fibrillation after mitral valve replacement is similar to that without operation (Selzer, et al., 1965).

A life-table analysis indicates that a substantial risk is associated with atrial fibrillation and organic heart disease. In a study of 3700 patients Gajewski and Singer (1979) noted an eightfold increase in mortality in patients with chronic atrial fibrillation. Atrial fibrillation associated with mitral valve stenosis carries a seventeenfold excess risk. Even paroxysmal atrial fibrillation in the latter setting suggested a substantial (thirteenfold) excess risk. Chronic atrial fibrillation in association with coronary artery disease or hypertension carried a sevenfold increased risk. Lone paroxysmal atrial fibrillation, in the absence of any associated heart disease, was, fortunately, without increased risk. Excess mortality caused by supervening heart failure appears to be the result of the associated heart failure, peripheral emboli, or sudden death rather than the rhythm disturbance itself (Aberg, 1969). This conclusion also applies to atrial fibrillation complicating acute myocardial infarction (Liberthson, et al., 1976; Hunt, et al., 1978). Patients who are able to maintain sinus rhythm after cardioversion have a survival advantage (Takkunen, et al., 1970).

Treatment

The therapeutic approach to atrial fibrillation depends on the clinical setting (Table 8-2).

General treatment approach Emergent treatment is indicated when hemodynamic embarrassment follows the onset of atrial fibrillation with rapid ventricular rates, usually in the setting of heart failure. The treatment of choice consists of a synchronized, direct current shock of 100-300 joules. Once sinus rhythm is restored, consideration is given to digitalization and oral maintenance therapy with antiarrhythmic drugs.

Urgent therapy is suggested for acute atrial fibrillation with rapid ventricular rates and hemodynamic compensation. In these cases a decision

Table 8-2 Treatment of irregular atrial arrhythmias*

Arrhythmia	Treatment of choice	Alternative	Remarks
Atrial fibrillation	Cardioversion	Digitalis to control ventricular rate	Propranolol or verapamil may help slow ventricular rate. Quinidine, disopyramide, or procainamide may be used for long-term suppression. Patients with Wolff-Parkinson-White syndrome may have adverse response to IV digitalis
Atrial flutter	Cardioversion; rapid atrial pacing	Digitalis	Same as atrial fibrillation
Multifocal atrial tachycardia (MAT)	Improvement of pulmonary insufficiency, heart failure, and infection	Beta blocking agents if not contraindicated Verapamil (?)	Avoid digitalis intoxication. A cardioselective beta blocker may be better tolerated in patients with bronchospastic pulmonary disease

*Modified from *Med. Lett.* 20:113, 1978

regarding drug therapy versus cardioversion is made clinically. Consideration is given to the possibility of early decompensation, underlying heart disease, the expected response to drug therapy, and suitability for and availability of electrical cardioversion and anesthesia. Intravenous verapamil or rapid digitalization is frequently the preferred initial management step. These drugs may on occasion also convert atrial fibrillation to sinus rhythm. If the ventricular rate continues to be rapid despite full digitalization, verapamil or propranolol (or other beta blockers) may be added either orally or in small intravenous increments. Verapamil should be used cautiously in this setting because it may cause an increase in digoxin levels and theoretically may potentiate the electrophysiologic (and toxic) effects of digitalis. Because of negative inotropism, propranolol is contraindicated if heart failure is not secondary to rapid rates alone. Verapamil should be used with caution when heart failure is not caused by the rapid ventricular response because it is a direct myocardial depressant (although its vasodilating properties may compensate for its direct action). As with digitalis and verapamil, the addition of propranolol may facilitate a return to sinus rhythm.

Chronic atrial fibrillation is initially treated with a digitalis glycoside (usually digoxin) if rate control is required. Here, the therapeutic goal includes resting ventricular rates of 60-90 beats/min and prevention of abnormal acceleration of rate early in exercise. If elective cardioversion is planned, consideration regarding anticoagulants and antiarrhythmic agents should be given. Large, loading regimens of antiarrhythmics, such as quinidine, are no longer recommended; however, conversion to sinus rhythm may occur with the addition of maintenance doses of quinidine, obviating the need for cardioversion (Sodermark, et al., 1975; Marriott and Myerburg, 1978).

Drug efficacy in atrial fibrillation (see Chapter 3) *Digitalis* Digitalis glycosides slow the ventricular rate in atrial fibrillation by an indirect, vagal effect on the AV node, as well as by a smaller, direct effect (Smith and Haber, 1963; Lown, 1967a; Mason, 1974). Digitalis also reduces the excessive rate of acceleration that is seen with exercise in atrial fibrillation (Benchimol, et al., 1965; Kaplan, et al., 1968). In most patients incremental digitalis allows satisfactory rate control without toxicity during acute management, and conversion to sinus rhythm is not uncommon (Jennings, et al., 1958). Maintenance therapy allows chronic rate control. Maintenance digitalis may not be required for all patients with chronic atrial fibrillation (Martin and Lamb, 1979). In contrast, therapeutic concentrations of digitalis may be insufficient to control the ventricular rate in very ill patients (Goldman, et al., 1975). Patients with hypokalemia, anemia, hyperthyroidism, and carditis are also unlikely to respond (Mason, 1974; Chopra, et al., 1977). Beta blockers may be useful in these situations (see the following section) (David, et al., 1979). Engel and

Gonzalez (1978) showed that ouabain narrows the zone of atrial vulnerability to electrophysiologic induction, suggesting that digitalis has a prophylactic effect against atrial fibrillation apart from its hemodynamic and rate effects. Digitalis is contraindicated in atrial fibrillation that has a slow ventricular response (50-80 beats/min) with the Wolff-Parkinson-White syndrome, and in cases of a rapid ventricular response (bypass tract conduction may accelerate) (Wolfson, et al., 1967). Digitalis toxicity should be suspected in the face of slow ventricular rates, regular ventricular rhythm (nonparoxysmal junctional tachycardia), and increased ventricular ectopy.

Verapamil Verapamil, a blocker of slow calcium currents, is a potent alternative drug for rate control in atrial fibrillation. Several studies have shown consistent results: a substantial decrease in ventricular rate, usually by one-third (or to less than 100 beats/min), and conversion to sinus rhythm (in over 10% of cases) follow intravenous verapamil therapy in patients with atrial fibrillation (Schamroth, et al., 1972; Heng, et al., 1975; Hagemeijer, 1978; Singh, et al., 1978). In rare cases AV block may be precipitated by verapamil. Oral verapamil may be used for maintenance therapy to sustain a slow ventricular response, but the prophylactic efficacy is unknown (Singh, et al., 1978). Klein and Kaplinsky (1982) have recently presented data suggesting the superiority of oral verapamil over digitalis in controlling ventricular response during exercise and improving exercise performance in atrial fibrillation. Verapamil may increase serum digoxin concentrations.

Beta-adrenergic blocking drugs The beta-adrenergic blocking drugs have proved to be of great value in facilitating rate control when digitalis is contraindicated or ineffective (Harrison, et al., 1965; Wolfson, et al., 1967; Frieden, et al., 1968; Lemberg, et al., 1970; Singh and Jewitt, 1974; David, et al., 1979). Propranolol is the only beta blocker currently approved for this use, but other beta blocking drugs appear to be equally efficacious (Singh and Jewitt, 1974; Yahalom, et al., 1977; Winchester, et al., 1978; Frishman, 1979; Williams, 1979). Incremental intravenous propranolol (0.5-1 mg every 2-5 minutes for a total dose of 0.05-0.15 mg/kg) usually results in prompt slowing and, less frequently, to conversion of atrial fibrillation (Harrison, et al., 1965; Lemberg, et al., 1970). Oral therapy (starting at 10-40 mg every 6 hours) is used electively and for maintenance. Propranolol has been used safely in acute myocardial infarction complicated by atrial fibrillation when rate control is the major hemodynamic problem (Lemberg, et al., 1970; Singh and Jewitt, 1974). Beta blockers alone are not as effective as quinidine in maintaining sinus rhythm after cardioversion (Szekely, et al., 1970; Levi, et al., 1973) but may be useful in combination (Byrne-Quinn and Wing, 1970; Fors, et al., 1971; Levi and Proto, 1972).

Quinidine, disopyramide, and procainamide The effectiveness of quinidine bisulfate in maintaining sinus rhythm after cardioversion from atrial fibrillation was 51%, as opposed to 28% in a control group, at 1 year in a randomized study of 176 patients (Sodermark, et al., 1975). Long-acting quinidine was significantly superior to the short-acting drug in maintaining sinus rhythm in another study, but whether differences were caused by variations in compliance or to blood concentrations of drug was not determined (Normand, et al., 1976). Quinidine therapy resulting in subtherapeutic concentrations, however, failed to increase the percentage of patients maintained in sinus rhythm from that of earlier studies (Hall and Wood, 1968; Szekely, et al., 1970). The addition of propranolol to quinidine may allow control of previously refractory arrhythmias or a reduction in excessive quinidine dosage (Byrne-Quinn and Wing, 1970; Fors, et al., 1971; Levi and Proto, 1972). Combined therapy with quinidine and beta blockers was effective in 65% of 122 patients with chronic atrial fibrillation who did not respond to quinidine alone and was less toxic than quinidine alone (Levi and Proto, 1972). The major concern with beginning quinidine therapy in atrial fibrillation relates to the small but significant risk of precipitating malignant ventricular arrhythmias, including ventricular tachycardia and fibrillation (Selzer and Wray, 1964; Reynolds and Vander Ark, 1976). The latter authors estimated the risk of quinidine syncope at 4% and of sudden death at 0.5%. Prolongation of the QT interval and potentiation of the effect of digitalis may be contributing factors (Reynolds and Vander Ark, 1976; Leahey, et al., 1978). Recently, an important interaction between quinidine and digitalis has been described (Kaplan, et al., 1973). The administration of quinidine to digitalized patients results in reduced digoxin clearance and approximate doubling of serum digoxin concentrations (Hager, et al., 1979). It thus appears prudent to reduce dosage or omit digoxin when quinidine is added, especially prior to cardioversion. Patients should be carefully observed for signs of digitalis intoxication, and blood sampling for the digoxin concentration is recommended. If only temporary antidysrhythmic therapy is anticipated in the postconversion period, consideration should be given to the use of procainamide or disopyramide, which do not interact to raise the digoxin concentration.

In one recent double-blind study disopyramide therapy resulted in maintenance of sinus rhythm 3 months after cardioversion of atrial fibrillation in 72% of patients, as opposed to 30% of placebo-treated controls (Hartel, et al., 1974). Acute atrial fibrillation (<7 days) was successfully returned to sinus rhythm by intravenous disopyramide in 50% of patients in another study (Luoma, et al., 1978). Disopyramide thus appears to be a useful alternative to quinidine in acute and maintenance therapy of both supraventricular and ventricular arrhythmias (Koch-Weser, 1979). It may, however, cause drug-induced myocardial depression.

Procainamide is also an effective agent in the prevention and treatment of supraventricular arrhythmias, including atrial fibrillation (Szekely, et al., 1970; Hoffman, et al., 1975; Lucchesi, 1977). Szekely and colleagues reported a 25% retention of sinus rhythm at the end of 10 months of 3 g/day of procainamide, as opposed to only 13% in patients treated with 60 mg/day of propranolol (Szekely, et al., 1970). Procainamide is a convenient agent for acute and short-term management because of the ease of both parenteral and oral administration, but its short half-life and tendency to precipitate drug-induced lupus erythematosus limit its usefulness in long-term maintenance (Lucchesi, 1977; Anderson, et al., 1978). A sustained-release procainamide preparation is now available.

Other agents Amiodarone, available outside of the United States, has been useful in the treatment of ventricular and supraventricular arrhythmias, especially those associated with the Wolff-Parkinson-White syndrome (Resnekov, 1974; Wellens, et al., 1976). Rosenbaum and colleagues (1976) noted successful "control" of recurrent paroxysmal atrial fibrillation and flutter with amiodarone in 29 out of 30 patients. Clonidine has been used successfully for rate control of acute atrial fibrillation in patients with chronic obstructive pulmonary disease, who were felt to be poor candidates for standard therapy (Cooper, et al., 1979a).

Other considerations In some instances sustained atrial fibrillation may be the rhythm of choice (Kowey, et al., 1979). Examples of this include paroxysmal atrial fibrillation despite antiarrhythmic therapy, with recurrent systemic emboli, or medically unmanageable atrial flutter. Discontinuation of antiarrhythmic drugs, adequate digitalization, and beta blockers, if needed, frequently allow sustained atrial fibrillation with controlled rates.

Patients with the bradycardia-tachycardia syndrome (see Chapter 6) and atrial fibrillation usually require the placement of a permanent pacemaker prior to antidysrhythmic therapy directed at the atrial fibrillation (Ferrer, 1974).

Patients with the Wolff-Parkinson-White syndrome (see Chapters 2 and 9) and refractory, recurrent atrial fibrillation may require experimental drug trials (i.e., amiodarone) or surgery for interruption of the anomalous bypass tract (Lemberg, et al., 1964; Rosenbaum, et al., 1976; Sealy, et al., 1977). In the latter case electrophysiologic testing, which includes provocative atrial stimulation, may characterize the bypass tract, including its ability to conduct rapidly in atrial fibrillation and its response to drug therapy (Wellens and Durrer, 1974; Campbell, et al., 1977; Denes, et al., 1979).

Electrocardioversion in Atrial Fibrillation

The most common elective use of the direct current cardioverter is for the conversion of atrial fibrillation (Lown, 1967a; Resnekov and McDonald, 1968). Widespread experience has been accumulated since the introduction of cardioversion by Lown in 1962 (Selzer, et al., 1966; Lown, 1967a; Resnekov and McDonald, 1968; Resnekov, 1976; Mancini and Goldberger, 1982). Some researchers recommend starting at 50 joules and increasing incrementally by 50 joules until a 200-400 joule maximum is reached or conversion occurs. One advantage of starting with 200 joules is that one shock is usually sufficient. Cardioversion for atrial fibrillation after cardiac surgery is best deferred until the patient has convalesced for several weeks (Selzer, et al., 1965).

Concomitant drug therapy Controversy exists regarding the use of quinidine prior to cardioversion (Marriott and Myerburg, 1978). Some investigators have suggested that it causes an increase in postshock arrhythmias, while other researchers indicate that it suppresses arrhythmias (Lemberg, et al., 1964; Lown, 1967a; Resnekov and McDonald, 1968; Hartel, et al., 1974; Resnekov, 1974). However, it is clear that a substantial proportion (15%-43%) of patients' fibrillations will convert to sinus rhythm precardioversion on standard doses of quinidine (Lown, 1967a; Sodermark, et al., 1975). This may be reason enough to recommend pretreatment with the drug. Commonly, quinidine sulfate or gluconate is begun 12-48 hours before conversion. Quinidine sulfate, 200 mg every 2 hours for three doses, may be given the night before cardioversion, and another dose may be given 1-2 hours before the procedure the following morning. Alternatively, doses every 4-6 hours may be given if treatment is begun 24 or 48 hours prior to conversion. Gastrointestinal tolerance is sometimes better with the gluconate salt (330 mg equals 200 mg of sulfate). Maintenance antiarrhythmic therapy is continued after cardioversion. We attempt to maintain postconversion patients on doses of quinidine that achieve therapeutic levels, usually the equivalent of 1.2-1.6 grams of quinidine sulfate. If recurrent cardioversion from atrial fibrillation is required, propranolol may be added to quinidine for prophylaxis (20-40 mg four times a day). Disopyramide appears to be a reasonable alternative drug to quinidine.

Duration of fibrillation and conversion The duration of atrial fibrillation before cardioversion is important prognostically. When fibrillation has been present for longer than 1 year, 90% reversion by 12 months can be expected, as compared to 65% reversion if fibrillation has been present for less than 1 year (Lown, 1967a). Cardioversion is rarely useful in patients who have had atrial fibrillation for over 5 years and is only occasionally useful in those patients who have had atrial fibrillation for more than 1 year.

Left atrial size and electrocardioversion Atrial fibrillation is uncommon in patients with a normal-sized left atrium and occurs more frequently in patients with left atrial enlargement (Henry, et al., 1975). In addition, patients who have echocardiographic evidence of severe left atrial enlargement are unlikely to maintain sinus rhythm over the long term, even if initial cardioversion is successful.

Digitalis and electrocardioversion It is well known that overdigitalization may predispose the patient to postconversion ventricular arrhythmias (Kleiger and Lown, 1966). The administration of quinidine is now known to increase the serum digoxin concentration acutely. For these reasons it appears prudent to discontinue digoxin from 24 to 48 hours before cardioversion. If digitalis intoxication is suspected, cardioversion should be deferred or, if it is absolutely necessary, very low initial energy settings (5-12.5 joules) should be used (Lown, 1967a; Hagemeijer and Van Houwe, 1975). If ventricular arrhythmias appear at these low settings, 100 mg of lidocaine are given as a prophylaxis before proceeding. If these arrhythmias recur despite the lidocaine, cardioversion attempts should be stopped. Hypokalemia should be corrected in patients prior to cardioversion, particularly if these patients have received digitalis. Electrocardioversion in stable patients on therapeutic doses of digitalis appears to present little excess risk.

Pulmonary edema and electrocardioversion Pulmonary edema develops in a small proportion of patients (1%-3%) in the immediate postconversion period (Lown, 1967a; Resnekov and McDonald, 1967; Budow, et al., 1971). This interesting and distressing result has been attributed to either atrial functional paralysis despite normal electrical activity or transient left ventricular dysfunction. Careful observation and ECG monitoring are, therefore, recommended for 24 hours after conversion.

Myocardial damage and electrocardioversion Animal studies have indicated that high-energy electrical shocks may produce myocardial damage. Elevation in muscle enzymes has been well described after cardioversion in humans. However, specific creatine-kinase-MB enzyme elevations in patients have been modest and inconsistent (Ehsani, et al., 1976). In most cases cardioversion, when applied as recommended, is felt to cause minimal myocardial necrosis.

Peripheral embolization and electrocardioversion The incidence of peripheral embolization consequent to cardioversion is 1%-2% (Lown, 1967a; Budow, et al., 1971). Restoration of the sinus rhythm, rather than the electric shock per se, is felt to be responsible because a similar incidence occurs after quinidine-induced cardioversion. Bjerkelund and Orning (1969) described a 2% incidence of embolic episodes in patients who received the anticoagulant sodium warfarin at the time of conversion, as opposed to a 7% incidence in patients who were not given anticoagulants. The use of anticoagulants prior to cardioversion is thus recommended whenever possible (Mancini and Goldberger, 1982). This is particularly true when atrial fibrillation is of more than 2 weeks duration or when it is associated with large left atria, low output states, recent myocardial infarction, or rheumatic mitral valve stenosis. If anticoagulants are used to prevent emboli, they should probably be started at least 2-3 weeks prior to conversion. Anticoagulants should be maintained for at least 1-4 weeks after cardioversion because this is the period of highest risk for reversion (Bjerkelund and Orning, 1969; Budow, et al., 1971). Continuous anticoagulation therapy should be strongly considered in those patients with previous embolic events and a high risk of recurrence.

Anticoagulation in Chronic Atrial Fibrillation

Atrial fibrillation and the risk of systemic arterial embolization A high risk of systemic embolization may be associated with fibrillation of any cause, especially mitral valve disease and ischemic heart disease. Systemic embolization is a dreaded complication of mitral valve stenosis and atrial fibrillation. It has been estimated that 25%-30% of untreated adults with rheumatic heart disease die from systemic arterial emboli, and a much higher percentage of patients are disabled (Askey, 1960). Frequently, embolization is the first sign of mitral valve disease, and the first embolism is fatal in one-sixth of patients.

Casella and colleagues (1964) observed systemic emboli in 179 out of 1337 patients who had mitral valve stenosis. Those patients with embolisms were older, had lower cardiac indexes, and much higher incidences of atrial fibrillation (86%) than those patients without embolisms (33%). Another study reviewed systemic arterial emboli in 839 cases of mitral valve disease (Coulshed, et al., 1970). Emboli occurred during observation in 32% of patients with mitral valve stenosis and atrial fibrillation, as opposed to only 8% of those patients without atrial fibrillation. Increasing age is also a predisposing factor to embolization. In another study the left atrial size was examined before and after mitral valve operation (Fleming and Bailey, 1971). These researchers concluded that left atrial enlargement predisposed the patient to atrial fibrillation. Atrial fibrillation plus a cardiac index less than 2 L/min/m^2 was associated with embolization in 50% of patients. Also noting the association between increased left atrial size and the onset of atrial fibrillation, Henry and colleagues (1975) argued for prophylactic anticoagulation therapy in patients over 40 years of age whose left atrial size was greater than 45 mm because of the high incidence of emboli occurring within 1 month of the onset of atrial fibrillation. Fleming and Bailey (1971) followed 500 cases of mitral valve disease for an average of 9½ years. Thirty percent of these patients developed systemic arterial emboli, 56% of which were cerebral, 20% were peripheral, and 14% were visceral. A threefold increased risk of emboli accompanied patients who were in atrial fibrillation. Fraser and Turner (1955) found left atrial clots in 40% of patients (43 out of 106) in atrial fibrillation, as opposed to 2% of patients (3 out of 144) in sinus rhythm coming to valvulotomy for mitral valve stenosis.

Hinton and colleagues (1977) studied 333 patients who manifested atrial fibrillation at the time of death. Autopsy evidence for systemic emboli was found in 41% of patients with mitral valve disease, 35% of patients with ischemic heart disease, 24% of patients with hypertensive heart disease, and 17% of patients with other diseases. In contrast, only 7% of patients with ischemic heart disease without atrial fibrillation showed signs of systemic emboli. Of note, 73% of embolization was to the brain. Szekely (1964) calculated a sevenfold excess risk for systemic emboli in patients with atrial fibrillation, irrespective of the degree of underlying mitral valve disease. Wolf and colleagues (1976) noted a sixfold increase in the risk of stroke with atrial fibrillation in the absence of rheumatic heart disease. Another study noted 26 emboli in 262 patients with atrial fibrillation associated with thyrotoxicosis, which is a higher prevalence than previously noted (Staffurth, et al., 1977).

In another larger autopsy series (642 cases of atrial fibrillation) systemic arterial emboli were found in association with ischemic, hypertensive, or valvular heart disease in 42%-52% of patients, as opposed to 18% of controls (Aberg, 1969). Seventy-seven percent of these emboli were cerebral. In consecutive surgical studies of peripheral arterial emboli atrial fibrillation was present in 73% of patients, 50% of whom had mitral valve disease and 50% coronary artery disease. Atrial fibrillation per se was thus emphasized as a risk factor (Darling, et al., 1967).

To summarize, overwhelming evidence has accumulated implicating atrial fibrillation both with and without associated mitral valve disease as a potent risk factor for systemic, particularly cerebral, embolization. As might be expected, a number of researchers have indicated the need for reevaluation of anticoagulant therapy to emphasize a more aggressive approach.

Anticoagulant therapy in atrial fibrillation Anticoagulation therapy with sodium warfarin (Coumadin) decreases the thromboembolic complications of atrial fibrillation, although supporting data are not extensive (Askey and Cherry, 1950; Freeman and Wexler, 1963; Owren, 1963; Szekely, 1964). In a Norwegian study patients who received anticoagulants after a first arterial embolism experienced one recurrence in 90 patient-years, as opposed to 22 recurrences in 81 patient-years in an untreated group (Owren, 1963). Fleming and Bailey (1971) reported one death from anticoagulant therapy in 649 patient-years (117 patients) and a 2.3% incidence of minor morbidity. Thus, the risk is felt to be sufficiently low to recommend therapy. Where anticoagulation can be safely administered, patients with atrial fibrillation who have experienced one embolism are candidates for long-term anticoagulation with sodium warfarin. A prothrombin time of 25%-30% of control is usually sought. Contraindications to anticoagulant therapy include a history of a bleeding disorder or major gastrointestinal or cerebral hemorrhage. A prothrombin time of 30%-50% is sometimes accepted when relative contraindications are present.

Controversy exists as to whether all patients with atrial fibrillation and mitral valve stenosis should receive anticoagulants even in the absence of a history of embolization. The high risk of embolization pointed up by the many studies discussed in this chapter has persuaded many centers, including our own, to administer anticoagulants to these patients prophylactically. Approximately a 1% per year incidence of mortality or serious morbidity caused by anticoagulants must be accepted. In addition, we give anticoagulants to patients with atrial fibrillation and low cardiac output, such as those with advanced heart failure resulting from ischemic or primary myocardial disease (DeMaria, et al., 1975). These patients are at risk for both pulmonary and peripheral emboli. We do not routinely administer anticoagulants to other patients with atrial fibrillation or mitral valve disease before the onset of atrial fibrillation. However, studies testing the risk:benefit ratio in these situations should be performed. Some researchers now recommend long-term anticoagulation therapy for patients with atrial fibrillation caused by coronary artery disease as well as by mitral valve disease (Fowler, 1977).

Antiplatelet agents (i.e., aspirin, dipyridamole, or sulfinpyrazone) are currently attracting attention as safer, alternative prophylactic agents for thromboembolism (Weiss, 1978). They have been used as alternative agents alone or in addition to sodium warfarin in several clinical settings with variable success to date. However, further prospective studies will be required to establish firmly the usefulness of these agents in preventing thromboembolism in patients with atrial fibrillation.

REFERENCES

Aberg, H. 1968. Atrial fibrillation. *Acta. Med. Scand.* 184:425.

Aberg, H. 1969. Atrial fibrillation. I. A study of atrial thrombosis and systemic embolism in a necropsy material. *Acta. Med. Scand.* 185:373.

Agarwal, B. L.; Agarwal, B. V.; and Agarwal, R. K. 1972. Atrial flutter, a rare manifestation of digitalis intoxication. *Br. Heart J.* 34:392.

Allessie, M. A.; Bouke, F. I. M.; and Schopman, F. J. G. 1976. Circus movement in rabbit atrial muscles as a mechanism of tachycardia. *Circ. Res.* 39:168.

Anderson, J. L.; Harrison, D. C.; Meffin, P. J., et al. 1978. Antiarrhythmic drugs: clinical pharmacology and therapeutic uses. *Drugs* 15:271.

Askey, J. M. 1960. Management of rheumatic heart disease in relation to systemic arterial emboli (a review). *Prog. Cardiovasc. Dis.* 3:220.

Askey, J. M.; Cherry, C. B. 1950. Continuous anticoagulant therapy. *J.A.M.A.* 114:97-100.

Bailey, G. W. H.; Braniff, B. A.; Hancock, W., et al. 1968. Relation of left atrial pathology to atrial fibrillation in mitral valvular disease. *Ann. Intern. Med.* 69:13.

Bellet, S. 1971. *Clinical disorders of the heart beat.* 3d ed. Philadelphia: Lea and Febiger. pp. 206-250.

Benchimol, A.; Lowe, H. M.; Alere, P. R. 1965. Cardiovascular response to exercise during atrial fibrillation and after conversion to sinus rhythm. *Am. J. Cardiol.* 16:31-41.

Berlinerblau, R.; and Feder, W. 1972. Chaotic atrial rhythm. *J. Electrocardiol.* 5(2):135-144.

Besoain-Santander, M.; Pick, A.; Langendorf, R. 1950. A-V conduction in auricular flutter. *Circulation* 2:604.

Bjerkelund, C. J.; and Orning, O. M. 1969. The efficacy of anticoagulant therapy in preventing pulmonary embolism related to (DC) electrical conversion of atrial fibrillation. *Am. J. Cardiol.* 23:208-216.

Braunwald, E.; Frey, R. L.; Aygen, M. M., et al. 1960. Studies on Starling's law of the heart. III. Observations in patients with mitral stenosis and atrial fibrillation on the relationships between left ventricular end-diastolic segment length, filling pressure, and the characteristics of ventricular contraction. *J. Clin. Invest.* 39:1874-1884.

Budow, J.; Natarojan, P.; and Kroop, I. 1971. Pulmonary edema following direct current cardioversion for atrial arrhythmias. *J.A.M.A.* 218:1803-1805.

Busby, D. E.; and Davis, A. W. 1976. Paroxysmal and chronic atrial fibrillation in airman certification. *Aviat. Space Environmental Med.* 47:185-186.

Buxton, A. E.; Rastor, J. A.; and Josephson, M. E. 1979. Role of P wave duration as a predictor of postoperative atrial arrhythmias. *Chest* 80(1): 68-73.

Byrne-Quinn, E.; and Wing, A. J. 1970. Maintenance of sinus rhythm after direct current reversion of atrial fibrillation. *Br. Heart J.* 32:370-376.

Campbell, M.; Neill, C.; and Suzman, S. 1957. Prognosis of atrial septal defect. *Br. Med. J.* 1:1375-1383.

Campbell, R. W. F.; Smith, R.; and Gallagher, J. J. 1977. Atrial fibrillation in the preexcitation syndrome. *Am. J. Cardiol.* 40:514-520.

Casella, L.; Abelmann, W.; and Ellis, L. 1964. Patients with mitral stenosis and systemic emboli. *Arch. Intern. Med.* 114:773-781.

Chopra, D.; Janson, P.; and Sawin, C. T. 1977. Insensitivity to digoxin associated with hypocalcemia. *N. Engl. J. Med.* 296:917-918.

Chung, E. K. 1971. Appraisal of multifocal atrial tachycardia. *Br. Heart J.* 33:500-504.

Chung, E. K. 1977. *Principles of cardiac arrhythmias.* Second ed. Baltimore: Williams and Wilkins, Co.

Clark, A. N. G. 1977. Multifocal atrial tachycardia (MAT), the misdiagnosed atrial arrhythmia of old age. *Gerontology* 23:445-451.

Class, R. N. 1957. Transient atrial fibrillation: a frequent occurrence in apparently normal hearts. *U.S. Armed Forces Med. J.* 8:1-13.

Cohen, S. I.; Lau, S. H.; Berkowitz, W. D., et al. 1970. Concealed conduction during atrial fibrillation. *Am. J. Cardiol.* 25:416-419.

Cooper, T. B.; Coghlan, H. C.; Plumb, V. J., et al. 1979a. Clonidine therapy for supraventricular tachyarrhythmias (abstract). *Am. J. Cardiol.* 43:430.

Cooper, T. B.; Griffith, M.; Plumb, V. J., et al. 1979b. Onset of classical atrial flutter—studies in man following open heart surgery (abstract). *Am. J. Cardiol.* 43:388.

Corazza, L. J.; and Pastor, B. H. 1958. Cardiac arrhythmias in chronic cor pulmonale. *N. Engl. J. Med.* 259:862-865.

Coulshed, N.; Epstein, E. J.; MacKendrick, C. C., et al. 1970. Systemic embolism in mitral valve disease. *Br. Heart J.* 32:26-34.

Cranefield, P. F. 1977. Action potentials, afterpotentials, and arrhythmias. *Circ. Res.* 41:415-423.

Daley, R.; McMillan, I. K. R.; and Gorlin, R. 1965. Mitral incompetence in experimental auricular fibrillation. *Lancet* 2:18.

Dalton, J. C.; Pearson, R. J.; and White, P. D. 1956. Constrictive pericarditis: a review and long-term follow-up of 78 cases. *Ann. Intern. Med.* 45:445-458.

Darling, R. C.; Austen, W. G.; and Linton, R. R. 1967. Arterial embolism. *Surg. Gynecol. Obstet.* 124:106-114.

Das, G.; Anand, K. M.; Ankineedu, K., et al. 1978. Atrial pacing for conversion of atrial flutter in digitalized patients. *Am. J. Cardiol.* 41:308-312.

David, D.; DiSegni, E.; Klein, H. O., et al. 1979. Inefficacy of digitalis in the control of heart rate in patients with chronic atrial fibrillation: beneficial effect of an added beta-adrenergic blocking agent. *Am. J. Cardiol.* 44:1378-1382.

D'Cruz, I. A.; Mehta, A. B.; Kelkar, P. N., et al. 1974. Benign repetitive multifocal ectopic atrial tachycardia: response to intracardiac atrial stimulation. *Am. Heart J.* 88:671-672.

DeMaria, A.; Lies, J.; King, J., et al. 1975. Echocardiographic assessment of atrial transport, mitral movement, and ventricular performance following electroversion of atrial arrhythmias. *Circulation* 51:273-282.

Denes, P.; Wu, D.; Amat-y-leon, F., et al. 1979. Paroxysmal supraventricular tachycardia induction in patients with Wolff-Parkinson-White syndrome. *Ann. Intern. Med.* 90:153-157.

DeSanctis, R. W.; Block, P.; and Hutter, A. M. 1972. Tachyarrhythmias in myocardial infarction. *Circulation* 45:681-702.

Desser, K. B.; DeSa'Neto, A.; and Benchimol, A. 1979. Hearts that go thump in the night. Positional atrial flutter in a patient with mitral valve prolapse. *N. Engl. J. Med.* 300:717-718.

Ehsani, A.; Ewy, G.; and Sobel, B. 1976. Effects of electrical countershock on serum creatine phosphokinase (CPK) isoenzyme activity. *Am. J. Cardiol.* 37:12-18.

Ellrodt, G.; Chew, C. Y. C.; and Singh, B. N. 1980. Therapeutic implications of slow-channel blockade in cardiocirculatory disorders. *Circulation* 62:669-679.

Engel, T. R.; and Gonzalez, A. D. C. 1978. Effects of digitalis on atrial vulnerability. *Am. J. Cardiol.* 42:570-576.

Evans, W.; and Swann, P. 1954. Lone auricular fibrillation. *Br. Heart J.* 16:189-194.

Ferrer, M. I. 1974. *The sick sinus syndrome.* New York: Futura Publishing Co.

Fleming, H. A.; and Bailey, S. M. 1971. Mitral valve disease, systemic embolism, and anticoagulants. *Postgrad. Med. J.* 47:599-604.

Forfar, J. C.; Miller, H. C.; and Toft, A. D. 1979. Occult thyrotoxicosis: a correctable cause of "idiopathic" atrial fibrillation. *Am. J. Cardiol.* 44:9-12.

Fors, W. J.; Vander Ark, C. R.; and Reynolds, F. W. 1971. Evaluation of propranolol and quinidine in treatment in quinidine-resistant arrhythmias. *Am. J. Cardiol.* 27:190-194.

Fosmoe, R. J.; Averill, K. H.; and Lamb, L. E. 1960. Electrocardiographic findings in 67,375 asymptomatic subjects. II. Supraventricular arrhythmias. *Am. J. Cardiol.* 6:84-95.

Fowler, N. O. 1977. *Cardiac arrhythmias, diagnosis and treatment.* Second ed. Maryland: Harper and Row, Inc. pp. 65-75.

Fraser, H. R. L.; and Turner, R. W. D. 1955. Auricular fibrillation. *Br. Med. J.* 2:1414-1418.

Freeman, I.; and Wexler, J. 1963. Anticoagulants for treatment of atrial fibrillation. *J.A.M.A.* 184:1007-1018.

Friedberg, C. K. 1966. *Diseases of the heart.* Third ed. Philadelphia: W. B. Saunders Co.

Frieden, J.; Rosenblum, R.; Enselberg, C. D., et al. 1968. Propranolol treatment of chronic intractable supraventricular arrhythmias. *Am. J. Cardiol.* 22:711-717.

Friedman, P. L.; Brugoda, P.; Kuck, K-H, et al. 1982. Inter- and intra-atrial dissociation during spontaneous atrial flutter: evidence for a focal origin of the arrhythmia. *Am. J. Cardiol.* 50:756-761.

Frishman, W. 1979. Efficacy of a new beta-adrenergic blocking agent (pindolol) in the acute and chronic therapy of supraventricular arrhythmia (abstract). *Am. J. Cardiol.* 43:431.

Fujiia, J.; Foster, J. R.; Mills, P. G., et al. 1978. Dual echocardiographic determination of atrial contraction sequence in atrial flutter and other related atrial arrhythmias. *Circulation* 58:314-321.

Gajewski, J.; and Singer, R. B. 1979. Mortality in atrial fibrillation (abstract). *Circulation* 60(4):II-52.

Goldman, S.; Probst, P.; Selzer, A., et al. 1975. Inefficacy of "therapeutic" serum levels of digoxin in controlling the ventricular rate in atrial fibrillation. *Am. J. Cardiol.* 35:651-655.

Gouaux, J. L.; and Ashman, R. 1947. Auricular fibrillation with aberration simulating ventricular paroxysmal tachycardia. *Am. Heart J.* 34:366-373.

Gould, W. L. 1957. Auricular fibrillation. Report of a study of a familial tendency. *Arch. Intern. Med.* 100:916-926.

Greenberg, M. A.; Herman, L. S.; and Cohen, M. V. 1979. Mitral valve closure in atrial flutter. *Circulation* 59:902-909.

Guiney, T. E.; and Lown, B. 1972. Electrical conversion of atrial flutter to atrial fibrillation. *Br. Heart J.* 34:1215-1224.

Hagemeijer, F. 1978. Verapamil in the management of supraventricular tachyarrhythmias occurring after a recent myocardial infarction. *Circulation* 57:751-755.

Hagemeijer, F.; and Van Houwe, E. 1975. Titrated energy cardioversion of patients on digitalis. *Br. Heart J.* 37:1303-1307.

Hager, W. D.; Fenster, P.; Mayersohn, M., et al. 1979. Digoxin-quinidine interaction. Pharmacokinetic evaluation. *N. Engl. J. Med.* 300:1238-1241.

Hall, J.; and Wood, D. 1968. Factors affecting cardioversion of atrial arrhythmias with special reference to quinidine. *Br. Heart J.* 30:84-90.

Harrison, D. C.; Griffin, J. R.; and Fiene, T. J. 1965. Effects of beta-adrenergic blockade with propranolol in patients with atrial arrhythmias. *N. Engl. J. Med.* 273:410-415.

Hartel, G.; Louhija, A.; and Konttinen, A. 1974. Disopyramide in prevention of recurrence of atrial fibrillation after electroconversion. *Clin. Pharmacol. Ther.* 15:551-555.

Harvey, R. N.; Ferrer, M. I.; Richards, D. W., et al. 1955. Cardiocirculatory performance in atrial flutter. *Circulation* 12:506-519.

Hecht, H. H. 1953. The mechanism of auricular fibrillation and flutter. *Circulation* 7:594-600.

Heng, M. K.; Singh, B. N.; Roche, A. H., et al. 1975. Effects of verapamil on cardiac arrhythmias and on the electrocardiogram. *Am. Heart J.* 90: 487-498.

Henry, W. L.; Morganroth, J.; Pearlman, A. S., et al. 1975. Relation between echocardiographically determined left atrial size and atrial fibrillation. *Circulation* 53:273-279.

Hinton, R. C.; Kistler, J. P.; Fallon, J. T., et al. 1977. Influence of etiology of atrial fibrillation on incidence of systemic embolism. *Am. J. Cardiol.* 40:509-513.

Hoffman, B. F.; Cranefield, P. F.; and Stuckey, J. H. 1961. Concealed conduction. *Circ. Res.* 9:194-203.

Hoffman, B. F.; Rosen, M. R.; and Wit, A. L. 1975. Electrophysiology and pharmacology of cardiac arrhythmias. VII. Cardiac effects of quinidine and procainamide. *Am. Heart J.* 89:804-808 and 90:117-122.

Homcy, C. J.; Lorell, B.; and Yurchak, P. M. 1979. Atrial flutter with exit block. *Circulation* 60:711-714.

Hunt, D.; Sloman, G.; and Penington, C. 1978. Effects of atrial fibrillation on prognosis of acute myocardial infarction. *Br. Heart J.* 40:303-307.

Hurst, J. W.; and Myerburg, R. J. 1968. Cardiac arrhythmias: evolving concepts. *Mod. Concepts Cardiovasc. Dis.* 37:73-78.

Hurst, J. W.; Paulk, E. A.; Proctor, H. D., et al. 1964. Management of patients with atrial fibrillation. *Am. J. Med.* 37:728-741.

Ikram, H.; Nixon, P. G. F.; and Arcan, T. 1968. Left atrial function after electrical conversion to sinus rhythm. *Br. Heart J.* 30:80-83.

Inone, H.; Matsuo, H.; Takayanayi, K., et al. 1981. Clinical and experimental studies of the effects of atrial extrastimulation and rapid pacing on atrial flutter cycle. *Am. J. Cardiol.* 48:623-631.

Jenkins, J. M.; Wu, D.; and Arzbaecher, R. C. 1979. Computer diagnosis of supraventricular and ventricular arrhythmias. A new esophageal technique. *Circulation* 60:977-985.

Jennings, P. B.; Makous, N.; and Vander Veer, J. B. 1958. Reversion of atrial fibrillation to sinus rhythm during digitalis therapy. *Am. J. Med. Sci.* 235:702-705.

Jewitt, D. E.; Balcon, R.; Raftery, E. D., et al. 1967. Incidence and management of supraventricular arrhythmias after acute myocardial infarction. *Lancet* 2:734-738.

Josephson, M. E.; and Kastor, J. A. 1977. Supraventricular tachycardia: mechanisms and management. *Ann. Intern. Med.* 87:346-358.

Julian, D. G.; Valentine, P. A.; and Miller, G. G. 1964. Disturbances of rate, rhythm, and conduction in acute myocardial infarction. *Am. J. Med.* 37:915-927.

Kahn, D. R.; Wilson, W. S.; Weber, W., et al. 1964. Hemodynamic studies before and after cardioversion. *J. Thoracic Cardiovasc. Surg.* 48:898-905.

Kannel, W. B.; Abbott, R. D.; Savage, D. D., et al. 1982. Epidemiologic features of chronic atrial fibrillation: the Framingham study. *N. Engl. J. Med.* 306:1018-1021.

Kaplan, M. A.; Gray, R. E.; and Iseri, L. T. 1968. Metabolic and hemodynamic responses to exercise during atrial fibrillation and sinus rhythm. *Am. J. Cardiol.* 22:543-549.

Kaplan, B. M.; Langendorf, R.; Lev, M., et al. 1973. Tachycardia-bradycardia syndrome (so-called "sick sinus syndrome"). *Am. J. Cardiol.* 31:497-508.

Katz, L. N.; and Pick, A. 1953. The mechanism of auricular flutter and auricular fibrillation. *Circulation* 7:601-606.

Katz, L. N.; and Pick, A. 1956. *Clinical electrocardiography. Part I: The arrhythmias.* Philadelphia: Lea & Febiger.

Kennelly, B. M.; and Lane, G. K. 1978. Electrophysiologic studies in four patients with atrial flutter and 1:1 atrioventricular conduction. *Am. Heart J.* 96:723-730.

Killip, T.; and Baer, R. A. 1964. Cardiac function before and after electrical conversion from atrial fibrillation to sinus rhythm. *Clin. Res.* 12:175-179.

Killip, T.; and Gault, J. H. 1965. Mode of onset of atrial fibrillation. *Am. Heart J.* 70:172-179.

Kleiger, R.; and Lown, B. 1966. Cardioversion and digitalis. II. Clinical studies. *Circulation* 33:878-887.

Klein, G. J.; Sealy, W. C.; Pritchett, E. L. C., et al. 1980. Cryosurgical ablation of the atrioventricular node-His bundle, long-term follow-up and properties of the junctional pacemaker. *Circulation* 61:8-15.

Klein, H. O.; and Kaplinsky, E. 1982. Verapamil and digoxin: their respective effects on atrial fibrillation. *Am. J. Cardiol.* 50:895-912.

Koch-Weser, J. 1979. Drug therapy: disopyramide. *N. Engl. J. Med.* 300: 957-962.

Kosowsky, B. D.; Scherlag, B. J.; and Damato, A. N. 1968. Reevaluation of the atrial contribution to ventricular function. Study using His bundle pacing. *Am. J. Cardiol.* 21:518-524.

Kowey, P. R.; DeSilva, R. A.; and Lown, B. 1979. Sustained atrial fibrillation as a rhythm of choice (abstract). *Circulation* 60(4):II-253.

Lamb, L. E.; and Pollard, L. W. 1964. Atrial fibrillation in flying personnel. Report of 60 cases. *Circulation* 29:694-701.

Langendorf, R.; and Pick, A. 1966. Cardiac arrhythmias in infants and children. In *Heart disease in children.* B. M. Gasul; R. A. Archilla; M. Lev, editors. Philadelphia: J. B. Lippincott Co. pp. 121.

Langendorf, R.; Pick, A.; and Winternitz, M. 1955. Mechanism of intermittent ventricular bigeminy. I. Appearance of ectopic beats dependent upon the length of the ventricular cycle, the "rule of bigeminy." *Circulation* 11:422-430.

Langendorf, R.; Pick, A.; and Katz, L. N. 1965. Ventricular response in atrial fibrillation. Role of concealed conduction in the AV junction. *Circulation* 32:69-75.

Leahey, E. B.; Reiffel, J. A.; Drusin, R. E., et al. 1978. Interaction between quinidine and digoxin. *J.A.M.A.* 240:533-544.

Lequime, J. 1942. Circulatory disturbance in pathologic conditions with high heart rates. *Cardiologica* 5:105-112.

Lemberg, L.; Castellanos, A.; and Swenson, J. 1964. Arrhythmias related to cardioversion. *Circulation* 30:163-170.

Lemberg, L.; Castellanos, A.; and Arcebal, A. G. 1970. The use of propranolol in arrhythmias complicating acute myocardial infarction. *Am. Heart J.* 80:479-487.

Levi, G. L.; and Proto, C. 1972. Combined treatment of atrial fibrillation with quinidine and beta-blockers. *Br. Heart J.* 34:911-914.

Levi, G.; Proto, C.; and Rovetta, A. 1973. Double-blind evaluation of practolol and quinidine in the treatment of chronic atrial fibrillation. *Cardiology* 58:364-368.

Lewis, T. 1918-20. Observations upon flutter and fibrillation. Theory of circus movement. *Heart* 7:293.

Liberthson, R. R.; Salisbury, K. W.; Hutter, A. M., et al. 1976. Atrial tachyarrhythmias in acute myocardial infarction. *Am. J. Med.* 60:956-960.

Lipson, J. J.; and Naimi, S. 1970. Multifocal atrial tachycardia (chaotic atrial tachycardia). *Circulation* 2:397-407.

Lister, J. W.; Gosselin, A. J.; Sayfre, E. J., et al. 1976. *Arrhythmia analysis by intracardiac electrocardiography*. Illinois: Charles C. Thomas Co., pp. 53.

Lown, B. 1967a. Electrical reversion of cardiac arrhythmias. *Br. Heart J.* 29:469-489.

Lown, B. 1967b. Unresolved problems in coronary care. *Am. J. Cardiol.* 20:494-508.

Lucchesi, B. R. 1977. *Antiarrhythmic drugs in cardiovascular pharmacology*. M. Antonaccio, editor. New York: Raven Press. pp. 269.

Luoma, P. V.; Kujala, P. A.; Juustila, H. J., et al. 1978. Efficacy of intravenous disopyramide in termination of supraventricular arrhythmias. *J. Clin. Pharmacol.* 18:293-301.

Mancini, G. B. J.; and Goldberger, A. L. 1982. Cardioversion of atrial fibrillation: consideration of embolization, anticoagulation, prophylactic pacemaker, and long-term success. *Am. Heart J.* 104:617-621.

Marriott, H. J. L.; and Sandler, J. A. 1966. Criteria, old and new, for differentiating between ectopic ventricular beats and aberrant ventricular conduction in the presence of atrial fibrillation. *Prog. Cardiovasc. Dis.* 9:18.

Marriott, H. J. L.; and Myerburg, R. J. 1978. *Recognition and treatment of cardiac arrhythmias and conduction disturbances in the heart.* Fourth ed. J. W. Hurst, editor. New York: McGraw-Hill Co.

Martin, A.; and Lamb, R. 1979. Maintenance digoxin. *Lancet* 1:825.

Mason, D. T. 1974. Digitalis pharmacology and therapeutics. *Ann. Intern. Med.* 80:520.

McIntosh, H. D.; Kong, Y.; and Morris, J. J. 1964. Hemodynamic effects of supraventricular arrhythmias. *Am. J. Med.* 37:712.

Meltzer, L. E.; and Kitchell, J. B. 1966. The incidence of arrhythmias associated with acute myocardial infarction. *Prog. Cardiovasc. Dis.* 9: 50-63.

Mirowski, M.; and Alkan, W. J. 1967. Left atrial impulse formation in atrial flutter. *Br. Heart J.* 29:299-304.

Mitchell, J. H.; and Shapiro, W. 1969. Atrial function and hemodynamic consequences of atrial fibrillation in man. *Am. J. Cardiol.* 23:556-567.

Moe, G. K.; and Abildskov, J. A. 1959. Atrial fibrillation as a self-sustaining arrhythmia independent of focal discharge. *Am. Heart J.* 58:59-70.

Moore, E. N.; Fisher, G.; Detweiler, O. K., et al. 1962. *The importance of atrial mass in the maintenance of atrial fibrillation. Proceedings of the International Symposium on Comparative Medicine.* New York: Eaton Labs. pp. 229-238.

Morris, J. J.; Entman, M. L.; North, N. C., et al. 1964. The changes in cardiac output with reversion of atrial fibrillation to sinus rhythm. *Circulation* 31:670-678.

Neporent, L. M. 1964. Atrial heart sounds in atrial fibrillation and flutter. *Circulation* 30:893-896.

Normand, J. P.; Legendre, M.; Kahn, J. C., et al. 1976. Comparative efficiency of short-acting and long-acting quinidine for maintenance of sinus rhythm after electrical conversion of atrial fibrillation. *Br. Heart J.* 38: 381-387.

Oram, S. 1963. Conversion of atrial fibrillation to sinus rhythm by direct current shock. *Lancet* 2:159-162.

Orlando, J.; Cassidy, J.; and Aronnow, W. S. 1977. High reversion of atrial flutter to sinus rhythm after atrial pacing in patients with pulmonary disease. *Chest* 71:580-582.

Ostrander, L. D.; Brandt, R. L.; Kjelsberg, M. O., et al. 1965. Electrocardiographic findings among the adult population of a total natural community, Tecumseh, Michigan. *Circulation* 31:888-898.

Owren, P. A. 1963. The results of anticoagulant therapy in Norway. *Arch. Intern. Med.* 111:240-247.

Pastelin, G.; Mendez, R.; and Moe, G. K. 1978. Participation of atrial specialized conduction pathways in atrial flutter. *Circ. Res.* 42:386-393.

Patton, R. D.; and Helfant, R. H. 1969. Atrial flutter with one-to-one conduction. *Chest* 55:250-252.

Peter, R. H.; Gracey, J. G.; and Beach, T. B. 1968. A clinical profile of idiopathic atrial fibrillation. *Ann. Intern. Med.* 68:1288-1295.

Phair, W. B. 1963. Familial atrial fibrillation. *Can. Med. Assoc. J.* 89: 1274-1276.

Phillips, J.; Spano, J.; and Burch, G. 1969. Chaotic atrial mechanism. *Am. Heart J.* 78:171-179.

Pittman, D. E.; Makar, J. S.; Kooros, K. S., et al. 1973. Rapid atrial stimulation: successful method of conversion of atrial flutter and atrial tachycardia. *Am. J. Cardiol.* 32:700-706.

Priest, M. F.; Cooper, T. B.; MacLean, W. A. H., et al. 1979. Nature of onset of atrial fibrillation in man (abstract). *Circulation* 60(4):II-254.

Prinzmetal, M. 1953. The mechanism of spontaneous auricular flutter and fibrillation in man. *Circulation* 7:607-611.

Reale, A. 1965. Acute effects of countershock conversion of atrial fibrillation upon right and left heart hemodynamics. *Circulation* 32:214-222.

Resnekov, L. 1967. Hemodynamic studies before and after electrical conversion of atrial fibrillation and flutter to sinus rhythm. *Br. Heart J.* 29:700-708.

Resnekov, L. 1974. Drug therapy before and after electroversion of cardiac dysrhythmias. *Prog. Cardiovasc. Dis.* 16:531-538.

Resnekov, L. R. 1976. Theory and practice of electroversion of cardiac dysrhythmias. *Med. Clin. North Am.* 60:325-342.

Resnekov, L.; and McDonald, L. 1967. Complications in 220 patients with cardiac dysrhythmias treated by phased direct current shock and indications for electrocardioversion. *Br. Heart J.* 29:926-936.

Resnekov, L.; and McDonald, L. 1968. Appraisal of electrocardioversion in treatment of cardiac dysrhythmias. *Br. Heart J.* 30:786-811.

Reynolds, E. W.; and Vander Ark, C. R. 1976. Quinidine syncope and the delayed repolarization syndromes. *Mod. Concepts Cardiovasc. Dis.* 45:117-122.

Ricci, D. R.; Orlick, A. E.; Reitz, B. A., et al. 1978. Depressant effect of digoxin on atrioventricular conduction in man. *Circulation* 57:898-903.

Rodman, T.; Pastor, B. H.; and Figueroa, W. 1966. Effect on cardiac output of conversion from atrial fibrillation to normal sinus mechanism. *Am. J. Med.* 41:249-258.

Rosen, K. M.; Lau, S. H.; and Damato, A. N. 1969. Simulation of atrial flutter by rapid coronary sinus pacing. *Am. Heart J.* 78:635-642.

Rosenbaum, M. B.; Chiale, P. A.; Halpern, M. S., et al. 1976. Clinical efficacy of amiodarone as an antiarrhythmic agent. *Am. J. Cardiol.* 38: 934-944.

Schaal, S. F.; and Leier, C. V. 1978. Atrial electrograms of coarse atrial fibrillation and flutter-fibrillation (abstract). *Am. J. Cardiol.* 41:443.

Schaeffer, A. H.; Greene, H. L.; Pendleton, A. R., et al. 1979. Comparative efficacy of aprindine in the management of refractory atrial fibrillation and flutter (abstract). *Am. J. Cardiol.* 43:430.

Schaffer, A. I.; Blumenfeld, S.; Pitman, E. R., et al. 1951. Procainamide: its effect on auricular arrhythmias. *Am. Heart J.* 42:115-123.

Schamroth, L. 1971. *The disorders of cardiac rhythm.* Philadelphia: F. A. Davis Co. pp. 58-62.

Schamroth, L.; Krikler, D. M.; and Garrett, C. 1972. Immediate effects of intravenous verapamil in cardiac arrhythmias. *Br. Med. J.* 1:660-662

Scherf, D. 1947. Studies on auricular tachycardia caused by aconitine administration. *Proc. Soc. Exper. Biol. Med.* 64:233-239.

Scott, M. E.; and Patterson, G. C. 1969. Cardiac output after direct current conversion of atrial fibrillation. *Br. Heart J.* 31:87-90.

Sealy, W. C.; Anderson, R. W.; and Gallagher, J. J. 1977. Surgical treatment of supraventricular arrhythmias. *J. Thoracic Cardiovasc. Surg.* 73: 511-522.

Selzer, A.; and Wray, H. W. 1964. Quinidine syncope. *Circulation* 30: 17-26.

Selzer, A.; Kelly, J. J.; Gerbode, F., et al. 1965. Treatment of atrial fibrillation after surgical repair of the mitral valve. *Ann. Intern. Med.* 62: 1213-1222.

Selzer, A.; Kelly, J. J.; Johnson, R. B., et al. 1966. Immediate and long-term results of electrical conversion of arrhythmias. *Prog. Cardiovasc. Dis.* 9:90-104.

Shapiro, W.; and Klein, G. 1968. Alterations in cardiac function immediately following electrical conversion of atrial fibrillation to normal sinus rhythm. *Circulation* 38:1074-1084.

Sherrid, M. V.; Clark, R. D.; and Cohn, K. 1979. Echocardiographic analysis of left atrial size before and after operation in mitral valve disease. *Am. J. Cardiol.* 43:171-178.

Shine, K. I.; Kastor, J. A.; and Yurchak, P. M. 1968. Multifocal atrial tachycardia. *N. Engl. J. Med.* 279:344-349.

Singh, B. N.; and Jewitt, D. E. 1974. Beta-adrenergic receptor blocking drugs in cardiac arrhythmias. *Drugs* 7:426-461.

Singh, B. N.; Ellrodt, G.; and Peter, C. T. 1978. Verapamil: a review of its pharmacological properties and therapeutic use. *Drugs* 15:169-197.

Skinner, N. S.; Mitchell, J. H.; Wallace, A. G., et al. 1963. Hemodynamic effects of altering the timing of atrial systole. *Am. J. Physiol.* 205:499-503.

Smith, T. W.; and Haber, E. 1963. Digitalis. *N. Engl. J. Med.* 289:945-1063.

Sodermark, T.; Jonsson, B.; Olsson, A., et al. 1975. Effect of quinidine on maintaining sinus rhythm after conversion of atrial fibrillation or flutter. *Br. Heart J.* 37:486-492.

Staffurth, J. S.; Gibberd, M. G.; and Fui, S. T. 1977. Arterial embolism in thyrotoxicosis with atrial fibrillation. *Br. Med. J.* 2:688-690.

Stemple, D. R. 1977. Benign slow paroxysmal atrial tachycardia. *Ann. Intern. Med.* 87:44-48.

Stessman, J.; and Bassan, M. M. 1979. Verapamil for atrial flutter/fibrillation. *Circulation* 60:964-965.

Sung, R. J.; Castellanos, A.; Mallon, S. M., et al. 1977. Mechanisms of spontaneous alternation between reciprocating tachycardia and atrial flutter-fibrillation in Wolff-Parkinson-White syndrome. *Circulation* 56: 409-416.

Szekely, P. 1964. Systemic embolism and anticoagulant prophylaxis in rheumatic heart disease. *Br. Med. J.* 1:1209-1212.

Szekely, P.; Sideris, A.; and Batson, G. 1970. Maintenance of sinus rhythm after atrial defibrillation. *Br. Heart J.* 32:741-746.

Takkunen, J.; Oilinki, O.; Salokannel, J., et al. 1970. Mortality of patients with atrial fibrillation of (DC) countershock therapy. *Acta Med. Scand.* 188:127-131.

Waldo, A. L.; MacLean, W. A. H.; Karp, R. B., et al. 1977. Entrainment and interruption of atrial flutter with atrial pacing: studies in man following open heart surgery. *Circulation* 56:737-745.

Wang, K.; Goldfarb, B. L.; Gobel, F. L., et al. 1977. Multifocal atrial tachycardia. *Arch. Intern. Med.* 137:161-164.

Watson, D. C.; Henry, W. L.; Epstein, S. E., et al. 1977. Effects of operation on left atrial size and the occurrence of atrial fibrillation in patients with hypertrophic subaortic stenosis. *Circulation* 55:178-181.

Watson, R. M.; and Josephson, M. E. 1980. Atrial flutter. I. Electrophysiologic substrates and modes of initiation and termination. *Am. J. Cardiol.* 45:732-741.

Weiss, H. J. 1978. Antiplatelet therapy. *N. Engl. J. Med.* 298:1344-1347.

Wellens, H. J. J.; and Durrer, D. 1974. Wolff-Parkinson-White syndrome and atrial fibrillation. *Am. J. Cardiol.* 34:777-782.

Wellens, H. J. J.; Lie, K. I.; Bar, F. W., et al. 1976. Effect of amiodarone in the Wolff-Parkinson-White syndrome. *Am. J. Cardiol.* 38:189-194.

Wellens, H. J. J.; Bar, F. W. H. M.; Gorgels, A. P., et al. 1978a. Electrical management of arrhythmias with emphasis on the tachycardias. *Am. J. Cardiol.* 41:1025-1034.

Wellens, H. J. J.; Bar, F. W. H. M.; Lie, K. I. 1978b. The value of the electrocardiogram in the differential diagnosis of a tachycardia with a widened QRS complex. *Am. J. Med.* 64:27-33.

Wells, J. L.; MacLean, W. A. H.; James, T. N., et al. 1979. Characterization of atrial flutter. *Circulation* 60:665-673.

Williams, D. B. 1979. Acebutolol. *Am. J. Cardiol.* 44:521-525.

Winchester, M. A.; Jackson, G.; Meltzer, R. S., et al. 1978. Intravenous atenolol and acebutolol in the treatment of supraventricular arrhythmias (abstract). *Circulation* 58(4):II-49.

Wit, A. L.; and Cranefield, P. F. 1977. Triggered and automatic activity in the canine coronary sinus. *Circ. Res.* 41:435-445.

Wolf, P. A.; Dowber, T. R.; Colton, T., et al. 1976. Epidemiologic assessment of atrial fibrillation as a risk factor for stroke. *Proc. Amer. Acad. Neurol.*

Wolfson, S.; Herman, M. V.; Sullivan, J. M., et al. 1967. Conversion of atrial fibrillation and flutter by propranolol. *Br. Heart J.* 29:305-309.

Wyndham, C. R. C.; Amat-y-leon, F.; Wu, D., et al. 1977. Effects of cycle length on atrial vulnerability. *Circulation* 55:260-267.

Yahalom, J.; Klein, H. O.; and Kaplinsky, E. 1977. Beta-adrenergic blockade as adjunctive oral therapy in patients with chronic atrial fibrillation. *Chest* 71:592-596.

9 Other Paroxysmal Supraventricular Tachycardias

Jay W. Mason, M.D.

Chief, Cardiology Division
University of Utah Medical Center
Salt Lake City, Utah

Although supraventricular tachycardias are lumped together under this single term, they are composed of a remarkably diverse miscellany of arrhythmias with varying clinical presentations, underlying mechanisms, and responses to treatment. Physicians have an unfortunate tendency to regard supraventricular tachycardia as a single entity. The purpose of this chapter is to "unlump" the supraventricular tachycardias so that the physician will better understand their underlying mechanisms and be able to select effective therapy for these arrhythmias in the clinical setting. The first section of this chapter will discuss the mechanisms and diagnosis of specific arrhythmias, and in the second section the basic concepts regarding the therapy of supraventricular arrhythmias will be covered. This information will enable the reader to better apply his or her understanding of these arrhythmias to clinical treatment.

MECHANISMS AND DIAGNOSIS OF THE SUPRAVENTRICULAR ARRHYTHMIAS

In this section the arrhythmias have been separated according to their origin in the sinoatrial (SA) node, the atrial myocardium, or the atrioventricular (AV) node or their use of an accessory pathway. Atrial flutter and fibrillation and multifocal atrial tachycardia were discussed in Chapter 8 and will not be covered in this chapter.

Tachycardias Arising from the Sinus Node Region

Sinus tachycardia can be considered an arrhythmia when there is no appropriate physiologic need for a rapid sinus rate. Abnormal sinus tachycardia is diagnosed when the usual physiologic causes, such as physical exertion, anxiety, fright, fever, and hyperthyroidism, are absent. The diagnostic characteristics of abnormal sinus tachycardia are as follows:

1. Normal P-wave axis and morphology
2. Sinus rate consistently above 100 beats/min
3. Expected physiologic variation in sinus rate (although at a higher-than-normal mean rate)
4. Failure to eliminate the tachycardia with rapid or premature stimulation or direct current cardioversion.

The etiology of abnormal sinus tachycardia is unknown, but it is a recognized syndrome. One explanation that has been considered is the coincidental location of an ectopic atrial focus very close to the SA node. However, such an ectopic focus might not show physiologic rate responses, as is seen in some (but not all) cases of abnormal sinus tachycardia. Other etiologic possibilities are autonomic imbalance or excess and the influence of unknown circulating hormones. A congenital, intrinsically abnormally rapid rate of phase 4 depolarization of otherwise normal sinus node cells is another possible etiology. This syndrome is usually not a cause of disability and is only moderately responsive to medical therapy.

SA nodal reentry tachycardia is the second recognized form of tachycardia arising from the sinus node region. This is one of the characteristically slower supraventricular tachycardias, its rate frequently between 115-140 beats/min. SA nodal reentry is similar to sinus tachycardia in that normal P-wave axis and morphology are retained. It differs, however, in that it is a paroxysmal rather than a constant tachyarrhythmia. As would be expected for a reentrant tachyarrhythmia, SA nodal reentry tachycardia can be terminated by properly timed premature or rapid atrial stimulation. The SA node is composed of a large proportion of cells that are dependent on the slow calcium current for depolarization, similar to the cells of the AV node. The tissue forming the approach to the SA node contains cells of a transitional type, having characteristics of both sodium-channel dependency and calcium-channel dependency, and these cells become more totally calcium-dependent as the center of the sinus node is approached. The presence of these transition cells is reminiscent of the variation in cellular electrophysiology around and within the AV node. The presence of calcium-dependent cells in the SA nodal region, capable of decremental conduction and of varying cellular electrophysiology, affords the necessary groundwork for the formation of reentrant circuits.

Tachyarrhythmias Arising from Atrial Myocardium

As mentioned previously, atrial flutter and atrial fibrillation were discussed in Chapter 8. The next most common tachycardia of atrial myocardial origin is ectopic atrial tachycardia. This type of tachycardia may be paroxysmal or virtually permanent. The paroxysmal ectopic atrial tachycardias can be divided further into those that occur relatively infrequently (from a few times a day to only a few times a year) and those that are present more often than not. Ambulatory ECG monitoring studies have shown that the former category of arrhythmias may occur in brief, asymptomatic paroxysms in many adults undergoing these recordings. The latter type of paroxysmal ectopic atrial tachycardia has been termed the Parkinson-Papp syndrome. As originally described, this syndrome consisted of very frequent paroxysms of tachycardia of brief duration, usually lasting less than 10 seconds (Parkinson and Papp, 1947). Although the original description did not specify the mechanism underlying the Parkinson-Papp syndrome, it now appears that the majority of cases are a result of ectopic atrial discharge. The variety of paroxysmal ectopic atrial tachycardia that is less repetitive is characterized by more sustained paroxysms and usually occurs in the presence of organic heart disease, while the Parkinson-Papp syndrome often occurs in the apparently normal heart.

The permanent form of ectopic atrial tachycardia is rare. Rates are commonly between 135 and 170 beats/min. There is little rate variation over time, and the usual physiologic responses, such as increased rate with physical exertion and fever, are absent or blunted. The P-wave axis and morphology are abnormal and distinctly different from that seen during normal sinus rhythm. This rhythm disturbance occurs most often in children, adolescents, and young adults. It is sometimes symptomatic, especially in older patients. It has been considered to cause cardiac dilatation and congestive heart failure, but in such cases the possibility of an underlying cardiomyopathy occurring concurrently with the arrhythmia or actually causing the tachyarrhythmia cannot be ruled out. As a group, the ectopic atrial tachycardias are difficult to treat.

Triggered automaticity (see Chapter 1) (Cranefield, 1977) may be the underlying mechanism in some, possibly many, cases of ectopic atrial rhythms. This is of considerable importance to the electrophysiologist because triggered automaticity mimics, in its inducibility, the reentrant arrhythmias.

Ectopic atrial tachycardia with AV block is of special interest because it may be a manifestation of digitalis glycoside toxicity (see Chapter 13). This possibility deserves consideration, especially when the ventricular response rate to atrial tachycardia, or the atrial rate itself, is relatively slow.

The existence of a reentry tachycardia mechanism confined to the atrial myocardium is unproven. However, atrial flutter and other atrial tachysystoles are frequently initiated by premature atrial stimulation and terminated in similar fashion, suggesting, but not proving, a reentry mechanism. That these atrial tachysystoles are often conducted with varying degrees of block to the ventricles provides circumstantial evidence of their being confined to the atrial myocardium. Intra-atrial reentry cannot be clinically distinguished from an ectopic atrial mechanism except by the findings of induction and termination by programmed stimulation.

Supraventricular Tachycardias Arising from the Atrioventricular Nodal Region

Abnormal automaticity may develop in the junctional tissues under a variety of conditions, the most common of which are the postoperative and other hyperadrenergic states and digitalis intoxication, resulting in ectopic junctional tachycardia. Automaticity is a normal characteristic of some of the cells within the AV nodal or junctional region. For this reason, junctional escape is the normal and most common rescue rhythm during failure of impulse formation from the SA node. In the adult junctional automaticity is abnormally rapid when its rate exceeds 60 beats/min in the resting state. As an aside, it is worthwhile to note here that two forms of junctional escape mechanisms exist: that which responds to normal physiologic stimuli and that which does not. Congenital complete heart block (see Chapter 6) is an example of the former type of junctional escape rhythm. In this condition complete or nearly complete AV block is present. The escape rhythm is characterized by a normal QRS complex and normal or nearly normal responsiveness to physiologic stimuli such as sleep and exercise. This type of junctional escape rhythm probably originates from cells of the AV node itself because these cells are well innervated and responsive to autonomic stimuli. Heart block with a narrow QRS escape rhythm that lacks responsiveness to physiologic stimuli is seen more commonly in adults. This rhythm probably arises from the His bundle itself, which is not as richly innervated as the AV node.

Ectopic junctional tachycardia may occur with or without AV dissociation or AV block. Thus, the P waves and QRS complexes may show no relationship to each other, or the P waves may occur consistently before, within, or after the QRS complexes. Junctional tachycardia is usually associated with narrow QRS complexes, but preexisting bundle branch block or functional block resulting from the rapid rate may produce wide QRS complexes. Automatic junctional rhythm should not be inducible or capable of being terminated by programmed stimulation. In addition, direct current cardioversion will fail to eliminate the arrhythmia.

AV nodal reentry tachycardia is a common arrhythmia that has gone under a variety of names. Excluding atrial fibrillation and flutter, it is the most frequent supraventricular tachycardia. It is seen in individuals with otherwise normal hearts and in patients with organic heart disease of virtually any etiology.

In its most common form AV nodal reentry tachycardia is characterized by rates of from 160 to 180 beats/min and the absence of a detectable P wave in the 12-lead ECG (Benditt, et al., 1979). However, rates may be as low as 100 beats/min, even in the absence of antiarrhythmic drug therapy, and as high as 240 beats/min. In addition, the P wave may be distinguished quite easily at the end of the QRS complex, and in certain circumstances might even be visible at the onset of the QRS complex. The mechanism for supraventricular tachycardia cannot be definitively diagnosed without a complete intracardiac electrophysiologic study.

AV nodal reentry tachycardia can usually be initiated by programmed atrial or ventricular extrastimulation. Initiation of the tachyarrhythmia is characterized by a critical degree of prematurity of the extrastimulus and a critical amount of delay between the extrastimulus and the first QRS complex of the tachycardia. The need for these critical intervals relates to the nature of the tachycardia circuit.

AV nodal reentry tachycardia is one of the best examples of a reentry circuit and will be used here to define the conceptual principles of reentry in circus-movement tachycardia (see Chapter 1). Figure 9-1 is a diagrammatic representation of the reentry circuit in the AV node. Two characteristics of the reentry pathway are assumed to exist. First, all parts of the circuit are electrically insulated from each other; thus, short-circuiting, which would destroy the circus movement, cannot occur. Second, conduction characteristics are not constant throughout the circuit. For the purposes of this discussion it is easiest to imagine two halves or limbs of the reentry circuit, as shown in Figure 9-1. One limb will be called the fast pathway and the other the slow pathway. It is generally true that the fast pathway has a longer effective refractory period than the slow pathway. With these assumptions it is easy to understand how this simplified reentry circuit can be induced to function and how the reentry can be extinguished. Figure 9-2 shows the introduction of premature atrial stimuli, which are conducted to the ventricle with some AV delay but which fail to initiate tachycardia because of insufficient

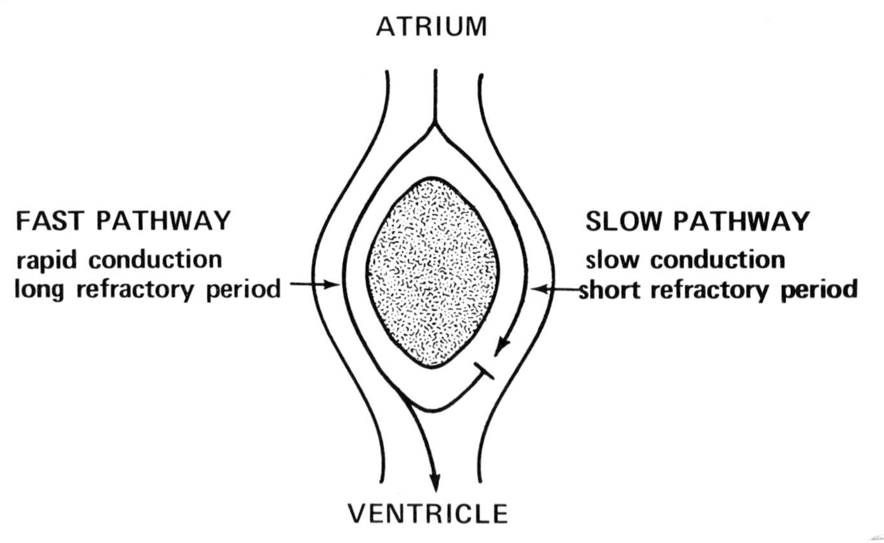

Figure 9-1 AV nodal reentry circuit. This is a schematic conceptualization of a reentry circuit within the AV node. The circuit consists of two pathways separated from each other by either anatomic or electrophysiologic barriers. The two pathways join each other at the atrial and ventricular ends of the AV node. The fast pathway conducts impulses more rapidly than the slow pathway, but has a longer effective refractory period. A normal sinus beat is shown traversing the reentry circuit. It enters both limbs of the circuit. The wavefront traversing the fast pathway emerges from the circuit first to excite the ventricles and also travels a short distance retrogradely in the slow pathway to collide with the antegrade impulse. Full-fledged reentry does not occur.

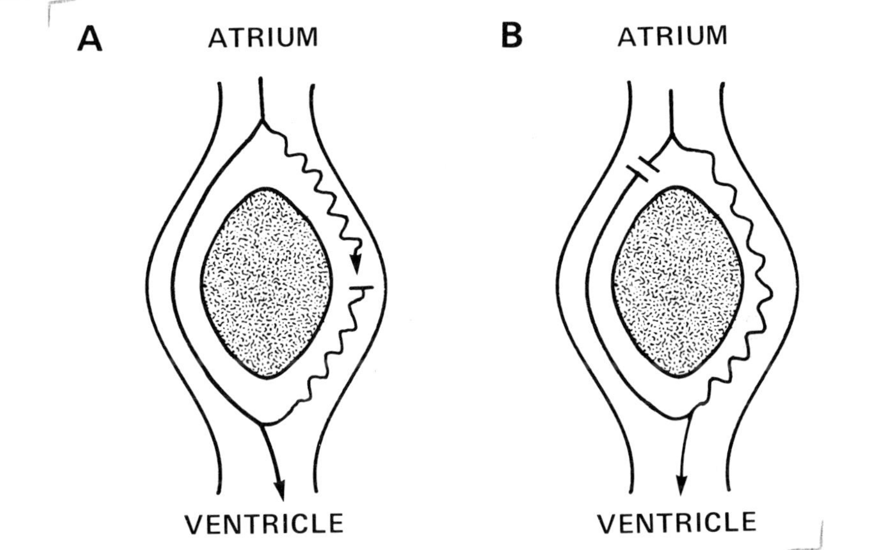

Figure 9-2 Premature beats that fail to induce reentry. In Panel A an atrial impulse enters the AV nodal reentry circuit prematurely. The impulse is not so premature that it blocks in the fast pathway. However, it is conducted with considerable delay in the slow pathway. As a result, the site of slow pathway collision moves retrogradely, but reentry does not occur. In Panel B the premature impulse is sufficiently early to encounter the effective refractory period of the fast pathway and be blocked. The antegrade impulse then reaches the His bundle through the slow pathway. The impulse also reenters the fast pathway and travels retrogradely. In this example the retrograde impulse encounters block in the same region where the antegrade fast pathway impulse was blocked. This occurs because the conduction delay in the slow pathway was not sufficient to allow full recovery in the region of block in the fast pathway.

prematurity. The next extrastimulus, shown in Figure 9-3, is sufficiently premature to initiate tachycardia. Note that this stimulus enters the fast pathway, which has a long refractory period, so early that it is blocked. However, the stimulus is propagated through the slow pathway because of its shorter effective refractory period. The slow conduction in the slow pathway delays the arrival of this stimulus, which propagates retrogradely into the fast pathway, sufficiently to allow the area of block in the fast pathway to recover excitability. As a result the propagating wavefront can reenter the slow pathway, completing and sustaining the reentry circuit. This reentry circuit can be expected to excite the ventricles and the atria each time the circuit is completely traveled. Note that the slow pathway is being used for forward, or antegrade, AV conduction while the fast pathway is utilized for backward or retrograde ventriculoatrial

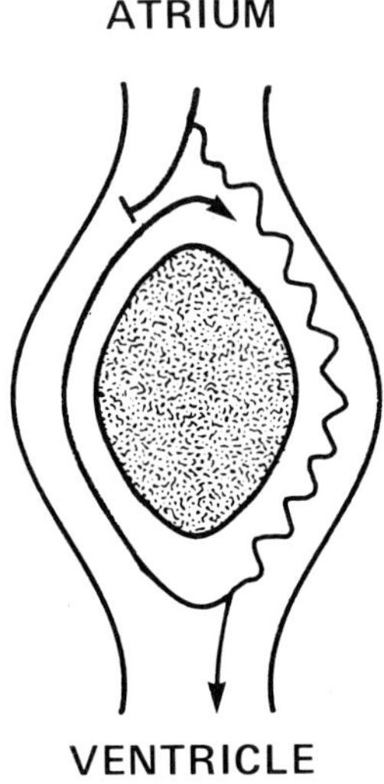

Figure 9-3 Successful AV nodal reentry. In this example the premature impulse is blocked in the fast pathway, as it was in Figure 9-2B. However, the impulse is more premature and thus encounters greater delay during antegrade propagation through the slow pathway. The result is that, when the wavefront reenters and travels retrogradely in the fast pathway, the region of block has recovered excitability, permitting the impulse to reengage the slow pathway and complete the circuit of reentry. Under proper conditions of conduction velocity and refractoriness this reentry could be maintained indefinitely.

conduction. This results in a long PR interval and a short RP interval during tachycardia. In most instances the RP interval is so short that the P wave becomes buried in the QRS complex. This occurs because the propagating impulse reaches the bottom of the reentry circuit and then must traverse the His-Purkinje system before the QRS complex is initiated. During the period of time consumed by travel through the His-Purkinje system and initial excitation of the ventricles the wavefront is also propagating retrogradely through the fast pathway to the atria. Conduction in the fast pathway is usually rapid enough to produce simultaneity of the P wave and QRS complex.

AV nodal reentry tachycardia usually results in narrow QRS complexes. However, if the rate is sufficiently rapid or if His-Purkinje system abnormalities exist, wide QRS complexes may result. It is extremely difficult to differentiate AV nodal reentry tachycardia with QRS aberrancy from ventricular tachycardia using surface electrocardiography. The morphology of the QRS complexes on 12-lead ECGs may be helpful in making the differential diagnosis (Wellens, et al., 1978). The most important hints are usually obtained from observations at the initiation or termination of the tachycardia, although these are not always captured on ECG recordings. Initiation of the tachycardia by premature atrial complexes is strong evidence in favor of a diagnosis of supraventricular tachycardia, although ventricular tachycardia can occasionally be initiated by atrial premature beats. The initial few complexes of an aberrantly conducted AV nodal reentry tachycardia are often narrow, which can serve as an important hint to the nature of the arrhythmias. Upon termination of the tachycardia, observation of a long delay before normal sinus rhythm is resumed indicates that the atrium was being captured during the tachycardia. This finding favors a diagnosis of supraventricular tachycardia, although retrograde atrial capture during ventricular tachycardia is not at all unusual. In some patients AV nodal reentry tachycardia terminates because of progressive delay during retrograde transmission through the fast pathway. This may become apparent on the surface ECG if the P wave emerges from the end of the QRS complex prior to tachycardia termination. This observation may also help distinguish the nature of the arrhythmia. Of course, clear identification of P waves dissociated from and slower than the QRS complexes strongly favors a diagnosis of ventricular tachycardia. However, the atria are not a required portion of the reentry circuit in AV nodal reentry and may not be captured retrogradely on a 1:1 basis. Thus, AV dissociation during a wide-complex tachycardia does not conclusively rule out AV nodal reentry with aberrant conduction.

In a sizable proportion of patients with AV nodal reentry tachycardia findings suggesting dual conduction pathways within the AV node can be elicited during electrophysiologic study (Denes, et al., 1975). It is best to consider dual pathways as a physiologic concept rather than an anatomic fact because histologic identification of separate AV nodal conduction pathways is not possible, and electrophysiologic proof of their function does not exist, and probably never will. The physiologic concept holds that separate conduction pathways within the AV node are electrically isolated from one another and have significantly different conduction characteristics. This concept is, in fact, very similar to the physiology depicted in Figure 9-1 describing AV nodal reentry. The difference here is that antegrade function of the two pathways can be demonstrated and there is a large, distinct difference between the two pathways: that is, their conduction characteristics do not form a continuum.

Dual pathways are usually recognized during atrial extrastimulation by the occurrence of a discontinuous conduction curve, as shown in Figures 9-4 and 9-5, which illustrate the technique of atrial extrastimulation and both normal and dual pathway-AV nodal function curves.

The dual-pathway curve shows a sudden change from one conduction pathway to the other. The clinician or electrocardiographer may occasionally see evidence for dual AV nodal pathways outside of the electrophysiology laboratory. Spontaneous alternation in the PR interval duration may occur in patients with dual-pathway physiology; marked differences in the PR interval resulting from premature atrial complexes of similar prematurity may also suggest the presence of dual pathways.

Dual AV nodal pathways may also occur in patients without paroxysmal supraventricular tachycardia. Supraventricular tachycardia caused by dual pathways is clinically indistinguishable from the AV nodal reentry tachycardia described above. Evidence supporting or suggesting the existence of three or more AV nodal pathways has appeared in the literature. For practical purposes, however, such tachycardia mechanisms are curiosities.

Some patients, primarily in the pediatric age group, have supraventricular tachycardia of a reentrant nature that constantly starts and stops with only short periods, often only a few sinus beats, in between paroxysms. This arrhythmia has been called permanent or incessant AV nodal reentrant tachycardia (Coumel, 1975). These patients are part of a very interesting, although uncommon, subgroup of individuals with supraventricular tachycardia caused by AV nodal reentry. The curious finding in this tachycardia is the presence of a short PR interval and a long RP interval during supraventricular tachycardia (Figure 9-6). The P waves are usually inverted in the inferior leads and show a vector that is typical of P waves generated by impulses traveling retrograde from the AV junction. Careful analysis of Holter monitoring studies shows that these tachycardias are initiated by modest accelerations in the sinus rate (Figures 9-6 and 9-7) rather than by premature atrial complexes, which are the usual initiators of the more common varieties of AV nodal reentry described above. Because the cardiac rate usually diminishes during sleep, patients with this form of tachycardia are often relatively free of the arrhythmia when sleeping (Figure 9-7).

Figure 9-4 Atrial extrastimulation. Recordings during AV nodal refractory period determinations by the extrastimulation technique are shown. Six surface ECG leads are displayed with high right atrial (HRA), right ventricular (RV), and His (HE) electrograms, as well as the aortic pressure (AO). Two beats during fixed-rate atrial pacing are shown on the left. In the second beat, just prior to the premature atrial stimulus, the atrial His and ventricular electrograms in the His electrogram lead are designated A_1, H_1, and V_1, respectively. The corresponding electrograms resulting from the subsequent programmed atrial premature extrastimulus are designated A_2, H_2, and V_2. Note that the AH interval on the premature stimulus (A_2H_2) is significantly longer than the AN interval during the preceding basic drive beat (A_1H_1). This is a normal finding and indicates that the premature atrial impulse has encountered the relative refractory period of the AV node.

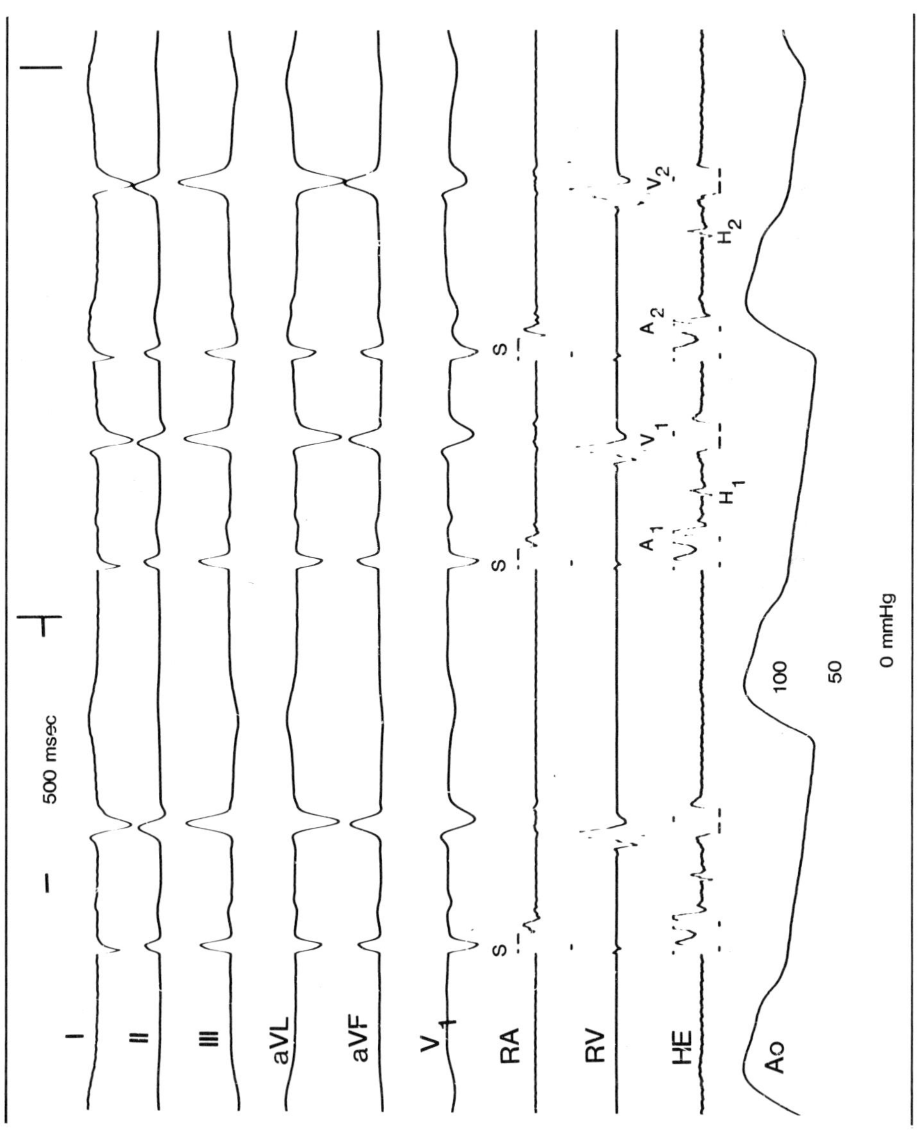
500 msec
I
II
III
aVL
aVF
V1
RA
RV
HE
Ao
S
S
S
A1
H1
V1
A2
H2
V2
100
50
0 mmHg

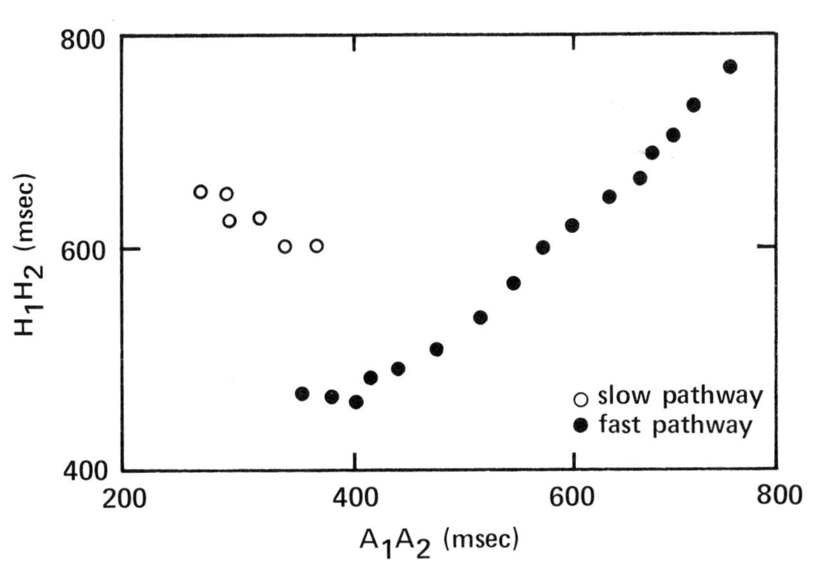

Figure 9-5 AV nodal refractory curve. Data from a series of premature atrial extrastimuli, as illustrated in Figure 9-4, were obtained from a patient with dual AV nodal physiology. $A_1 A_2$ intervals are graphed against $H_1 H_2$ intervals. Toward the left side of the graph the $H_1 H_2$ intervals become prolonged compared to the $A_1 A_2$ intervals, as illustrated in Figure 9-4. Then a sudden jump in the length of the $H_1 H_2$ interval occurs. This sudden increase is thought to result from a shift in antegrade conduction from a fast pathway to a slow pathway.

A mechanism for this tachycardia is described, as follows. Some investigators believe that this rhythm disturbance is not a result of AV nodal reentry, but rather a result of circus movement utilizing an accessory pathway. For our purposes this controversy is not important. As one would expect from the relationship of the P wave and the QRS complexes during this tachycardia, a fast pathway appears to be utilized

Figure 9-6 Incessant AV nodal reentry tachycardia. This two-channel Holter monitor recording was obtained from a patient with nearly permanent tachycardia. Note that on the right and left-hand sides of the recording an inverted P wave can be seen approximately 180 milliseconds before each QRS complex during tachycardia. Thus, this tachycardia is characterized by a short PR and a long RP interval. In the middle of the recording the tachycardia spontaneously terminates. After termination, four beats occur, which are apparently of sinus origin. The first two, with an RR interval of 800 milliseconds, are not associated with reinitiation of tachycardia. The subsequent two beats have an interbeat interval of 700 milliseconds and are associated with reinitiation of the tachycardia.

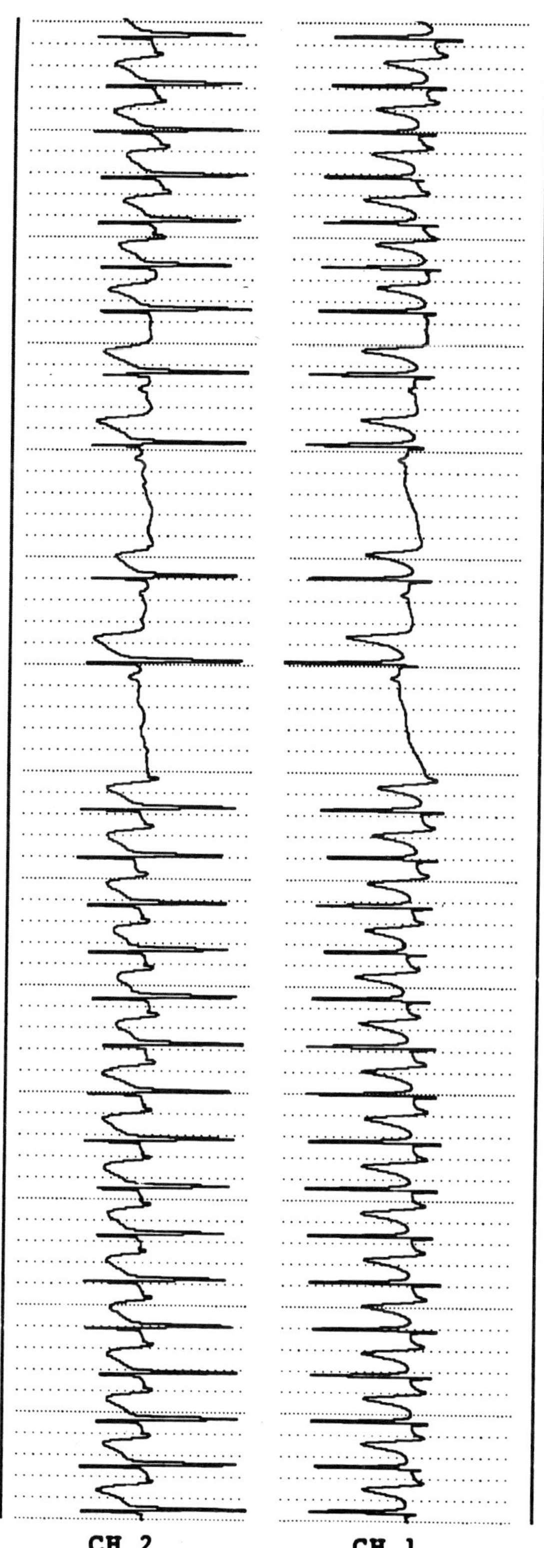
CH 2
CH 1

for antegrade conduction from atrium to ventricle and a slow pathway for retrograde conduction from ventricle to atria, which is exactly opposite to the direction of circus movement in the usual form of AV nodal reentry. The mechanism that appears to permit reentry to occur is permanent antegrade conduction block in the slow pathway. The only missing ingredient for reentry, then, is sufficient conduction delay in the circuit to slow arrival of the reentering wavefront until after excitability has recovered at the origin of the antegrade fast pathway. This requirement is easily met by simple acceleration of the cardiac rate, producing the necessary delay in AV nodal conduction time. Thus, the tachycardia can be expected to start up whenever the heart rate exceeds a certain limit.

Paroxysmal Supraventricular Tachycardia Caused by Accessory Pathways of Conduction

A number of anomalous pathways of conduction, most of them connecting the atria with the ventricles, have either been physically identified or electrophysiologically inferred. Figure 9-8 illustrates these fibers diagrammatically. The fiber most frequently responsible for cardiac arrhythmias has been called the Kent bundle, which connects the atria with the ventricles, usually over the AV grooves. James fibers connecting the atria to various sites on the AV node or the tricuspid annulus may exist normally but are only infrequently responsible for abnormal electrophysiology. The fibers of Mahaim have also been termed nodoventricular bypass fibers. These fibers may connect the AV node with the ventricles or may form abnormal connections between the His bundle or the left bundle branch and the ventricles. The fibers of Brechenmacher establish connections between the atria and the His bundle or proximal bundle branches. Although anatomic studies have suggested the existence of the latter three types of fibers, proof of their contribution to cardiac conduction and abnormal electrophysiology has necessarily been indirect (Mason, 1980). Indirect evidence has also been presented suggesting the existence

Figure 9-7 Chronology of the incessant tachycardia. This figure is a plot of the RR interval against time, obtained in the patient who was described in Figure 9-6. Each dot represents an RR interval. The tachycardia, which has a cycle length of 400 milliseconds, is almost continuously present. The sinus beats are represented by the dots that appear above the 400-millisecond level. Note that while the patient is asleep (the left-hand portion of the figure), he is spending much more time in sinus rhythm, probably in part because of a decrease in the spontaneous sinus rate when the tachycardia stops. At 6:30 A.M. the patient awakens. Not only is the arrhythmia more easily reinitiated during the wakeful state, but spontaneous terminations are much less frequent. Autonomic influences may well be involved in this phenomenon.

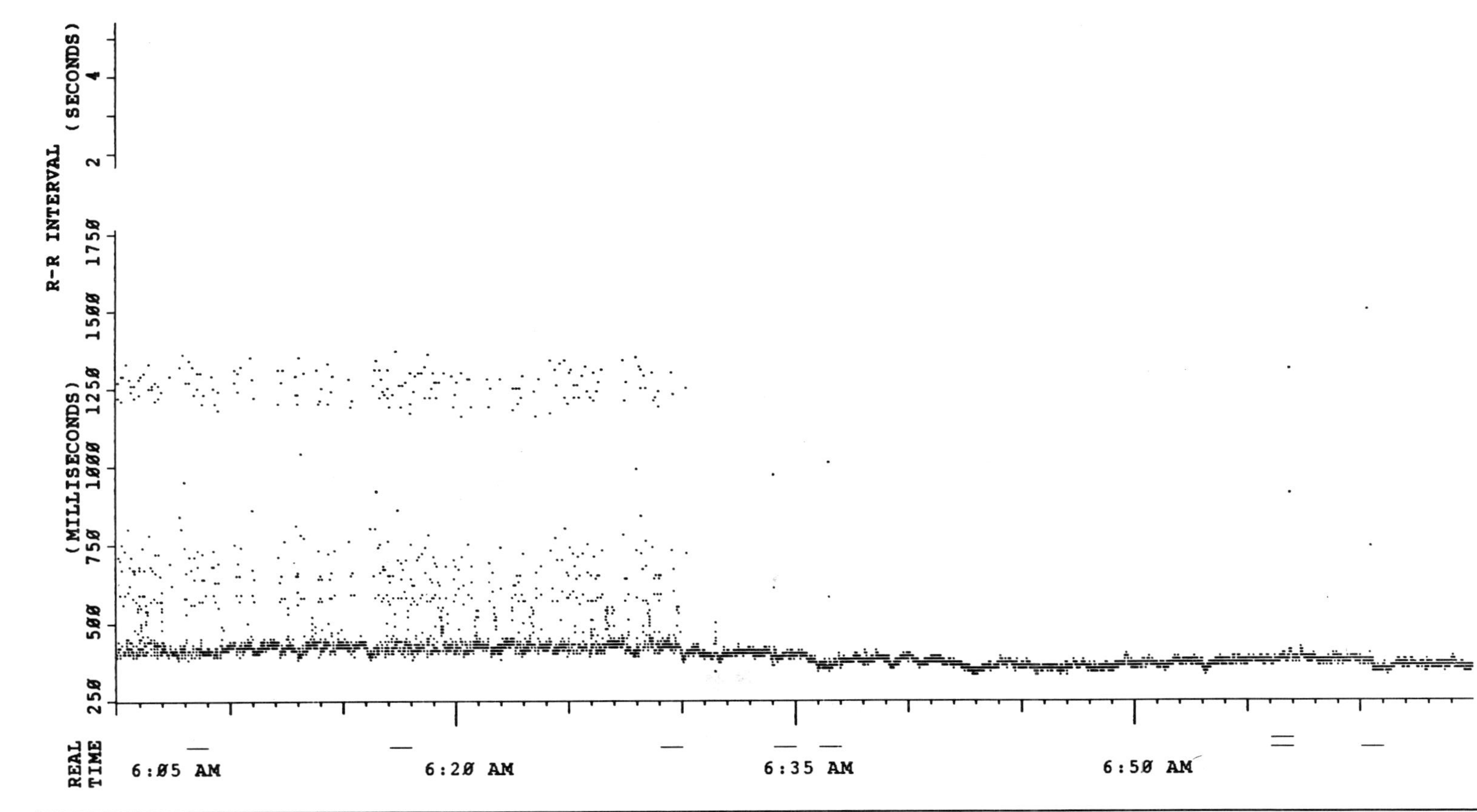
R-R INTERVAL
(SECONDS)
2
4
(MILLISECONDS)
25Ø
5ØØ
75Ø
1ØØØ
125Ø
15ØØ
175Ø
REAL TIME
6:Ø5 AM
6:2Ø AM
6:35 AM
6:5Ø AM

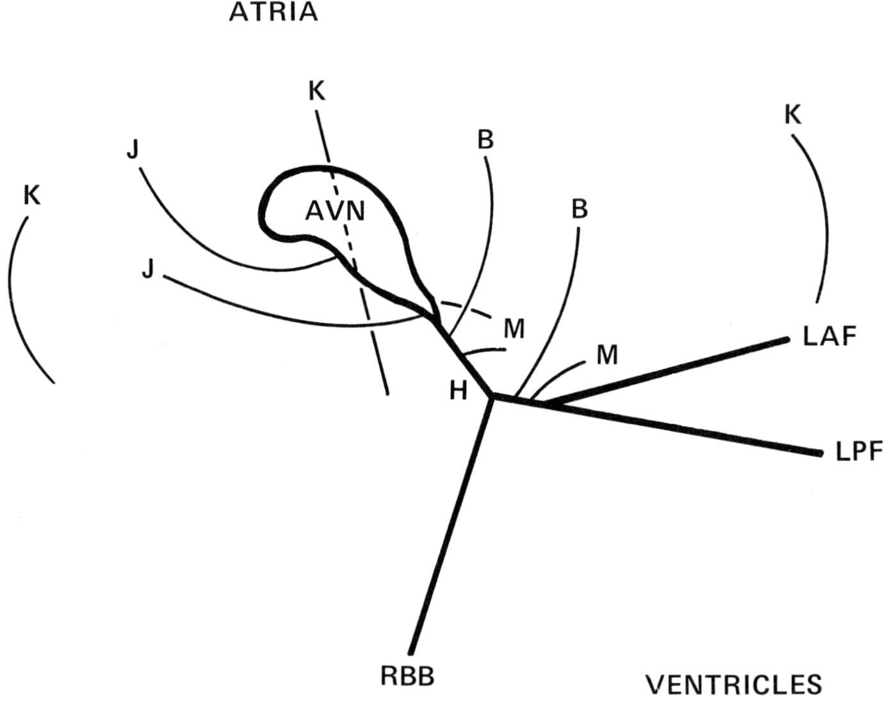

Figure 9-8 Accessory pathways of conduction. The AV node (AVN), bundle of His (H), right bundle branch (RBB), left anterior fascicle of the left bundle branch (LAF), and the left posterior fascicle (LPF) are shown diagrammatically. Kent bypass fibers (K) course between the atrium and ventricle either along the AV grooves or in the septum. James fibers (J) arise in the atrium and connect with the AV node at various levels. (Fibers described by James that course from the atrium to the region of the tricuspid valve are not shown here.) Brechenmacher fibers (B) connect the atrium with the His bundle or the left bundle branch. Mahaim fibers (M) connect the distal AV node, the His bundle, or the proximal left bundle branch with the ventricular septal myocardium.

of bypass fibers connecting the atria and ventricles, similar to the Kent fibers but with a long conduction time caused either by the unusually long physical length of the fibers or slow conduction velocity. Most Kent bypass fibers can be recognized or suspected by examining the surface ECG, which will show shortening of the PR interval, a slurred onset of the QRS complex (a delta wave), or both of these. However, these bypass fibers need not necessarily function in the antegrade direction. They may conduct only retrogradely from ventricle to atrium, making their recognition from the surface ECG essentially impossible. Bypasses that function only retrogradely are called concealed bypasses. The most important anomalous pathways of conduction to be aware of are the Kent bundles, which are responsible for the Wolff-Parkinson-White syndrome, and the James fibers, which may be responsible for the Lown-Ganong-Levine syndrome.

The Wolff-Parkinson-White syndrome As originally described, the Wolff-Parkinson-White syndrome included all preexcitation phenomena. Current usage limits the term to preexcitation caused by Kent bundles. In fact, considerable controversy exists regarding the proper name for these AV connections. In most of the world the word Kent is used to refer to the fibers associated with the Wolff-Parkinson-White syndrome.

Kent bypass fibers may be located anywhere around the circumferences of the right and left AV annuli. The majority of bypass fibers are found coursing between atrium and ventricle in the left AV groove, although none have been found in the anterior left AV groove just to the left of the septum. Less frequently, bypass fibers can be found in the right AV groove or in the anterior or posterior septal regions. The surface ECG cannot be used reliably to predict the exact location of Kent bundles. The use of the "A" and "B" ECG classification scheme of the Wolff-Parkinson-White syndrome is not very useful because it ignores septal bypass fibers and the relative inaccuracy of ECG localization. One ECG criterion for bypass fiber localization is reasonably reliable. If the first 20-millisecond QRS vector during beats showing preexcitation (a delta wave) is directed rightward, the bypass fiber is almost invariably located somewhere along the left AV groove (Tonkin, et al., 1975). In these cases the ECG will show initially negative delta waves in frontal leads 1 and aVL. In the absence of this finding the bypass fiber will be located either along the right AV groove or in the septum.

Patients with the Wolff-Parkinson-White syndrome are subject to two major arrhythmic complications: circus-movement tachycardia utilizing the accessory pathway and atrial fibrillation with a rapid ventricular response caused by transmission over the accessory pathway. The former arrhythmia is the only human arrhythmia in which a functioning circuit of reentry is proven beyond a reasonable doubt. In over 90% of instances the reentry circuit utilizes the AV node and normal His-Purkinje conduction pathways for antegrade conduction. The circuiting impulse then enters ventricular myocardium, after which it enters the Kent bundle and is propagated retrogradely to the atria. The AV node is then reentered, completing the circuit. This common form is referred to as orthodromic circus-movement tachycardia. The direction of circus movement will occasionally be reversed, with retrograde conduction through the AV node and antegrade conduction over the Kent fiber; this is referred to as antidromic circus-movement tachycardia. It is important to recognize that during orthodromic reentry, which is the most common form of tachycardia in the Wolff-Parkinson-White syndrome, the QRS complexes are usually normal in appearance. That is, they are narrow and the delta waves seen during sinus rhythm are absent. This is because antegrade preexcitation during the tachycardia is eliminated since the Kent bundle is utilized for the retrograde limb of the reentry circuit. Disappearance of delta waves during supraventricular tachycardia supplies strong evidence for the Wolff-Parkinson-White syndrome in cases where the diagnosis is uncertain. Because the circuiting impulse traverses and depolarizes ventricular myocardium before entering the Kent fiber and reentering the atria, P waves usually occur after the end of the QRS complex. The occurrence of such late P waves in an adult patient with paroxysmal supraventricular tachycardia should suggest the possibility of a Kent bundle (either manifest or concealed) as the retrograde limb of the reentry circuit.

As is the case with any supraventricular tachycardia, functional right or left bundle branch block may develop. This may be helpful in making the diagnosis in the Wolff-Parkinson-White syndrome. If the bundle branch involved in functional block is on the same side as the bypass tract, the tachycardia rate will be reduced because the circuiting impulse will be delayed in arriving at the accessory pathway. Thus, in the case of a left free-wall bypass fiber spontaneous development of functional left bundle branch block during tachycardia will increase the tachycardia cycle length by perhaps 40 or 50 milliseconds, while the spontaneous development of right bundle branch block would not alter the rate of the tachycardia. Spontaneous right or left bundle branch block in AV nodal reentry supraventricular tachycardia will also not alter the tachycardia rate.

It is important to remember that patients with Kent bundles and obvious delta waves may also have typical AV nodal reentry supraventricular tachycardia, or they may have multiple bypass fibers and reentry circuits involving antegrade conduction over one bypass fiber and retrograde conduction over another bypass fiber, such that the AV node is not part of the tachycardia circuit.

The second major arrhythmic complication in the Wolff-Parkinson-White syndrome is atrial fibrillation (Figure 9-9). For unknown reasons the incidence of atrial fibrillation is higher in patients with the Wolff-Parkinson-White syndrome than in the normal population. In a minority of patients with atrial fibrillation the effective refractory period of the Kent fiber is so short that life-threatening rapid ventricular rates can be achieved. This is a particularly challenging therapeutic problem.

Electrophysiologic study may be required in patients with the Wolff-Parkinson-White syndrome (see Chapter 2). There are three major indications for electrophysiologic study. First, when the diagnosis is uncertain but required, electrophysiologic study provides the only definitive diagnostic technique. Second, whenever the arrhythmias accompanying the syndrome are sufficiently symptomatic to require therapy, electrophysiologic study should be performed to evaluate the anticipated therapy, especially with regard to its potential adverse effects on the accessory pathway. Third, when surgery for ablation of the bypass fiber is to be done (see Chapter 11), preoperative electrophysiologic study is required to rule out other diagnostic possibilities, to attempt to rule out the possibility of multiple accessory pathways, to evaluate the most effective means for inducing and maintaining supraventricular tachycardia, and to approximate the location of the bypass fiber. A list of the information obtained during electrophysiologic study of patients with the Wolff-Parkinson-White syndrome can be found in Chapter 2.

The Lown-Ganong-Levine syndrome This syndrome can be defined succinctly as the concurrence of recurrent supraventricular tachycardia and a baseline ECG showing a short PR interval (less than 0.12 seconds) with normal, narrow QRS complexes (that is, no delta waves). The cause of this syndrome is unknown. There are two possible explanations for the shortened AV transmission time. The first is an anomalous pathway that bypasses a portion or all of the AV node but communicates with the normal conduction system above the bifurcation of the His bundle. James described the common presence of fibers passing from the lower right atrium to the AV junction or the tricuspid valve region. These are referred to as James fibers and are a convenient possible explanation for a short AV transmission time. The second conceivable explanation is enhanced AV nodal conduction. That is, the AV node may have unusually rapid conduction characteristics. This latter possibility could be caused by a physically small AV node, altered autonomic input to the node, or intrinsic cellular properties. Patients with James physiology or enhanced AV nodal function have a short PR interval and a short AH interval, show a minimal increase in AV nodal conduction time during rapid atrial pacing, and have a short AV nodal effective refractory period. Recurrent supraventricular tachycardia in patients with James physiology appears to be caused by reentry in the junctional region.

TREATMENT OF PAROXYSMAL SUPRAVENTRICULAR TACHYCARDIA

The physician who is aware of the mechanisms underlying the various forms of supraventricular tachycardia should be able to treat these arrhythmias effectively given adequate information regarding the various forms of therapy that are available. This section of the chapter will cover the three principal forms of treatment for supraventricular tachycardias: drugs, pacemakers, and surgery.

Drug Therapy

Specific drug therapy can be applied to all forms of supraventricular tachycardia, including automatic and reentrant arrhythmias and arrhythmias arising from the SA node, the atrial myocardium, or the AV nodal region. The following five characteristics of the agent to be used must be considered:

1. Which cardiac cells are most susceptible to the drug's direct effects?
2. What is the drug's effect on phase 4 depolarization (or automaticity)?
3. What is the drug's effect on conduction velocity?
4. What is the drug's effect on refractoriness?
5. What is the drug's effect on the cardiac autonomic nervous system?

If the physician understands the mechanisms underlying the supraventricular tachyarrhythmia to be treated and can answer these questions regarding the available antiarrhythmic agents, he or she can make a reasonable antiarrhythmic drug selection to either terminate established supraventricular tachycardia or prevent recurrences of supraventricular tachycardia. Of course, a rational drug selection does not guarantee successful therapy, but it does improve the chances for success and reduce the likelihood of an adverse effect.

The automatic tachycardias, although often difficult to treat, are best treated with agents that have a powerful depressant effect on phase 4 (or the period of diastolic depolarization) of the action potential. Quinidine, procainamide, and disopyramide are the most effective such agents currently available in the United States. When the automatic focus is located in the upper portion of the AV node, the atrium, or the SA nodal

Figure 9-9 Atrial fibrillation in the Wolff-Parkinson-White syndrome. Six surface ECG leads are displayed simultaneously with high right atrial (HRA), distal coronary sinus (CS_d), proximal coronary sinus (CS_p), low right atrium (LRA), right ventricle (RV), and His bundle (HE) electrograms. One sinus beat with mild preexcitation is shown, followed by a two-second period of rapid atrial stimulation indicated by the arrows. Varying degrees of preexcitation are seen during rapid stimulation. At the cessation of rapid stimulation atrial fibrillation is present. This ECG recording illustrates a period of ventricular excitation via the accessory pathway in the middle of the tracing, followed by a period of conduction over the normal conduction pathway with an absence of preexcitation. Alternating conduction through the normal and abnormal pathways is common in atrial fibrillation associated with the Wolff-Parkinson-White syndrome. The shortest RR interval during preexcitation in this patient was 350 milliseconds. This corresponds to a maximum ventricular response rate of 171 beats/min, which does not represent a potentially life-threatening problem.

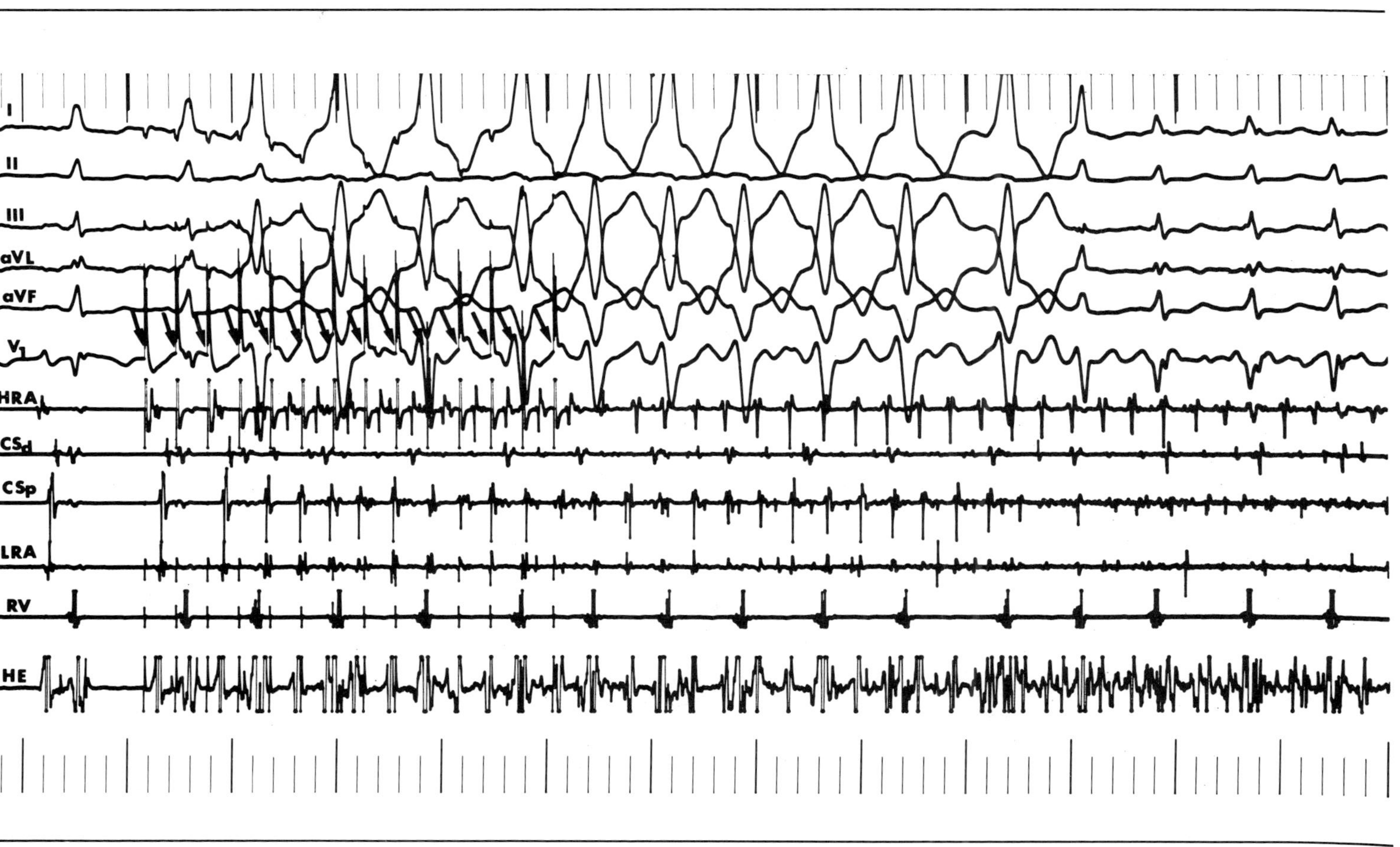

I
II
III
aVL
aVF
V_1
HRA
CS_d
CS_p
LRA
RV
HE

region, the patient's symptoms may also be relieved by agents promoting block in the AV node, thereby reducing the ventricular response rate. The most appropriate class of drugs with which to achieve the goal of depressing AV nodal transmission is the calcium antagonist group (see Chapter 3). The best known agent in this group is verapamil (Isoptin or Calan) 5-25 mg intravenously or 40-120 mg orally every 6-8 hours. The cells in the AV node that are responsible for verapamil's conduction-delaying properties depend on the slow inward current (also known as the calcium current) for depolarization. Verapamil specifically blocks this inward current and, therefore, has potent effects on the AV node. Verapamil is the agent of choice in the treatment of a number of supraventricular arrhythmias. In patients with AV reentry verapamil terminates the tachycardia by its depressant effect on the AV node. In some studies the effect has been primarily on antegrade AV nodal function (Rinkenberger, et al., 1980), but in others retrograde conduction has also been altered (Sung, et al., 1980). In patients with supraventricular tachycardia caused by an accessory pathway the drug terminates the arrhythmia by altering only AV nodal conduction. Verapamil and other calcium antagonists may also be used to treat tachyarrhythmias caused by triggered automaticity, which also depend on calcium. Other agents that can depress AV nodal function include the beta blocking agents (such as propranolol and metoprolol) and digoxin, which exert both direct and autonomically mediated AV nodal depressant effects.

In the treatment of reentrant supraventricular tachycardias choice of the proper agent depends on the location of the reentry circuit and the drug's ability to affect conduction velocity or refractoriness of cardiac tissue in that region. For reentrant arrhythmias arising from the AV or SA nodal regions verapamil remains the drug of choice because of its selective effects on the calcium current, which cells in these locations depend on. However, if verapamil is contraindicated, many other agents can be selected on a rational basis. Drugs capable of increasing tissue refractoriness can be used to promote block in an AV nodal reentry circuit. Both digoxin and propranolol have this capability. Some drugs, such as procainamide, may exert their major effect by depressing retrograde conduction over the AV nodal fast pathway (Wu, et al., 1978).

In attempting to determine what effects a given drug will have on the reentry circuit both its direct and autonomically mediated actions must be considered. For example, digoxin's vagotonic effects work in concert with its direct depressant effects on the SA and AV nodal regions. However, digitalis shortens atrial refractory periods by an autonomic mechanism; thus, it could enhance some reentry phenomena in atrial muscle. Quinidine, procainamide, and disopyramide have competing direct and autonomic nervous system-mediated influences. Therefore, while these drugs depress AV nodal conduction and prolong AV nodal refractoriness by their direct actions, they have prominent vagolytic effects that usually (but not always) override, or at least counteract, the direct effects. Hence, they would not be a good choice to suppress AV nodal reentry unless the correct balance of direct versus autonomically mediated actions could be achieved.

A distinction should be made between prophylaxis against and termination of ongoing paroxysmal supraventricular tachycardia. The autonomic nervous system can be used to the clinician's advantage for interruption of established reentrant tachycardias utilizing the SA or AV nodes. Edrophonium (Tensilon), given as an intravenous bolus of 5-10 mg, can terminate most supraventricular reentrant tachycardias by promoting brief but intense vagal influences on the reentry circuit. Vagal maneuvers without the aid of drugs may also terminate such tachycardias. The Valsalva maneuver, carotid sinus massage, eyeball pressure, gagging, and immersing the face in ice water are all methods for promoting intense vagal discharge. Supraventricular tachycardias caused by reentry mechanisms can also be interrupted by elevating the systemic blood pressure by pressor agents such as phenylephrine (Neo-Synephrine), which results in reflex vagotonia as a response to the induced hypertension.

Most of the previously mentioned drugs used for prophylaxis against reentrant paroxysmal supraventricular tachycardia can also be used successfully to terminate the rhythms. Verapamil is unquestionably the preferred agent for this purpose.

Reentrant supraventricular tachycardias (as well as atrial fibrillation) can also be terminated by externally applied direct current cardioversion. These rhythms (except for atrial fibrillation) often respond to relatively small doses of current (<100 joules). Cardioversion is not useful in treating the automatic arrhythmias.

The reader has probably noticed that essentially all available antiarrhythmic drugs (except lidocaine and bretylium) and some nonantiarrhythmic drugs have been mentioned for termination of or prophylaxis against paroxysmal supraventricular tachycardia caused by reentry in the SA or AV nodal regions. All of these agents actually do have one or another helpful attribute.

Drug therapy of circus-movement tachycardia in the Wolff-Parkinson-White syndrome requires special consideration. The drugs mentioned above that promote block in the AV node may be valuable because the AV node forms a portion of the reentry circuit. The Kent bundle itself can also be the target of therapy, however. Quinidine, procainamide, disopyramide, and a variety of new antiarrhythmic drugs all have the desirable ability to slow conduction velocity and prolong refractoriness in the Kent bundle in the majority of patients. Thus, they are first-line agents in the United States for the treatment of circus-movement tachycardia

tachycardia in the Wolff-Parkinson-White syndrome. On the other hand, digitalis preparations should be avoided. Even though digitalis may promote desirable AV nodal delay or block, it may also improve refractoriness in the Kent bundle, much as it decreases ventricular refractory periods. If atrial fibrillation were to occur, which is a common event in the Wolff-Parkinson-White syndrome, the ventricular rate achieved by conduction over the Kent bundle could be increased to a lethal extent. Verapamil may also cause undesirable facilitation of conduction over the bypass fiber during atrial fibrillation; however, this has not yet been unequivocally established. For reasons that are unclear even quinidine, procainamide, and disopyramide may improve Kent bundle refractoriness in rare cases; therefore, we recommend electrophysiologic study to assess drug effects on the Kent bundle whenever antiarrhythmic drug therapy is applied to patients with the Wolff-Parkinson-White syndrome.

The ability to induce reentrant supraventricular tachyarrhythmias by programmed extrastimulation has afforded a new technique for antiarrhythmic drug selection in paroxysmal supraventricular tachycardia. The hypothesis behind this technique is that inducibility of the tachyarrhythmia indicates continued functional integrity of the reentry circuit. On the other hand, a lack of inducibility of supraventricular tachycardia implies functional disability of the circuit. The study protocol is as follows: supraventricular tachycardia is initiated using one or more programmed atrial or ventricular premature extrastimuli with a special stimulator, as described in Chapter 2. The induced supraventricular tachycardia can then be terminated by pacing in most cases. After that an antiarrhythmic drug, expected to be effective on the basis of the considerations discussed above, is administered intravenously in a full loading dose. Tachycardia induction is then attempted once more. Prospective studies have shown that if the tachycardia is not inducible, the antiarrhythmic drug will provide effective prophylaxis against supraventricular tachycardia during long-term oral administration.

Pacemaker Therapy

Except for the rare ectopic atrial tachycardia initiated during long atrial diastoles, which is potentially amenable to atrial demand pacing, pacemaker therapy in paroxysmal supraventricular tachycardia is restricted to the reentrant tachyarrhythmias, predominantly those involving the AV node or an accessory pathway. Pacemaker therapy in paroxysmal supraventricular tachycardia may be prophylactic or interruptive; that is, the pacing modality may be used either to prohibit occurrence of the tachyarrhythmia or to interrupt or terminate an established tachyarrhythmia.

Prophylaxis against AV nodal reentry supraventricular tachycardia may be achieved with AV sequential or atrial-synchronous ventricular pacing or with rapid atrial pacing. Efficacy of the former technique has only recently been recognized (Spurrel and Sowton, 1976; Akhtar, et al., 1979). All of these techniques depend on interruption of the reentry circuit by promoting block in one or both of its limbs. AV sequential or atrial-synchronous ventricular pacing causes premature retrograde entry into the reentry circuit, resulting in block in the retrograde limb of the circuit. Rapid continuous atrial pacing promotes antegrade block in either or both limbs of the circuit. This latter technique was applied successfully in one of our patients with AV nodal reentry tachycardia that could not be eliminated by standard and investigational agents. The combination of rapid right atrial continuous pacing at 180 beats/min and sufficient doses of digoxin and propranolol to promote 3:1 block totally eliminated tachycardia recurrence. Rapid atrial pacing would not be applicable for prophylaxis in patients with the Wolff-Parkinson-White syndrome and a bypass fiber with antegrade function unless its refractory period was long.

Interruptive atrial pacing consists of introducing either programmed individual extrastimuli during established tachycardia or rapid atrial stimulation (overdrive or burst pacing) during the tachycardia. Interruptive pacing can be provided by implanted pacemaker systems that require the patient to initiate the pacing or by systems that automatically initiate pacing by electronically recognizing the tachyarrhythmia. Patient-initiated interruptive pacing requires that the patient be able to accurately recognize the presence of the tachyarrhythmia and not be disabled by the arrhythmia. Although pacemakers can be made to order with a variety of magnet-activated pacing capabilities, the greatest experience with interruptive pacing in paroxysmal supraventricular tachycardia has been attained using a radio frequency-triggered pacing system in which a compact external radio transmitter is used to stimulate the heart inductively at a selectable rate through an implanted receiver-lead system (Peters, et al., 1978). Regardless of the specific techniques employed, the mechanism of pacing termination of reentrant paroxysmal supraventricular tachycardia is by premature entry into the circuit, which induces block within it (Figure 9-10). Recent experience with an automatic tachycardia-terminating system has documented the feasibility of electronic recognition and automatic termination of supraventricular tachycardias (Griffin, et al., 1980). This system was discussed in detail in Chapter 7.

Surgical Therapy

Both automatic and reentrant supraventricular tachycardias are amenable to surgical therapy in certain cases. For automatic tachycardias two operative approaches are possible. In the first approach electrical sequence mapping is used in the operating room to identify the location of the ectopic focus. The focus can then simply be excised or electrically isolated from the remainder of the atria by an encircling incision. Alternately, when the ectopic focus resides above the AV node, or when the ventricular rate during atrial fibrillation or atrial flutter cannot be adequately controlled, the normal AV transmission system can be interrupted, either by surgical incision, by cryothermal destruction, or by a percutaneous catheter technique (Gallagher, et al., 1982). While the latter two techniques do not eliminate the arrhythmia itself, they do eliminate the symptoms and the potential risk of rapid ventricular response. Although there is some uncertainty with regard to the exact location of the lesions that successfully interrupt AV nodal transmission, the interruption appears to occur at the distal end of the AV node or in the His bundle itself because patients are left with a narrow complex escape rhythm with His bundle potentials preceding the QRS complexes (Klein, et al., 1980). Thus, these ablative procedures are effective in preventing AV nodal reentry.

Patients with the Wolff-Parkinson-White syndrome have provided the most extensive experience in surgical therapy of reentrant supraventricular tachyarrhythmias (Gallagher, et al., 1978). Epicardial and endocardial mapping for accurate identification of Kent bypass fiber location and surgical techniques for interrupting bypass fibers have been developed to the point of sufficient efficacy and safety; thus, consideration for surgery should be given to any patient who has symptomatic arrhythmias caused by Kent bypass fibers. While it can still be debated whether patients who have not yet failed all medical regimens should be offered surgery, most investigators agree that atrial fibrillation with life-threateningly rapid ventricular response rates and circus-movement tachycardia that is resistant to antiarrhythmic drug therapy are indications for surgical ablation of a bypass fiber. This will be discussed in detail in Chapter 11.

Figure 9-10 Automatic tachycardia termination. This Holter monitor recording was obtained in a patient with an implanted automatic tachycardia-terminating pacemaker (Cybertach-60, Intermedics, Inc.). In the middle strip an episode of supraventricular tachycardia with an average rate of 150 beats/min occurs. After the eighth short atrial cycle detected by the pacemaker, a rapid burst of atrial stimuli (206 pulses/min for 4 seconds) is delivered to the atrium, resulting in termination of the tachycardia and eventual resumption of normal sinus rhythm.

DL

REFERENCES

Akhtar, M.; Gilbert, C. J.; Al-houri, M., et al. 1979. Electrophysiologic mechanisms for modification and abolition of atrioventricular junctional tachycardia with simultaneous and sequential atrial and ventricular pacing. *Circulation* 60:1443.

Benditt, D. G.; Pritchett, E. L. C.; Smith, W. M., et al. 1979. Ventriculo-atrial intervals: diagnostic use in paroxysmal supraventricular tachycardia. *Ann. Intern. Med.* 91:161-166.

Coumel, P. 1975. Junctional reciprocating tachycardia. The permanent and paroxysmal forms of AV nodal reciprocating tachycardias. *J. Electrocardiol.* 8:79.

Cranefield, P. F. 1977. Action potentials, afterpotentials, and arrhythmias. *Circ. Res.* 41:415-423.

Denes, P.; Wu, D.; Dhingra, R. C., et al. 1975. Dual AV nodal pathways. *Br. Heart J.* 37:1069.

Gallagher, J. J.; Pritchett, E. L. C.; Sealy, W. C., et al. 1978. The preexcitation syndromes. *Prog. Cardiovasc. Dis.* 20:285-327.

Gallagher, J. J.; Svenson, R. H.; Kasell, J. H., et al. 1982. Catheter technique for closed chest ablation of the atrioventricular conduction system. *N. Engl. J. Med.* 306:194-200.

Griffin, J. C.; Mason, J. W.; and Calfee, R. V. 1980. Clinical use of an implantable automatic tachycardia-terminating pacemaker. *Am. Heart J.* 100:1093.

Klein, G. J.; Sealy, W. C.; Pritchett, E. L. C., et al. 1980. Cryosurgical ablation of the atrioventricular node-His bundle: long-term follow-up and properties of the junctional pacemaker. *Circulation* 61:8.

Mason, J. W. 1980. Evidence for a unidirectional retrograde communication between distal His bundle and atria. *Br. Heart J.* 43:600-604.

Parkinson, J.; and Papp, C. 1947. Repetitive paroxysmal tachycardia. *Br. Heart J.* 9:241-262.

Peters, R. W.; Shafton, E.; Frank, S., et al. 1978. Radio frequency-triggered pacemakers: use and limitations. *Ann. Intern. Med.* 88:17.

Rinkenberger, R. L.; Prystowsky, E. N.; Heger, J. J., et al. 1980. Effects of intravenous and chronic oral verapamil administration in patients with supraventricular tachyarrhythmias. *Circulation* 62:996-1010.

Spurrell, R. A. J.; and Sowton, E. 1976. An implanted atrial synchronous pacemaker with a short atrioventricular delay for the prevention of paroxysmal supraventricular tachycardia. *J. Electrocardiol.* 9:89.

Sung, R. J.; Elser, B.; and McAllister, R. G. 1980. Intravenous verapamil for termination of reentrant supraventricular tachycardias. *Ann. Intern. Med.* 93:682-689.

Tonkin, A. M.; Wagner, G. S.; Gallagher, J. J., et al. 1975. Initial forces of ventricular depolarization in the Wolff-Parkinson-White syndrome. *Circulation* 52:1030-1036.

Wellens, H. J. J.; Bär, F. W. H. M.; and Lie, K. I. 1978. The value of the electrocardiogram in the differential diagnosis of a tachycardia with a widened QRS complex. *Am. J. Med.* 64:27-33.

Wu, D.; Denes, P.; Bauernfeind, R., et al. 1978. Effect of procainamide on atrioventricular nodal reentrant paroxysmal tachycardia. *Circulation* 57:1171.

10 Ventricular Arrhythmias

Roger A. Winkle, M.D.
Associate Professor of Medicine
Cardiology Division
Stanford University School of Medicine
Stanford, California

Jay W. Mason, M.D.
Chief, Cardiology Division
University of Utah Medical Center
Salt Lake City, Utah

VENTRICULAR ECTOPIC BEATS

Diagnosis, Incidence, and Prognostic Significance

Ventricular ectopic beats result from an abnormal ventricular depolarization. Electrocardiographically, they appear as QRS complexes, which are usually premature; however, they may occasionally be late and may even follow a P wave and result in fusion beats. Ventricular ectopic beats are usually wide (≥0.12 seconds), and their morphology is different from sinus beats. It is important to distinguish ventricular ectopic beats from supraventricular premature beats with aberration. The following is a list of the characteristics of aberration:

1. Preceding P′ wave present
2. Right bundle branch block pattern
3. Triphasic (RSR′) in lead V_1
4. Initial QRS vector identical to sinus beats
5. Second in a group
6. Noncompensatory pause
7. In irregular rhythms aberration tends to occur after long preceding cycles (unless bigeminy exists)—Ashman phenomenon
8. In the presence of varying aberration the beats with the shortest coupling interval show the greatest aberration

Occasional ventricular ectopic beats are common in all age groups. Frequent (>30/hr) ventricular ectopic beats are uncommon in younger subjects but are seen occasionally in older patients. Frequent and complex ventricular ectopic beats are even more prevalent in patients with cardiac diagnoses such as coronary artery disease, mitral valve prolapse, and hypertrophic cardiomyopathy (Winkle, 1980). Frequent and complex ventricular ectopic beats detected by short periods of ambulatory ECG monitoring identify patients who are at high risk in the first 6 months to 1 year after a myocardial infarction (Moss, et al., 1979; Ruberman, et al., 1977 and 1981). Ventricular ectopic beats are considered benign when they occur in apparently healthy subjects (Hinkle, et al., 1969 and 1974). The prevalence and prognostic significance of ventricular ectopic beats were discussed in greater detail in Chapter 4.

Mechanism

The mechanism by which ventricular ectopic beats occur remains uncertain. The most widely proposed theories are those of reentry and abnormal automaticity. The classical theory holds that parasystolic ventricular ectopic beats result from a protected automatic focus and that fixed, coupled premature ventricular ectopic beats result from reentry. However, Moe and colleagues (1977) recently showed that it can be difficult to distinguish reentry from parasystole because the latter may occur with fixed coupling as a result of the electrotonic effects of normal beats on its discharge rate. The discovery of calcium-dependent after-depolarizations suggests yet another mechanism by which ventricular ectopic beats can occur (see Chapter 1).

Indications for Therapy

The majority of people with premature ventricular ectopic beats are unaware of their cardiac irregularity or experience only minor palpitations. Occasional patients may be aware of all or many of their ventricular ectopic beats and may experience considerable anxiety at the thought that their heart is skipping beats. In the absence of organic heart disease reassuring the patient is often the most valuable initial therapy. For some patients reassurance is inadequate and they desire to try antiarrhythmic therapy even when they realize that some risk of serious toxicity exists. The need for therapy of asymptomatic frequent and complex ventricular ectopic beats, when they occur in the presence of organic heart disease, remains controversial. In the setting of a recent myocardial infarction these arrhythmias do identify high-risk patients (see Chapter 4), and many experts recommend long-term suppression with antiarrhythmic drugs even though there are no data to indicate that such therapy is beneficial. A rational approach is to attempt therapy with membrane-active antiarrhythmic agents and, if the drugs suppress the repetitive and other complex forms without side-effects, to continue therapy for at least 6 months. However, if arrhythmias are not easily suppressed or if drugs produce considerable side-effects, it is wisest to abandon long-term therapy. During the next decade there should be a number of controlled trials performed to determine whether suppression of these frequent complex ventricular ectopic beats reduces the risk of sudden cardiac death.

Therapy

Although a large number of antiarrhythmic drugs are capable of suppressing ventricular ectopic beats, few data are available to aid in choosing the drug that is most likely to suppress these arrhythmias in an individual patient. While quinidine, procainamide, and disopyramide can suppress ventricular ectopic beats in many patients, their poor pharmacokinetic properties and high incidence of side-effects do not make them ideal for long-term treatment. Newer drugs (see Chapter 3), such as encainide, lorcainide, propafenone, and flecainide, are extremely efficacious for the long-term suppression of ventricular ectopic beats. Other drugs, such as tocainide, mexiletine, amiodarone, and, occasionally, propranolol, are also effective for suppressing ventricular irritability in some patients. Coronary artery bypass surgery has been assessed carefully as a potential treatment for ventricular ectopic beats but has no effect on these arrhythmias (Tilkian, et al., 1976; de Soyza, et al., 1978; Lehrman, et al., 1979). Based on current knowledge, the presence of frequent and/or complex ventricular ectopic beats is not an indication for more aggressive management such as electrophysiologic study, coronary artery bypass grafting, or myocardial resection.

VENTRICULAR TACHYCARDIA

Diagnosis

Clinical findings If a wide QRS complex tachycardia is hemodynamically well tolerated, clinicians tend to consider it more likely to be supraventricular tachycardia with aberration than ventricular tachycardia. However, the clinical status of the patient is not a reliable guide for differentiating these two arrhythmias because the amount of hemodynamic embarrassment precipitated by a tachycardia is more a function of the underlying cardiac disease and the tachycardia rate than of the arrhythmia's origin. Rapid supraventricular tachycardias may cause hemodynamic compromise in a severely diseased heart, and ventricular tachycardia may be well tolerated for hours or even days in a patient with good myocardial function. Some clinicians use the response to therapy as a clue as to whether an arrhythmia is supraventricular tachycardia with aberration or ventricular tachycardia. They consider that a rhythm that fails to respond to lidocaine or that responds to verapamil is more likely to be supraventricular tachycardia with aberration. These observations, however, are also frequently misleading. Many patients with sustained ventricular tachycardia will not respond to intravenous lidocaine, and ventricular tachycardia may sometimes be terminated by intravenous verapamil.

The clinical setting in which the arrhythmia occurs often provides a clue to the diagnosis of ventricular tachycardia. Wide QRS complex tachycardia occurring in a patient with the Wolff-Parkinson-White syndrome is more likely to be reciprocating AV tachycardia with bundle branch block than ventricular tachycardia, whereas a similar rhythm occurring in a patient with coronary artery disease and a previous myocardial infarction is more likely to be ventricular tachycardia. The most helpful clue to the diagnosis of ventricular tachycardia on physical examination is a varying intensity of the first heart sound, reflecting AV dissociation. The presence of this finding strongly suggests ventricular tachycardia. However, this finding may be absent in patients with 1:1 retrograde conduction during sustained ventricular tachycardia.

Surface ECG and esophageal leads Although there are no findings on the surface ECG that are absolutely diagnostic of ventricular tachycardia, careful examination of a 12-lead ECG will yield the proper diagnosis in the majority of cases. Because helpful findings are often missed on a single-lead rhythm strip, we cannot emphasize too strongly the value of obtaining 12-lead ECGs whenever the patient's clinical status permits a delay in therapy for the few minutes required to obtain such a recording. The ECG should be carefully inspected to determine the relationship between atrial and ventricular activation. In supraventricular tachycardia with aberration or circus-movement tachycardia utilizing a bypass fiber a 1:1 relationship between atria and ventricles almost always exists. However, atrial activation is often buried in the QRS complex or T wave and may not be readily apparent on the surface ECG. Because one-quarter to one-third of patients with ventricular tachycardia have retrograde 1:1 ventriculoatrial conduction, the finding of AV association does not confirm a diagnosis of supraventricular tachycardia with aberration. Although a few cases of supraventricular tachycardias with dissociation of the atria and ventricles have been reported (Josephson and Kastor, 1976), the finding of AV dissociation strongly favors a diagnosis of ventricular tachycardia. AV dissociation is most easily recognized when complete dissociation exists with easily identifiable P waves that march through the QRS complexes. During some ventricular tachycardias intermittent ventriculoatrial conduction may occur, resulting in irregularities of the PP intervals. In other instances retrograde ventriculoatrial conduction with block (such as 2:1 or 3:2) may exist, which is a finding that also strongly favors a diagnosis of ventricular tachycardia. Because surface ECG monitoring frequently fails to identify P waves during ventricular tachycardia, we have found esophageal ECG recordings to be of great value for documenting AV dissociation (Figure 10-1). Esophageal recordings may be made from a small bipolar electrode, which is placed in a gelatin capsule and swallowed by the patient (Arzbaecher, 1973) (see Chapter 4). The electrode is attached to a thin wire, which passes through the patient's mouth without discomfort. After the signal is filtered to exclude respiratory artifacts caused by changes in intrathoracic pressure the esophageal ECG is displayed simultaneously with surface lead II using a three-channel ECG recorder.

In some patients with sustained ventricular tachycardia occasional sinus beats will capture the ventricle, causing early, narrower QRS complexes on the surface ECG. Other sinus beats may partially capture the ventricle and result in QRS complexes that are intermediate between sinus beats and the ventricular tachycardia QRS morphology. Such capture or fusion beats are virtually diagnostic of ventricular tachycardia.

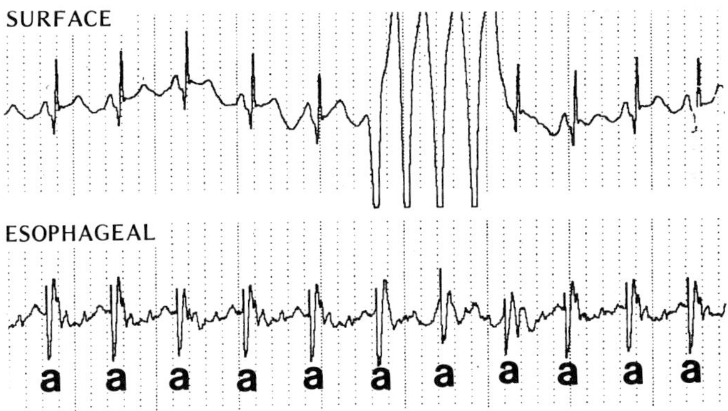

Figure 10-1 Esophageal recording made using a two-channel 24-hour ambulatory ECG recorder. The upper strip shows a surface ECG recording made on channel 1 of the ambulatory ECG recorder. It demonstrates sinus rhythm and a four-beat run of a wide QRS complex tachyarrhythmia at a rate of 150 beats/min. P-wave activity is not identifiable during this four-beat salvo on the surface lead. The simultaneously recorded esophageal recording is shown in the bottom strip. A large atrial ECG can be seen corresponding to the P-wave activity on the surface lead. During the four-beat salvo of wide QRS complex tachycardia atrial activity proceeds uninterrupted. This documentation of AV dissociation strongly suggests that this tachyarrhythmia was a run of ventricular tachycardia. Using the pill electrode, these esophageal recordings can be made in most patients for periods of 24 hours or longer (see Chapter 4).

Unfortunately, they occur in a small percentage of patients with sustained ventricular tachycardia.

Wellens and colleagues (1978) assessed the value of tachycardia rate, axis, and surface ECG morphology for distinguishing ventricular tachycardia from supraventricular tachycardia with aberration. They found that most episodes of ventricular tachycardia in patients not receiving antiarrhythmic drugs consisted of rates between 130 and 170 beats/min, whereas the largest number of episodes of supraventricular tachycardia with aberration consisted of rates between 170 and 200 beats/min. These researchers found that left-axis deviation favored a diagnosis of ventricular tachycardia, while right-axis deviation in the presence of right bundle branch block favored a diagnosis of supraventricular tachycardia with aberration. There were, however, many exceptions to these generalizations. In their study all tachycardias with a QRS duration greater than 140 milliseconds were ventricular. However, a number of episodes of ventricular tachycardia had narrower QRS complexes. The ECG morphology in leads V_1 and V_6 were most helpful in distinguishing supraventricular tachycardia with aberration from ventricular tachycardia (Figure 10-2). With a right bundle branch block pattern the finding of a triphasic rsR′ or an rSR′ favored a diagnosis of supraventricular tachycardia, whereas Rsr′ and other configurations favored a diagnosis of ventricular tachycardia. In lead V_6 a terminal conduction delay typical of right bundle branch block favored a diagnosis of supraventricular tachycardia with aberration. The surface morphology in left bundle branch block tachycardias was less helpful in distinguishing between supraventricular tachycardia and ventricular tachycardia. Wellens and colleagues noted that both supraventricular and ventricular tachycardia may have irregular cycle lengths occasionally, but this finding favors a diagnosis of ventricular tachycardia slightly. Disease of the His-Purkinje system may reduce the diagnostic accuracy of these criteria.

Intracardiac recordings The use of intracardiac electrode catheters facilitates an accurate diagnosis of ventricular tachycardia (Kastor, et al., 1981). Three catheters are usually used to record from the high right atrium, the right ventricle, and the region of the His bundle. These recordings not only facilitate evaluation of the relationship between atrial and ventricular depolarization but also permit the assessment of electrograms in the region of the His bundle. As previously mentioned, the presence of AV dissociation strongly suggests a diagnosis of ventricular tachycardia, and this finding is detected most reliably by intracardiac recording. The strongest finding supporting a diagnosis of ventricular tachycardia is dissociation of the His bundle electrogram and the ventricular electrogram, although this finding is only rarely noted. In most cases of ventricular tachycardia the His bundle region is depolarized retrogradely, the His electrogram is buried in the ventricular electrogram, and

RBBB QRS MORPHOLOGY

Lead V_1

QRS Complex	SVT with Aberrancy	Ventricular Tachardia
1	–	12
2	7	9
3	12	2
4	28	2
5	–	4
6	1	12
7	–	4
	48	45

Lead V_6

QRS Complex	SVT with Aberrancy	Ventricular Tachardia
1	31	2
2	15	10
3	2	18
4		11
5		3
6		1
	48	45

LBBB QRS MORPHOLOGY

Lead V_1

QRS Morphology

not very helpful

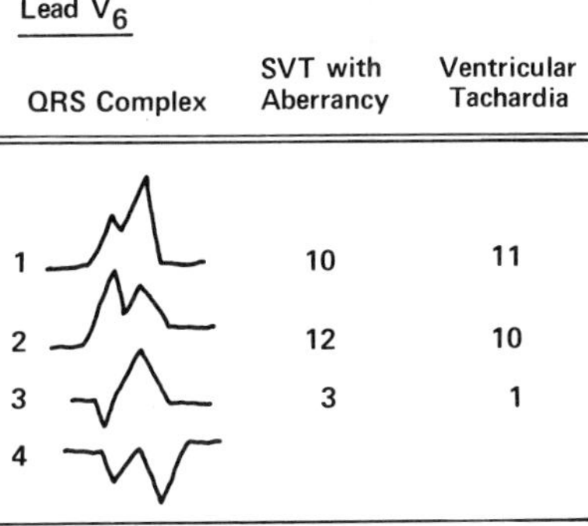

Lead V_6

QRS Complex	SVT with Aberrancy	Ventricular Tachardia
1	10	11
2	12	10
3	3	1
4		

Figure 10-2 The value of the surface ECG morphology in distinguishing supraventricular tachycardia with aberration from ventricular tachycardia. These data were obtained by Wellens and colleagues (1978) in patients who were not taking antiarrhythmic medications and who did not have bundle branch block during sinus rhythm. Assessment of morphology in leads V_1 and V_6 is valuable in distinguishing supraventricular tachycardia with aberration from ventricular tachycardia for patients with wide QRS complex tachyarrhythmias showing right bundle branch block morphology. For left bundle branch block morphology the surface ECG is not as valuable but limited information can be obtained from lead V_6. (*Source:* Wellens, H. J. J.; Bar, F. W. H. M.; and Lie, K. I. 1978. The value of the electrocardiogram in the differential diagnosis of a tachycardia with a widened QRS complex. *Am. J. Med.* 64:27-33.)

His spikes are absent. When examining intracardiac recordings, His electrogram identification must be made during sinus rhythm or after atrial depolarization during ventricular tachycardia because the absence of His spikes during ventricular tachycardia may be related to improper positioning of the His catheter rather than a true absence of His electrograms. A ventricular tachycardia focus in the upper septal myocardium or in the proximal His-Purkinje conduction system or ventricular tachycardia caused by bundle branch reentry will result in a His spike preceding each QRS complex. In the former region the HV interval is usually shorter, while in the latter case it is usually longer than that noted during sinus rhythm or during supraventricular capture beats.

Mechanism

The two most widely proposed mechanisms for sustained ventricular tachycardia are abnormal automaticity and reentry (Wellens, 1975). In the case of automaticity the mechanism is presumed to be abnormal tissue taking control of the ventricles because the spontaneous diastolic depolarization of this tissue reaches threshold faster than the sinus pacemaker. It is thought that premature beats neither initiate nor terminate an automatic focus tachycardia. Premature beats introduced during tachycardia may reset the focus and result in a noncompensatory pause; however, if the focus is protected by entrance block, premature beats may capture the rest of the ventricle but have no effect on the tachycardia cycle length. Rapid pacing may cause transient overdrive suppression without termination of an automatic tachycardia.

Recent experimental and clinical evidence suggests that some ventricular tachycardias may be caused by triggered automaticity (see Chapter 1). This type of automaticity is caused by delayed after-depolarizations that are more prominent after premature beats or at faster heart rates. These after-depolarizations may reach threshold and initiate a sustained tachycardia. A clue to the presence of triggered automaticity is the finding of a shorter time from the initiating premature beat to the first beat of the tachycardia as the coupling interval of the premature beat is decreased. Abnormal automaticity may also occur in myocardium with a low resting diastolic potential as a result of ischemia or other causes.

Available evidence favors reentry as the mechanism for most recurrent sustained ventricular tachycardias (Josephson, et al., 1978), especially in patients with coronary artery disease in the first few minutes after myocardial infarction or in the postinfarction phase beginning several days later. Reentrant ventricular tachycardia may be initiated by premature beats that are completely blocked in one portion of the ventricle and are conducted with delay in another portion. If the conduction delay is sufficient, the tissue in which conduction block occurred may recover sufficiently so that retrograde conduction is possible and a sustained reentrant circuit may be established. Classically, such arrhythmias may be terminated by appropriately timed premature ventricular stimuli. The reentry circuit may be confined to a small area or may involve an aneurysm (Mason, et al., 1981), a part of the normal His-Purkinje conduction system (Spurrell, et al., 1973), or another anatomic structure, resulting in macro-reentry.

In our experience determining the actual mechanism of ventricular tachycardia in a given patient can be difficult. Often even detailed intraoperative epicardial and endocardial mapping fails to clearly elucidate the mechanism of ventricular tachycardia. It is our opinion that, while considering the commonly proposed mechanisms may help the clinician in dealing with some cases of ventricular tachycardia, further study is needed before we will understand completely the various mechanisms of ventricular tachycardia.

Clinical Setting

Ventricular tachycardia occurs in a variety of clinical settings. In all situations a careful history and physical exam and the indicated diagnostic tests should be performed to define the underlying cardiac pathology clearly. Potentially reversible causes of the arrhythmia, such as electrolyte imbalance (especially hypokalemia), digitalis intoxication, hypoxia, foreign bodies, such as catheters, and acute myocardial infarction, must be excluded.

Most ventricular tachycardia is nonsustained and typically lasts for only three or four consecutive beats. Nonsustained ventricular tachycardia may be seen occasionally in apparently healthy subjects. It is uncommon in younger individuals but may occur in 3%-5% of apparently healthy middle-aged patients and in up to 15% or more of patients with coronary heart disease, especially 1-3 weeks after myocardial infarction (Winkle, 1980 and 1981). Other commonly associated conditions include congestive cardiomyopathies, hypertrophic cardiomyopathies (Savage, et al., 1979), and the mitral valve prolapse syndrome (Winkle, et al., 1975; DeMaria, et al., 1976). Nonsustained ventricular tachycardia usually occurs in association with frequent, isolated premature ventricular beats and complex ventricular ectopy. The limited data available indicate that these brief salvos may identify high-risk subgroups among patients with coronary disease (Bigger, et al., 1981) and hypertrophic cardiomyopathies (Maron, et al., 1981). The exact indication for long-term suppression of ventricular tachycardia remains uncertain, but most clinicians treat this arrhythmia, especially when it occurs in patients with organic heart disease.

Longer episodes of self-terminating ventricular tachycardia, lasting from six beats to 20 or 30 seconds, are observed less frequently. The rate of these paroxysms may vary considerably, and although occasional patients are completely asymptomatic, most individuals experience palpitations that may be disabling and may result in syncope or presyncope. This form of ventricular tachycardia generally requires long-term suppressive therapy.

Sustained ventricular tachycardia occurs considerably less frequently than nonsustained ventricular tachycardia. These episodes generally last 1 minute or longer and usually require pharmacologic or electrical termination. Five to ten percent of patients with sustained ventricular tachycardia have no evidence of organic heart disease, although a few of the patients previously diagnosed as having ventricular tachycardia associated with a normal heart may actually have had arrhythmogenic right ventricular dysplasia, a condition that has only recently been characterized (Marcus, et al., 1982). Patients with this condition have dysplasia of all or a portion of the right ventricular myocardium with replacement by fatty and fibrous tissue. There is a male predominance, and the ventricular tachycardia has a left bundle branch block morphology. The physical exam is usually normal. The heart is moderately enlarged and two-dimensional echocardiograms show an increased right ventricular diastolic diameter. Right ventricular angiography shows an enlarged chamber with segmental wall motion abnormalities.

Approximately two-thirds of our patients with recurrent sustained ventricular tachycardia are diagnosed as having coronary heart disease and most have had one or more previous myocardial infarctions. The remainder of our patients have myocardial or valvular disease. Most patients with sustained ventricular tachycardia are severely disabled by this arrhythmia. The severity of symptoms is influenced by the rate and duration of the tachycardia, as well as by the degree of left ventricular dysfunction. Patients commonly complain of severe palpitations, dizziness, lightheadedness, chest pain, dyspnea, diaphoresis, presyncope, or syncope. Rapid, sustained ventricular tachycardia may result in immediate cardiac arrest or may be initially well tolerated by the patient, whose condition later deteriorates. Sustained ventricular tachycardia may occur many times a day or only infrequently. Because of the severe symptoms and hemodynamic embarrassment often associated with this rhythm, immediate or urgent termination and long-term preventive therapy are usually required.

Termination of Ventricular Tachycardia

Clinical assessment The mode of treatment used to terminate sustained ventricular tachycardia depends on the clinical status of the patient. Conscious patients with suspected ventricular tachycardia should undergo a rapid but careful clinical assessment, including blood-pressure measurement, examination of the neck veins and lungs for evidence of left or right ventricular failure, and cardiac auscultation with special attention paid to the intensity of the first heart sound. An overall assessment of the degree of clinical distress noted by the patient is most important. Patients who complain of severe dyspnea or chest pain or have clinical evidence of shock require immediate termination of the arrhythmia. Patients who are in sustained ventricular tachycardia require frequent careful clinical reassessment to be certain that they are not showing evidence of hemodynamic deterioration. A 12-lead ECG should be obtained in all patients who lack severe hemodynamic compromise. Twelve-lead ECG recordings are superior to rhythm strips because the multiple leads often aid in distinguishing ventricular tachycardia from supraventricular tachycardia with aberration. These tracings may be used later on, if the patient undergoes initiation of ventricular tachycardia during electrophysiologic studies, to determine if induced and spontaneous arrhythmias are similar morphologically. Many patients tolerate their ventricular tachycardias well enough to permit the recording of atrial activity from esophageal electrograms, which can be obtained in 10 minutes or less. Some patients may be stable enough to permit the recording of intracardiac electrograms or even the performance of a full intracardiac electrophysiologic study. The latter is useful not only to confirm a diagnosis of ventricular tachycardia but to permit termination of ventricular tachycardia by pacing (see the section on pacing techniques). Patients with ventricular tachycardias that lead to a loss of consciousness will require immediate termination by cardioversion. All patients who are receiving chronic antiarrhythmic therapy or digitalis when the ventricular tachycardia occurs should have blood drawn for drug plasma concentration determinations.

Pharmacologic therapy Ventricular tachycardias that do not result in an immediate loss of consciousness may be amenable to pharmacologic conversion (see Chapter 3). The initial drug used is usually intravenous lidocaine. A bolus of lidocaine, ranging from 50 to 150 mg, may be given over a period of 3-5 minutes. In this situation termination of the tachycardia may be more dependent on the peak blood levels achieved rather than the total dose given. The clinician should be alert during administration of lidocaine for signs of minor toxicity such as lethargy, tremor, slurred speech, or ringing in the ears. These signs of minor toxicity virtually always precede more serious toxic side-effects such as grand mal seizures or respiratory arrest. The more serious side-effects usually occur when a large lidocaine bolus is given too rapidly. Little information is available about the kinetics of lidocaine administration during acute ventricular tachycardia, and the clinician should remember that many of these patients probably have a low output state and a reduced volume of distribution that may result in high plasma levels. The major advantage of lidocaine is its lack of adverse hemodynamic effects, although it may occasionally accelerate the rate of a ventricular tachycardia. Lidocaine is the most convenient agent for terminating ventricular tachycardia because it may be administered over a relatively short period of time. If lidocaine terminates the ventricular tachycardia, a continuous infusion should be initiated. Although intravenous bretylium tosylate (5-10 mg/kg may also be given rapidly, we generally avoid intravenous bretylium for the termination of hemodynamically stable ventricular tachycardia because of the drug's potential adverse hemodynamic effects. Bretylium may cause significant hypotension either immediately or 15-30 minutes after administration. This is an especially serious problem if the drug fails to terminate the arrhythmia because a previously well-tolerated episode of ventricular tachycardia may then become poorly tolerated. If lidocaine fails and termination is needed urgently, we prefer the use of cardioversion to bretylium. Bretylium can be used when ventricular tachycardia rapidly and repeatedly recurs despite lidocaine therapy. In this setting the initial bretylium loading dose may be followed by an intravenous infusion of 0.5-2 mg/min. Moderate bretylium-induced hypotension is usually well tolerated by supine patients, but severe postural hypotension, causing syncope, can occur if the patient attempts to ambulate while receiving a bretylium infusion. This side-effect may be ameliorated by concomitant administration of a tricyclic antidepressant.

A number of other intravenous antiarrhythmic agents may be given in an attempt to terminate ventricular tachycardia (see Chapter 3). The next most frequently used drug is procainamide (750-1000 mg), but mexiletine, encainide, lorcainide, and a variety of other agents may also be effective. A major problem with procainamide is that it cannot generally be given safely at a rate exceeding 50 mg/min; therefore, 20-45 minutes are required for infusion of an adequate dose. Procainamide should only be used for termination of ventricular tachycardia if the rhythm is well tolerated and if the patient is likely to remain stable long enough for infusion of an adequate dose. Many of these drugs result in significant slowing of the tachycardia when they do not terminate it and this may improve the patient's hemodynamic status. Some, however, also cause peripheral vasodilatation and may worsen the patient's overall clinical status.

Pacing techniques Sustained ventricular tachycardia can often be terminated by pacing techniques (Fisher, et al., 1978 and 1982). Most arrhythmias that are susceptible to pace termination are caused by reentry. During pace termination a portion of the reentry circuit is depolarized by premature beats introduced to the ventricle via a pacing catheter. This alters the circuit in such a manner as to interrupt the reentry and terminate the tachycardia. Single premature beats are effective in terminating ventricular tachycardia when the rate of the ventricular tachycardia is slow. The ability of a single premature beat to terminate tachycardias depends on refractoriness, conduction, and the amount of tissue between the catheter and the reentry circuit. For many ventricular tachycardias (especially those with faster rates), single premature beats may capture part or all of the ventricles but fail to penetrate the reentry circuit with sufficient prematurity. In such instances pairs or trains of critically timed beats may terminate the ventricular tachycardia. The technique that is most often effective in terminating sustained ventricular tachycardia is a burst of rapid ventricular pacing at a cycle length shorter than that of the tachycardia. In many instances pacing will change the morphology and the rate of the tachycardia transiently with either subsequent termination or change to a different, stable morphology. The major danger associated with termination of ventricular tachycardia by pacing techniques is acceleration to a faster ventricular tachycardia or degeneration to ventricular fibrillation (Figure 10-3), requiring defibrillation. Acceleration may occur unexpectedly despite several previous successful attempts.

In some patients with frequent episodes of ventricular tachycardia requiring cardioversion we have used an automatic antitachycardia pacemaker (see Chapter 7) attached to a temporary transvenous pacing wire

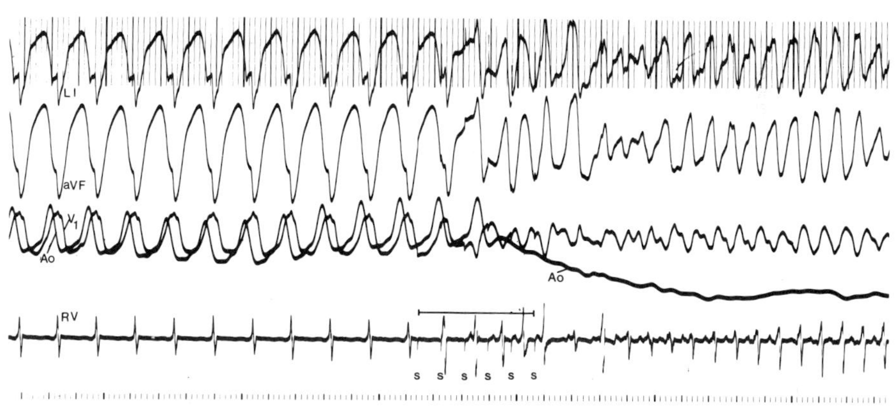

Figure 10-3 Acceleration of ventricular tachycardia during attempted pace termination. This figure shows three surface leads, I, aVF, and V_1, and a simultaneous right ventricular bipolar electrogram, labeled RV. The aortic (Ao) pressure is also shown. The left-hand portion of the figure shows a stable ventricular tachycardia that maintains adequate arterial pressure. In the center of the figure a train of six stimuli (S) are introduced in an attempt to pace-terminate the ventricular tachycardia. This burst accelerates the rhythm to ventricular flutter with an immediate fall in blood pressure. This ventricular flutter required cardioversion for termination. (*Source:* Mason, J. W.; and Winkle, R. A. 1978. Electrode-catheter arrhythmia induction in the selection and assessment of antiarrhythmic drug therapy for recurrent ventricular tachycardia. *Circulation* 58:971-985.)

in the intensive care unit to successfully pace-terminate multiple episodes of ventricular tachycardia. This is a temporizing measure to be used while antiarrhythmic therapy is being initiated and only where prompt intervention by nursing personnel can provide successful conversion to sinus rhythm if acceleration is induced by the pace-termination attempts.

Cardioversion Cardioversion is the most uniformly successful method for terminating ventricular tachycardia and should be employed immediately when a loss of consciousness or severe hemodynamic embarrassment occurs. It should also be utilized when a patient shows clinical deterioration during attempts at pharmacologic conversion or after reasonable attempts at pharmacologic conversion have failed. Although low energy, such as 10 or 20 watt-seconds, terminates ventricular tachycardia, we generally prefer to begin with at least 100 watt-seconds of delivered energy. Lower energies increase the risk of depolarizing insufficient quantities of myocardium to convert the rhythm successfully and may result in ventricular fibrillation. Ventricular tachycardia should always be cardioverted with the defibrillator in the synchronized mode. In circumstances where a cardioversion terminates ventricular tachycardia briefly (several sinus beats are noted) and then resumes a repeat cardioversion is unlikely to be successful in maintaining sinus rhythm and should be repeated only after drug therapy has been initiated.

Prevention

The clinician must always look for reversible causes of ventricular tachyarrhythmias. If no reversible cause is found, the patient will require long-term suppressive therapy. Pharmacologic therapy is generally the initial treatment, and more aggressive surgical and pacing techniques should be reserved for those patients whose arrhythmias are resistant to drugs. The selection of a specific antiarrhythmic drug is empiric. The process of drug selection is often protracted and may involve many trials of single drugs and drug combinations before arrhythmia control is achieved. Patients should be counseled about the possibility of prolonged hospitalization and the need for intensive follow-up. Careful consideration of the clinical pharmacology of each antiarrhythmic drug is important (see Chapter 3), as is the measurement of drug plasma concentrations with many drugs. By and large, however, the end point of antiarrhythmic therapy should be the prevention of ventricular tachycardia rather than the attainment of a therapeutic drug plasma concentration. Drug level determinations may be useful in identifying patients who require unusually large or small doses of an agent and for evaluating drug compliance and the potential for toxic side-effects. The widespread availability of elaborate ECG monitoring techniques and intracardiac electrophysiologic studies has minimized strict reliance on drug plasma concentrations for adjusting the drug dose.

ECG monitoring techniques Brief, frequent salvos of ventricular tachycardia are often best managed by using continuous ambulatory or in-hospital ECG monitoring (see Chapter 4). In selected patients exercise testing may assist in the selection of effective therapy. In most instances patients should be withdrawn from all antiarrhythmic drugs and adequate baseline ECG monitoring performed to characterize the frequency with which the arrhythmia occurs, as well as its relationship to the patient's symptoms. Antiarrhythmic therapy is then started and the response followed with further ECG monitoring. The end point of therapy is usually complete suppression of all runs of ventricular tachycardia.

Electrophysiologic drug testing In most patients with recurrent sustained ventricular tachycardia the arrhythmia can be initiated in the electrophysiology laboratory (Wellens, et al., 1972; 1974; and 1976; Mason, et al., 1982b) (see Table 10-1). Although ventricular tachycardia is occasionally initiated by rapid atrial pacing or atrial premature beats, ventricular pacing techniques are generally required for initiation. We introduce one, two, or three extrastimuli during sinus rhythm and during ventricular pacing at one or more cycle lengths, as well as rapid bursts of ventricular pacing. The pacing combination that is most often successful is two or three extra ventricular beats given during ventricular pacing. Although a third extrastimulus is required in many patients to induce the clinically occurring ventricular tachycardia, the use of three or more extrastimuli can induce nonsustained polymorphic salvos in many individuals who lack a prior history of serious ventricular arrhythmias. Such "junk" rhythms should only be considered as relevant when strong supporting clinical data exist. Some patients with exercise-induced ventricular tachycardia can only have their arrhythmias induced during isoproterenol infusion (Figure 10-4). Although most sustained ventricular tachycardias

Table 10-1 Arrhythmia inducibility: nature of induced arrhythmia

Clinical arrhythmia	N total	Induced arrhythmia			
		Sustained VT	Unsustained VT	VF	None
Sustained VT	(n = 241)	76%	8%	6%	7%
Unsustained VT	(n = 42)	19%	36%	7%	38%
VF	(n = 28)	14%	18%	36%	29%
Sudden death	(n = 104)	58%	12%	15%	15%

VT = ventricular tachycardia.

VF = ventricular fibrillation.

may be initiated using right ventricular apical pacing (especially if three extrastimuli are used), occasional patients may require stimulation of the right ventricular outflow tract or left ventricle (Robertson, et al., 1981). The morphology of the induced ventricular tachycardia is usually similar to that which has occurred clinically, but other morphologies of ventricular tachycardia that have not been previously documented clinically may also be induced. Induced ventricular tachycardias are terminated using pacing techniques or direct current cardioversion and are then reinitiated two or more times to document the reproducibility of induction. Antiarrhythmic drugs are then administered and a repeat attempt is made to induce the ventricular tachycardia. If sustained ventricular tachycardia is no longer inducible, the drug is likely to prevent recurrence of sustained ventricular tachycardia (Mason and Winkle, 1978 and 1980; Horowitz, et al., 1978) (Figure 10-5). With increasing understanding of the pharmacology of antiarrhythmic drugs, it is apparent that many have active metabolites, and we now prefer to administer most drugs orally until maximally tolerated steady-state drug levels are achieved before testing efficacy using ventricular stimulation techniques.

These invasive tests frequently create life-threatening ventricular rhythm disturbances and should only be carried out by highly trained physician and nursing personnel (see Chapter 2). Although some centers perform follow-up drug tests on the general ward or in the intensive care unit, we prefer to perform them in a dedicated electrophysiology laboratory. They are often carried out with arterial pressure monitoring, and always with full resuscitation capabilities immediately available. These electrophysiologic tests are usually well accepted by the patients, who often return to the laboratory on a number of occasions.

If a drug prevents the induction of sustained ventricular tachycardia, there is an increased likelihood of long-term prevention of ventricular tachycardia or sudden death with that drug. If a drug fails to prevent the induction of sustained ventricular tachycardia, it is more likely that the patient will experience a recurrence of the ventricular tachycardia or sudden death if treated with that drug on a chronic basis. Although the inducibility or noninducibility of a ventricular tachycardia is a strong, independent predictor of long-term mortality on antiarrhythmic therapy,

Figure 10-4 The use of isoproterenol to facilitate ventricular tachycardia induction. These tracings were made in a 16-year-old male with a history of exercise-induced QRS complex tachycardia. Panel A shows six surface ECG leads, right atrial electrogram (RA), right ventricular electrogram (RV), His bundle recordings (HB), and arterial pressure tracings (BP). The introduction of up to three ventricular extrastimuli, labeled V_2, V_3, and V_4, during ventricular drive (V_1) failed to induce any ventricular arrhythmias. When pacing is terminated, sinus rhythm resumes. Panel B shows tracings obtained during the infusion of isoproterenol. In this tracing a single premature beat, labeled V_2, given during

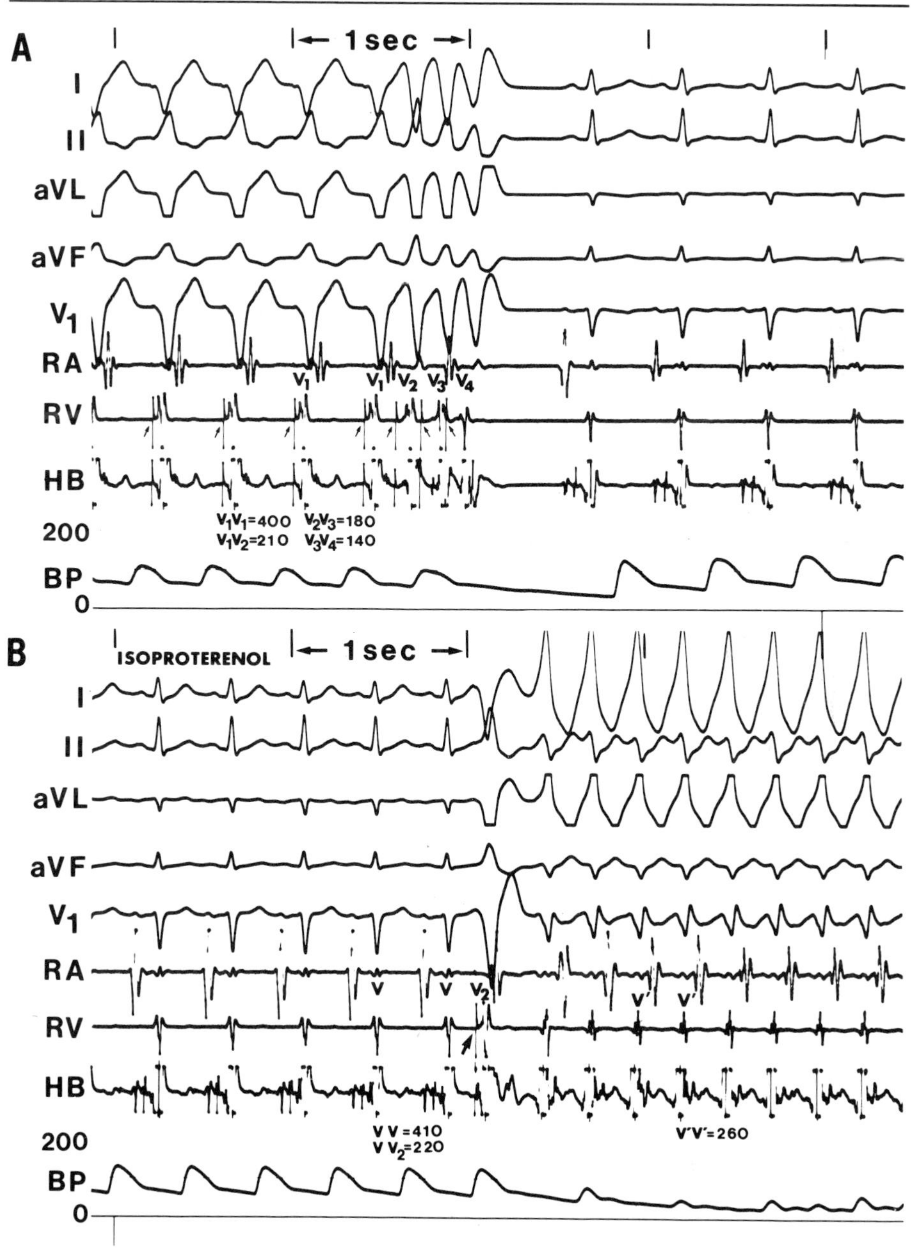

sinus rhythm initiates a sustained ventricular tachycardia, the morphology of which was identical to the rhythm that was precipitated during exercise treadmill testing. This patient was subsequently treated with propranolol and has been arrhythmia-free.

it is not as important as the severity of heart failure for predicting outcome (Swerdlow, et al., 1982). Amiodarone may be the one exception to this generalization that the results of electrophysiologic study predict long-term outcome. However, in our experience, most patients whose ventricular tachycardia remains inducible on amiodarone will have a clinical recurrence during long-term treatment.

A variety of definitions of drug success using electrophysiologic testing exist. Although we have previously required that a drug convert sustained ventricular tachycardia to fewer than six inducible beats or totally prevent nonsustained ventricular tachycardia before we declare it effective, a more recent analysis of our follow-up data indicates that a cut-off of 10-15 beats may be more appropriate (Swerdlow, et al., 1982b). The clinical relevance of making a ventricular tachycardia harder to induce (e.g., two extrastimuli required for induction in the control state but three extrastimuli needed after drug administration) remains uncertain (Swerdlow, et al., 1982c).

Early experience with electrophysiologic testing using intravenous drug administration or those drugs that permitted rapid oral loading gave promise that the technique could rapidly screen antiarrhythmic drugs for efficacy (Mason and Winkle, 1978). However, with the realization that oral drug therapy must be tested in most patients and the increasing number of antiarrhythmic drugs with long loading periods, the drug selection process has become considerably lengthened despite the use of electrophysiologic testing. In our experience any single antiarrhythmic drug will be effective in only approximately 9%-25% of patients (Mason, et al., 1982b) (Table 10-2), and even when multiple drugs are tested in an individual patient, a drug that effectively blocks the induction of ventricular tachycardia can be found in only approximately one-third of patients. Because a large number of the patients who are subjected to serial electrophysiologic testing will not have an effective antiarrhythmic drug determined, it would be desirable to identify in advance those patients most likely to benefit from these tests. We have found that the patients who are most likely to have an effective drug found are those without evidence of organic heart disease or those with fewer coronary

Figure 10-5 Evaluation of antiarrhythmic drug therapy using programmed stimulation. Figure 10-5A shows recordings obtained in a patient with a history of recurrent sustained ventricular tachycardia. Surface ECG leads I, aVF, and V_1 are displayed with a right atrial electrogram (RA), a right ventricular electrogram (RV), and a His bundle electrogram (HE). Ao and bl represent the aortic pressure tracing and the baseline for pressure calibration. The right ventricle is being driven at a basic cycle length of 600 milliseconds. After the last basic drive beat (V_1), two programmed extrastimuli (V_2 and V_3) are introduced and ventricular tachycardia ensues. Figure 10-5B shows a similar tracing made in this patient after the

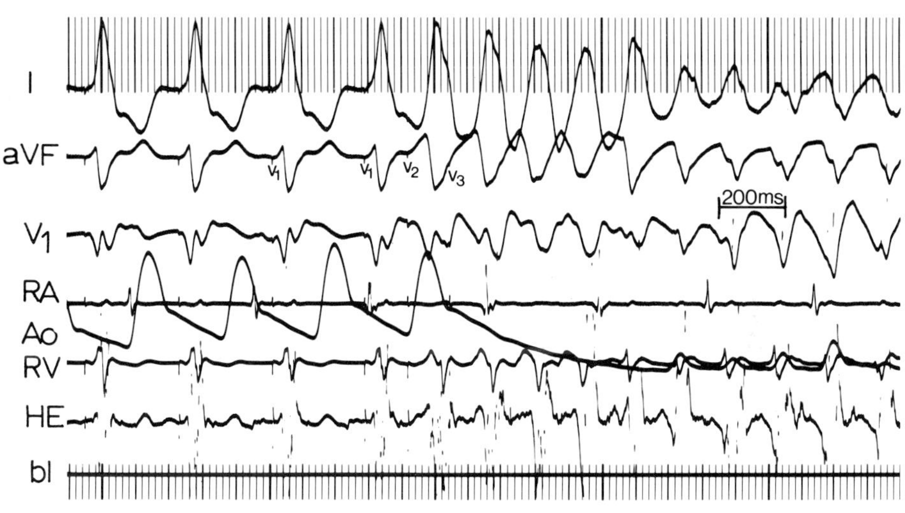

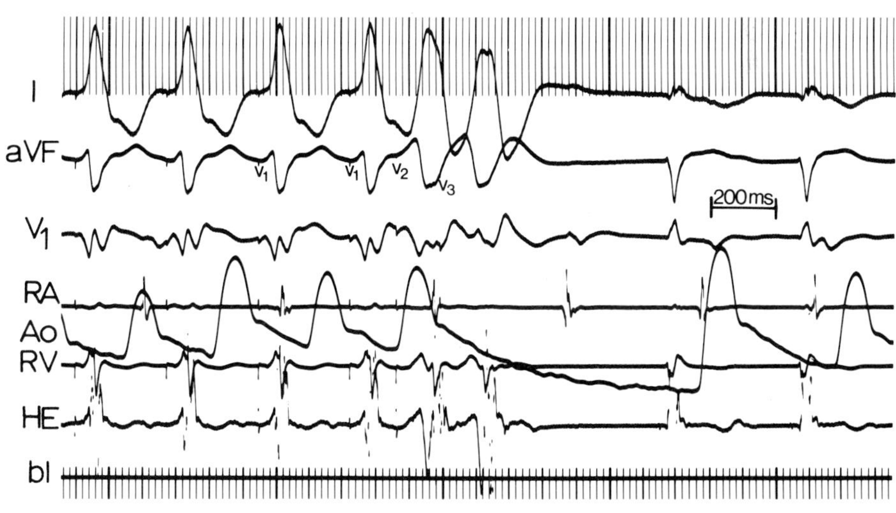

infusion of 10 mg/kg of quinidine gluconate. Ventricular tachycardia could no longer be initiated after V_1, V_2, and V_3 stimulation. This protection against induced ventricular tachycardias indicates that there is a high likelihood the drug will be effective during long-term oral therapy. (*Source:* Mason, J. W.; and Winkle, R. A. 1978. Electrode-catheter arrhythmia induction in the selection and assessment of antiarrhythmic drug therapy for recurrent ventricular tachycardia. *Circulation* 58:971-985.

Table 10-2 Efficacy of antiarrhythmic drugs at electrophysiologic study

Drug	No. of patients tested	No. of patients with effective trial	Efficacy rate
Lidocaine	136	18	13%
Quinidine	97	21	22%
Procainamide	66	13	20%
Propranolol	20	5	25%
Disopyramide	12	4	33%
Phenytoin	7	1	14%
All other drugs	203	18	9%
Investigational drugs	155	14	9%
Excluding amiodarone	118	11	9%

stenoses, females, those without left ventricular aneurysms, those having failed the fewest number of empiric drug trials before electrophysiologic testing, and those with the least severe arrhythmias (Swerdlow, et al., 1983). Patients who are predicted to be unlikely to have an effective drug found by serial electrophysiologic testing could be considered for amiodarone, endocardial mapping with endocardial ablation, or a defibrillator implantation early in their hospital course and avoid serial electrophysiologic drug testing.

Chronic pacing techniques Pacing techniques were discussed in Chapter 7, and the role of chronic pacing for prevention or termination of ventricular tachycardia will only be summarized here. Although a number of cases of chronic pacing used to treat ventricular tachycardia have been reported, the overall proportion of patients for whom this form of treatment is effective is small (Fisher, et al., 1982). Overdrive pacing at rates that are 10-20 beats faster than the sinus rate is occasionally effective for preventing recurrences of sustained ventricular tachycardia. Some patients with permanent pacemakers can terminate ventricular tachycardia by converting their pacemaker to the asynchronous mode using a magnet; however, this technique works only in patients in whom the ventricular tachycardia is slow, well tolerated, and terminated by single premature beats. Although pairs and bursts of pacing are more frequently effective for ventricular tachycardia termination, the danger of acceleration limits the number of cases in which this technique may be useful on a long-term basis. In patients with hemodynamically well-tolerated ventricular tachycardia a patient-activated, radiofrequency-triggered pacemaker may be used (Figure 10-6). In such instances it is safest for the patient to proceed to an emergency room where the pacemaker can be triggered under careful ECG monitoring so that if acceleration occurs, it can be treated promptly by medical personnel.

Operative management This topic will be covered in detail in Chapter 11 and only a few points will be made here. Patients who are candidates for surgical management of ventricular tachycardia are generally those who have failed multiple attempts at medical therapy (Horowitz, et al., 1980; Mason, et al., 1982a). Such patients should have enough residual cardiac function to survive cardiac surgery. The ventricular tachycardia in these patients should be either continuously present or reliably inducible using electrical stimulation techniques. The best candidates for surgical mapping and ablation are those patients with ventricular tachycardia of stable morphology with discrete onset of the QRS complexes. Those patients who have rapid, sinusoidal ventricular tachycardia morphologies often prove difficult to map in the operating room because it is difficult to determine whether electrical activity is early or late.

Atrial RF Pacer for VT

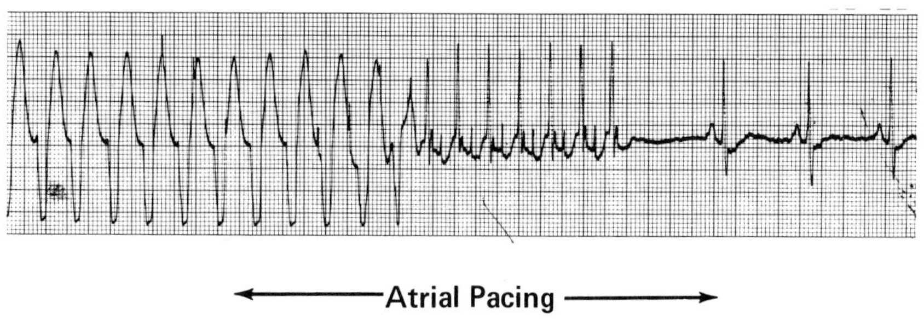

Figure 10-6 Use of an atrial radiofrequency pacemaker to terminate ventricular tachycardia. This patient had an unusual type of recurrent sustained ventricular tachycardia that could be initiated and terminated by rapid atrial pacing. A permanent atrial radiofrequency pacemaker was implanted. An episode of sustained ventricular tachycardia is shown on the left-hand side of the strip. Rapid atrial pacing is initiated, which eventually results in supraventricular capture of the ventricle. When atrial pacing is terminated, sinus rhythm ensues. This patient's ventricular tachycardia is hemodynamically well tolerated, and when episodes occur he goes to the local emergency room where the ventricular tachycardia is terminated under direct ECG monitoring using the radiofrequency pacemaker.

A preoperative endocardial catheter map can be attempted (Josephson, et al., 1982) in patients who are being considered for intraoperative mapping and ablation of ventricular tachycardia. Preoperative catheter maps occasionally provide useful information but we have found that they have a number of significant limitations. In many patients the ventricular tachycardia is hemodynamically poorly tolerated and no more than a few sites can be mapped. In such cases intravenous administration of antiarrhythmic drugs to slow the tachycardia may be helpful. Another serious limitation is that one is frequently unable to manipulate the catheter successfully within the left ventricular cavity. Even when the catheter can be freely manipulated within the left ventricle, estimation of its exact anatomic position by fluoroscopy is often impossible. The technique is also plagued by several problems common to intraoperative endocardial mapping. These include multiple morphologies of induced ventricular tachycardia, difficulties in distinguishing early from late electrical activity, and the inability to determine intramyocardial electrical activation. Endocardial catheter maps have been useful in selected cases for determining a right ventricular origin of ventricular tachycardia, and a good preoperative map may be of great value when the rhythm cannot be initiated in the operating room.

ATYPICAL VENTRICULAR TACHYCARDIAS

Drug-Induced Ventricular Arrhythmias

A number of drugs can produce ventricular arrhythmias de novo or can aggravate preexisting ventricular arrhythmias (Vladimir, et al., 1982). The drugs that are commonly implicated include digoxin, the psychotropic drugs (especially phenothiazines and tricyclic antidepressants), and the membrane-active antiarrhythmic agents. While all membrane-active antiarrhythmic agents can aggravate arrhythmias, exacerbation occurs uncommonly with lidocaine, tocainide, and mexiletine. Drug-induced worsening of ventricular arrhythmias may occur either as an increase in the frequency and duration of preexisting ventricular tachyarrhythmia or as the appearance of new ventricular tachycardia. In many instances it is difficult to distinguish drug-induced arrhythmias from a spontaneous degeneration in the patient's clinical status. The mechanism of drug-induced exacerbation of ventricular arrhythmias is unknown.

Drug-induced ventricular tachyarrhythmias often take the form of atypical or polymorphic ventricular tachycardia (Sclarovsky, et al., 1979). These may be self-terminating and present as recurrent syncopal episodes and often occur in association with an excessively long QT interval. The polymorphic rhythm sometimes assumes a classical torsade de pointes (Krikler and Curry, 1976; Smith and Gallagher, 1980) morphology with alternation of the major electrocardiographic QRS axis (Figure 10-7).

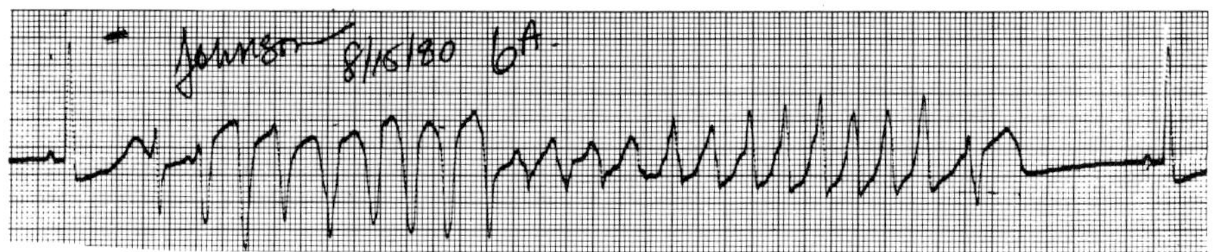

Figure 10-7 Example of torsade de pointes associated with the use of quinidine. The first QRS complex on this strip shows a sinus beat with an extremely long QT interval (greater than 0.64 seconds). A premature beat falling on the down-slope of the T wave initiates a paroxysm of ventricular tachyarrhythmia. During the first portion of the tachyarrhythmia the initial QRS forces are predominately negative, but during the episode a torsade de pointes occurs and the predominant QRS forces become positively directed. The episode self-terminates and sinus rhythm ensues.

The introduction of this term, however, has caused considerable semantic confusion. In many instances multiple simultaneous ECG leads recorded during atypical ventricular tachycardia may show classical torsade de pointes in some leads and polymorphic ventricular tachycardia in others. Internists and cardiologists are most likely to encounter drug-induced arrhythmias in patients who are receiving membrane-active agents for suppression of asymptomatic ventricular ectopic beats or for treatment of supraventricular arrhythmias. The patient typically experiences new syncopal or presyncopal episodes several days or weeks after the drug is started. These drug-induced rhythms may also first appear after many months or years of therapy. It is important to recognize the drug-induced nature of these ventricular arrhythmias because the addition of other antiarrhythmic drugs to control them may lead to further clinical deterioration. The preferred method of treatment is to withdraw all antiarrhythmic drugs and treat the patient with rapid overdrive pacing. Rates of 130-150 beats/min may be required initially to control the runs of polymorphic ventricular tachycardia. As the drug effect dissipates the pacing rate may be gradually slowed. Isoproterenol infusion may occasionally control these arrhythmias. Drug-induced ventricular tachyarrhythmias may occur either as an idiosyncratic reaction to small or standard doses of the drugs or as a toxic reaction to excessive doses. Patients whose arrhythmias are aggravated by one drug may or may not react in the same way to other antiarrhythmic drugs.

The Long QT Syndrome

Patients with the long QT syndrome usually present with a history of syncope or presyncope and recurring paroxysms of self-terminating polymorphic ventricular tachycardia or classical torsade de pointes in association with a long QT interval (Romano, et al., 1963; Ward, 1964). The long QT interval may be continuously present or may occur only intermittently. The repolarization abnormality is frequently not strictly limited to the QT interval but involves bizarre repolarization abnormalities with prominent U waves. These repolarization changes may sometimes occur or become more prominent in response to emotional stress or other stimuli. Although many cases are sporadic, the condition does occur in families (Garza, et al., 1970) and may be associated with congenital deafness (Jervell and Lange-Neilson, 1957). Many patients are diagnosed as having idiopathic epilepsy before it is recognized that their seizures are caused by ventricular tachyarrhythmia. These patients' arrhythmias may be worsened by membrane-active antiarrhythmic agents. Propranolol and phenytoin are the drugs of choice for managing these arrhythmias. Patients whose arrhythmias are not controlled by drug therapy may be candidates for surgical excision of the left cervicothoracic sympathetic ganglia. The rationale for this operation is that the QT prolongation and subsequent arrhythmias in this condition arise from an imbalance in cardiac autonomic input from the left and right sympathetic ganglia with either overstimulation from the left or understimulation from the right stellate ganglion (Crampton, 1979). This operation may control the occurrence of the arrhythmias without fully normalizing the QT interval.

VENTRICULAR FIBRILLATION

In-Hospital Ventricular Fibrillation

Most episodes of ventricular fibrillation in the hospital occur in association with acute myocardial infarction. Other instances of in-hospital ventricular fibrillation are caused by drug toxicities, electrolyte imbalance (usually hypokalemia), hypoxia or other respiratory or metabolic abnormalities, or the postcardiac surgical state. Ventricular fibrillation requires immediate, nonsynchronized defibrillation generally starting with 200 watt-seconds (see Chapter 14). It is important to emphasize that, if some time has elapsed from the onset of cardiac arrest until defibrillation is attempted, adequate oxygenation and closed-chest massage may be necessary before successful defibrillation is possible. When defibrillation is initially unsuccessful, it may ultimately be successful after the administration of intravenous epinephrine, lidocaine, or bretylium. When in-hospital ventricular fibrillation occurs in association with a reversible cause, only temporary preventive therapy may be needed. When no reversible cause can be found for the ventricular fibrillation, it should be managed as outlined below.

Out-of-Hospital Ventricular Fibrillation

Clinical setting and predisposing factors Many of the same factors that predispose the patient to in-hospital ventricular fibrillation also predispose him or her to out-of-hospital ventricular fibrillation. However, in the majority of cases of out-of-hospital cardiac arrest no acute, reversible factors are identifiable. Although approximately 75% of cardiac arrest patients have coronary artery disease, less than 50% have cardiac arrest in association with an acute myocardial infarction (Cobb, et al., 1980a and 1980b). Other patients experience this arrhythmia in the setting of myocardial disease (either congestive or hypertrophic cardiomyopathy), in association with the mitral valve prolapse syndrome or other valvular heart disease (especially aortic stenosis), and in the absence of apparent organic heart disease in rare cases.

Until recently, out-of-hospital ventricular fibrillation was uniformly fatal. The increased teaching of cardiopulmonary resuscitation (CPR) and the availability of excellent paramedic units in many communities have resulted in a large number of patients surviving out-of-hospital ventricular fibrillation. Both survival rates and the number of patients without significant brain damage can be increased by extensive teaching of CPR to the lay public (Thompson, et al., 1979). Those patients who have ventricular fibrillation in association with acute myocardial infarction or other temporary or reversible situations appear to have an excellent long-term prognosis (Cobb, et al., 1975). However, follow-up studies of individuals who experience ventricular fibrillation outside of the hospital without a recognizable acute predisposing factor indicate a 30% recurrence rate over the next 1-2 years (Liberthson, et al., 1974; Schaffer and Cobb, 1975).

Prevention Because of the high recurrence rate among patients surviving out-of-hospital ventricular fibrillation, aggressive management techniques have evolved to minimize the chance of subsequent recurrences. Using intracardiac electrophysiologic studies similar to those described above for patients with recurrent sustained ventricular tachycardia, approximately two-thirds of these patients can have ventricular arrhythmias initiated in the laboratory. Although many patients are in ventricular fibrillation when found by the paramedics, the rhythm most commonly induced in these patients is a hemodynamically unstable, rapid ventricular tachycardia. If this rhythm were not terminated promptly, it would rapidly degenerate into ventricular fibrillation. An occasional patient will have a polymorphic ventricular tachycardia that rapidly degenerates into ventricular fibrillation or ventricular fibrillation that is itself initiated by ventricular stimulation. Serial electrophysiologic drug testing may be performed in these patients, and if a drug can be found that prevents the induction of the malignant tachyarrhythmia, the drug has an excellent chance of preventing a recurrence of ventricular fibrillation (Ruskin, et al., 1980). Although some studies have suggested efficacy of routine coronary artery bypass surgery in such patients, there are no controlled trials to prove that this therapy is valuable. Antiarrhythmic drug therapy directed at suppressing all repetitive forms and R on T premature beats has also been reported to be effective (Lown and Graboys, 1977; Graboys, et al., 1982).

Automatic implantable defibrillator After 10 years of developmental work (Mirowski, et al., 1978) the automatic implantable defibrillator has begun clinical trials in humans (Mirowski, et al., 1980 and 1981). This device consists of a subcutaneously implanted generator unit that is attached to the heart via a transvenous rod-shaped electrode placed in the superior vena cava and a rectangular patch electrode sutured directly to the pericardium or epicardial surface of the heart (Figure 10-8). This unit monitors continuously for the presence of ventricular tachycardia or fibrillation and, after times ranging from approximately 13 to 20 seconds, will deliver a 25-30 joule defibrillation shock (Figure 10-9). If this initial shock is unsuccessful, the device will deliver up to three additional shocks,

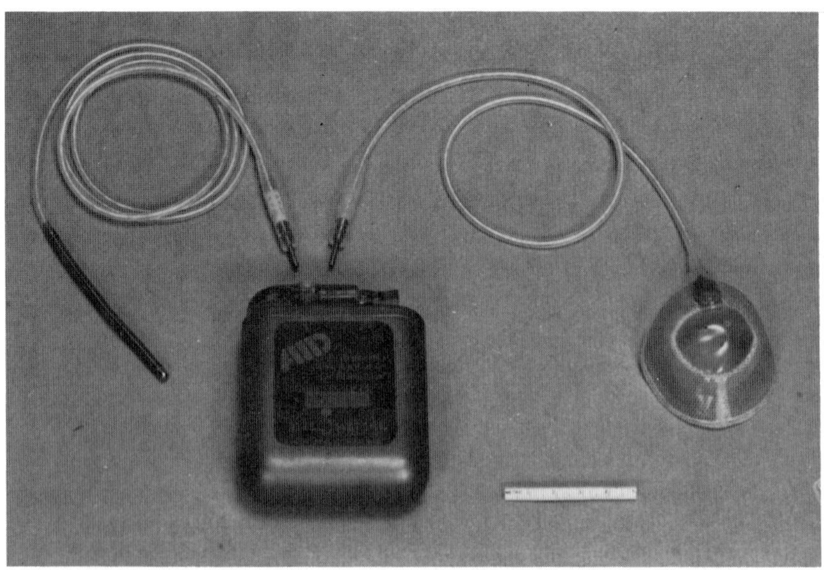

Figure 10-8 The automatic implantable defibrillator. The left-hand electrode is the rod-shaped electrode that is placed in the superior vena cava. On the right-hand side is an apical patch electrode. All implanted apical electrodes to date have actually been rectangular patches rather than this cone-shaped type of patch. The generator is shown in the center. The length of the small ruler is 5 cm.

the last one of somewhat higher energy. This device was designed for and worked exceedingly well in patients with ventricular fibrillation. It was not initially designed to sense hemodynamically unstable ventricular tachycardia. Changes in the device's sensing capability to include bipolar electrogram sensing for accurate rate detection have made the unit useful in patients with hemodynamically unstable ventricular tachycardia (Winkle, et al., 1982). These changes essentially convert the unit from an automatic implantable defibrillator to an automatic implantable cardioverter. Although initially reserved for patients who have failed medical management, after improvements in the device increasing numbers of individuals are now candidates for its use.

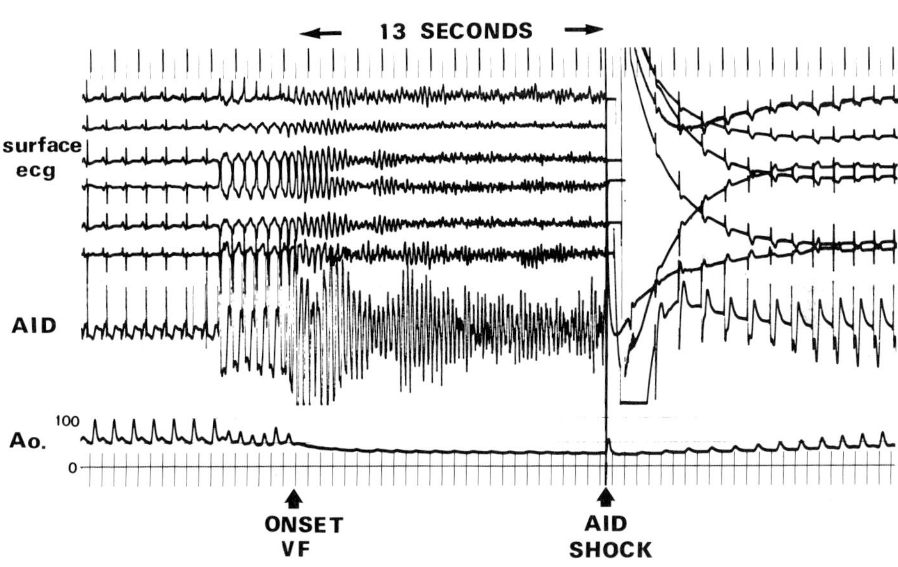

Figure 10-9 Successful termination of ventricular fibrillation using the automatic implantable defibrillator. This recording was made from a 12-year-old male with a nonobstructive hypertrophic cardiomyopathy. He had experienced several out-of-hospital cardiac arrests caused by ventricular fibrillation. This recording was made during electrophysiologic testing at the time of implantation of his automatic implantable defibrillator. Shown are six surface ECG leads. The lead labeled AID is a bipolar electrogram recorded between the rod-shaped electrode in the superior vena cava and the apical epicardial patch (see Figure 10-8). The aortic blood pressure (Ao) is also shown. The first seven beats on the left-hand side of the figure are sinus rhythm. This is followed by a brief period of six beats of ventricular paced rhythm and three premature extrastimuli. This induces ventricular fibrillation with an immediate fall in blood pressure. After 13 seconds the ventricular fibrillation is successfully converted by the AID shock of 24.8 joules and blood pressure gradually returns towards normal.

REFERENCES

Arzbaecher, R. 1973. A pill electrode for the study of cardiac arrhythmias. *Med. Instr.* 12:277-281.

Bigger, J. T., Jr.; Weld, F. M.; and Rolnitzky, L. M. 1981. Prevalence, characteristics, and significance of ventricular tachycardia (three or more complexes) detected with ambulatory electrocardiographic recording in the late hospital phase of acute myocardial infarction. *Am. J. Cardiol.* 48:815-823.

Cobb, L. A.; Baum, R. S.; Alvarex, H., III, et al. 1975. Resuscitation from out-of-hospital ventricular fibrillation: 4 years follow-up. *Circulation* 51 and 52 (*Suppl.* III):III-223-235.

Cobb, L. A.; Werner, J. A.; and Trobaugh, G. B. 1980a. I. A decade's experience with out-of-hospital resuscitation. *Mod. Concepts Cardiovasc. Dis.* 49:31-36.

Cobb, L. A.; Werner, J. A.; and Trobaugh, G. B. 1980b. II. Outcome of resuscitation: management and future directions. *Mod. Concepts Cardiovasc. Dis.* 49:37-42.

Crampton, R. 1979. Preeminence of the left stellate ganglion in the long QT syndrome. *Circulation* 59:769-778.

De Maria, A. N.; Amsterdam, E. A.; Vismara, L. A., et al. 1976. Arrhythmias in the mitral valve prolapse syndrome: prevalence, nature, and frequency. *Ann. Intern. Med.* 84:656-660.

de Soyza, N.; Murphy, M. L.; Bissett, J. K., et al. 1978. Ventricular arrhythmia in chronic stable angina pectoris with surgical or medical treatment. *Ann. Intern. Med.* 89:10-14.

Fisher, J. D.; Mehra, R.; and Furman, S. 1978. Termination of ventricular tachycardia with bursts of rapid ventricular pacing. *Am. J. Cardiol.* 41: 94-102.

Fisher, J. D.; Kim, S. G.; Furman, S., et al. 1982. Role of implantable pacemakers in control of recurrent ventricular tachycardia. *Am. J. Cardiol.* 49:194-206.

Garza, L. A.; Vick, R. L.; Nora, J. J., et al. 1970. Heritable QT prolongation without deafness. *Circulation* 41:39-48.

Graboys, T. B.; Lown, B.; Podrid, P. J., et al. 1982. Long-term survival of patients with malignant ventricular arrhythmia treated with antiarrhythmic drugs. *Am. J. Cardiol.* 50:437-443.

Hinkle, L. E.; Carver, S. T.; and Stevens, M. 1969. The frequency of asymptomatic disturbances of cardiac rhythm and conduction in middle-aged men. *Am. J. Cardiol.* 24:629-650.

Hinkle, L. E.; Carver, S. T.; and Argyros, D. C. 1974. The prognostic significance of ventricular premature contractions in healthy people and in people with coronary heart disease. *Acta Cardiol.* (*Suppl.*) 18:5-23.

Horowitz, L. N.; Josephson, M. E.; Farshidi, A., et al. 1978. Recurrent sustained ventricular tachycardia: 3. Role of the electrophysiologic study in selection of antiarrhythmic regimens. *Circulation* 58:986-997.

Horowitz, L. N.; Harken, A. H.; Kastor, J. A., et al. 1980. Ventricular resection guided by epicardial and endocardial mapping for treatment of recurrent ventricular tachycardia. *N. Engl. J. Med.* 302:589-628.

Jervell, A.; and Lange-Neilson, F. 1957. Congenital deaf mutism, functional heart disease with prolongation of the QT interval, and sudden death. *Am. Heart J.* 54:59-68.

Josephson, M. E.; and Kastor, J. A. 1976. Paroxysmal supraventricular tachycardia: is the atrium a necessary link? *Circulation* 54:430-435.

Josephson, M. E.; Horowitz, L. N.; Farshidi, A., et al. 1978. Sustained ventricular tachycardia: evidence for protected localized reentry. *Am. J. Cardiol.* 42:416-424.

Josephson, M. E.; Horowitz, L. N.; Spielman, S. R., et al. 1982. Role of catheter mapping in the preoperative evaluation of ventricular tachycardia. *Am. J. Cardiol.* 49:207-220.

Kastor, J. A.; Horowitz, L. N.; Harken, A. H., et al. 1981. Clinical electrophysiology of ventricular tachycardia. *N. Engl. J. Med.* 304:1004-1020.

Krikler, D. M.; and Curry, P. V. L. 1976. Torsade de pointes, an atypical ventricular tachycardia. *Br. Heart J.* 38:117-120.

Lehrman, K. L.; Tilkian, A. G.; Hultgren, H. N., et al. 1979. Effect of coronary arterial bypass surgery on exercise-induced ventricular arrhythmias. *Am. J. Cardiol.* 44:1056-1061.

Liberthson, R. R.; Nagel, E. L.; Hirschman, J. C., et al. 1974. Prehospital ventricular defibrillation: prognosis and follow-up course. *N. Engl. J. Med.* 291:317-321.

Lown, B.; and Graboys, T. B. 1977. Management of patients with malignant ventricular arrhythmias. *Am. J. Cardiol.* 39:910-918.

Marcus, F. I.; Fontaine, G. H.; Guiraudon, G., et al. 1982. Right ventricular dysplasia: a report of 24 adult cases. *Circulation* 65:384-398.

Maron, B. J.; Savage, D. D.; Wolfson, J. K., et al. 1981. Prognostic significance of 24-hour ambulatory electrocardiographic monitoring in patients with hypertrophic cardiomyopathy: a prospective study. *Am. J. Cardiol.* 48:252-257.

Mason, J. W.; and Winkle, R. A. 1978. Electrode-catheter arrhythmia induction in the selection and assessment of antiarrhythmic drug therapy for recurrent ventricular tachycardia. *Circulation* 58:971-985.

Mason, J. W.; and Winkle, R. A. 1980. Accuracy of the ventricular tachycardia-induction study for predicting long-term efficacy and inefficacy of antiarrhythmic drugs. *N. Engl. J. Med.* 303:1073-1077.

Mason, J. W.; Stinson, E. B.; Winkle, R. A., et al. 1981. Mechanisms of ventricular tachycardia: wide, complex ignorance. *Am. Heart J.* 102: 1083-1087.

Mason, J. W.; Stinson, E. B.; Winkle, R. A., et al. 1982a. Surgery for ventricular tachyarrhythmias: efficacy of left ventricular aneurysm resection compared to operation guided by electrical activation mapping. *Circulation* 65:1148-1155.

Mason, J. W.; Swerdlow, C. D.; Winkle, R. A., et al. 1982b. Ventricular tachyarrhythmia induction for drug selection: experience with 311 patients. National Institutes of Health symposium on antiarrhythmic drug therapy. New York: Raven Press.

Mirowski, M.; Mower, M. M.; Langer, A., et al. 1978. A chronically implanted system for automatic defibrillation in active conscious dogs. *Circulation* 58:90-94.

Mirowski, M.; Reid, P. R.; Mower, M. M., et al. 1980. Termination of malignant ventricular arrhythmias with an implanted automatic defibrillator in human beings. *N. Engl. J. Med.* 303:322-324.

Mirowski, M.; Reid, P. R.; Watkins, L., et al. 1981. Clinical treatment of life-threatening ventricular tachyarrhythmias with the automatic implantable defibrillator. *Am. Heart J.* 102:265-270.

Moe, G. K.; Jalife, J.; Mueller, W. J., et al. 1977. A mathematical model of parasystole and its application to clinical arrhythmias. *Circulation* 56: 968-979.

Moss, A. J.; Davis, H. T.; DeCamilla, J., et al. 1979. Ventricular ectopic beats and their relation to sudden and nonsudden cardiac death after myocardial infarction. *Circulation* 60:998-1003.

Robertson, J. F.; Cain, M. E.; Horowitz, L. N., et al. 1981. Anatomic and electrophysiologic correlates of ventricular tachycardia requiring left ventricular stimulation. *Am. J. Cardiol.* 48:263-268.

Romano, C.; Gemme, G.; and Pongiglione, R. 1963. Aritmie cardiache rare dell'eta pediatrica. *Clin. Pediatr.* 45:656-683.

Ruberman, W.; Weinblatt, E.; Goldberg, J. D., et al. 1977. Ventricular premature beats and mortality after myocardial infarction. *N. Engl. J. Med.* 297:750-757.

Ruberman, W.; Weinblatt, E.; Goldberg, J. D., et al. 1981. Ventricular premature complexes and sudden death after myocardial infarction. *Circulation* 64:297-305.

Ruskin, J. N.; DiMarco, J. P.; and Garan, H. 1980. Out-of-hospital cardiac arrest: electrophysiologic observations and selection of long-term anti-arrhythmic therapy. *N. Engl. J. Med.* 303:607-613.

Savage, D. D.; Seides, S. F.; Maron, B. J., et al. 1979. Prevalence of arrhythmias during 24-hour electrocardiographic monitoring and exercise testing in patients with obstructive and nonobstructive hypertrophic cardiomyopathy. *Circulation* 59:866-875.

Schaffer, W. A.; and Cobb, L. A. 1975. Recurrent ventricular fibrillation and modes of death in survivors of out-of-hospital ventricular fibrillation. *N. Engl. J. Med.* 293:259-262.

Sclarovsky, S.; Strasberg, G.; Lewin, R. F., et al. 1979. Polymorphous ventricular tachycardia: clinical features and treatment. *Am. J. Cardiol.* 44:339-344.

Smith, W. M.; and Gallagher, J. J. 1980. "Les torsades de pointes": an unusual ventricular arrhythmia. *Ann. Intern. Med.* 93:578-584.

Spurrell, R. A. J.; Sowton, E.; and Deuchar, D. C. 1973. Ventricular tachycardia in 4 patients evaluated by programmed electrical stimulation of heart and treated in 2 patients by surgical division of anterior radiation of left bundle-branch. *Br. Heart J.* 35:1014-1025.

Swerdlow, C. D.; Blum, J.; Winkle, R. A., et al. 1982a. Decreased incidence of antiarrhythmic drug efficacy at electrophysiologic study associated with use of a third extrastimulus. *Am. Heart J.* 104:1004-1010.

Swerdlow, C. D.; Echt, D. S.; Winkle, R. A., et al. 1982b. Determinants of survival in patients with ventricular tachyarrhythmias (VTA) (abstract). *Circulation* 66 (*Suppl.* II):II-25.

Swerdlow, C. D.; Winkle, R. A.; and Mason, J. W. 1982c. Prognostic significance of ten and fewer induced beats during assessment of therapy for ventricular tachycardia (VT) (abstract). *Circulation* 66 (*Suppl.* II):II-80.

Swerdlow, C. D.; Gong, G.; Echt, D. S., et al. 1983. Clinical factors predicting successful electrophysiologic-pharmacologic study in patients with ventricular tachycardia. *J. Am. Coll. Cardiol.* (in press).

Thompson, R. G.; Hallstrom, A. P.; and Cobb, L. A. 1979. Bystander-initiated cardiopulmonary resuscitation in the management of ventricular fibrillation. *Ann. Intern. Med.* 90:737-740.

Tilkian, A. G.; Pfeifer, J. F.; Barry, W. H., et al. 1976. The effect of coronary bypass surgery on exercise-induced ventricular arrhythmias. *Am. Heart J.* 92:707-714.

Vladimir, V.; Podrid, P.; Lown, B., et al. 1982. Aggravation and provocation of ventricular arrhythmias by antiarrhythmic drugs. *Circulation* 65: 886-894.

Ward, O. 1964. New familial cardiac syndrome in children. *J. Irish Med. Assoc.* 54:103-106.

Wellens, H. J. J. 1975. Pathophysiology of ventricular tachycardia in man. *Arch. Intern. Med.* 135:473-479.

Wellens, H. J. J.; Schuilenburg, R. M.; and Durrer, D. 1972. Electrical stimulation of the heart in patients with ventricular tachycardia. *Circulation* 46:216-226.

Wellens, H. J. J.; Lie, K. I.; and Durrer, D. 1974. Further observations on ventricular tachycardia as studied by electrical stimulation of the heart. *Circulation* 49:647-653.

Wellens, H. J. J.; Durrer, D. R.; and Lie, K. I. 1976. Observations on mechanisms of ventricular tachycardia in man. *Circulation* 54:237-244.

Wellens, H. J. J.; Bar, F. W. H. M.; and Lie, K. I. 1978. The value of the electrocardiogram in the differential diagnosis of a tachycardia with a widened QRS complex. *Am. J. Med.* 64:27-33.

Winkle, R. A. 1980. Ambulatory electrocardiography and the diagnosis, evaluation, and treatment of chronic ventricular arrhythmias. *Prog. Cardiovasc. Dis.* 23:99-128.

Winkle, R. A.; Lopes, M. G.; Fitzgerald, J. W., et al. 1975. Arrhythmias in patients with mitral valve prolapse. *Circulation* 52:73-81.

Winkle, R. A.; Peters, F.; and Hall, R. 1981. Characterization of ventricular tachyarrhythmias on ambulatory ECG recordings in post-myocardial infarction patients: arrhythmia detection and duration of recording, relationship between arrhythmia frequency and complexity, and day to day reproducibility. *Am. Heart J.* 102:162-169.

Winkle, R. A.; Imran, M.; and Bach, S. M., Jr. 1982. The implantable defibrillator: accurate detection of ventricular tachyarrhythmias by a new bipolar rate detection circuit (abstract). *Circulation* 66 (*Suppl.* II): II-217.

11 Surgical Treatment of Cardiac Arrhythmias

Edward B. Stinson, M.D.
Professor of Cardiovascular Surgery
Stanford University School of Medicine
Stanford, California

Jay W. Mason, M.D.
Chief, Cardiology Division
University of Utah Medical Center
Salt Lake City, Utah

This chapter reviews the surgical treatment of cardiac arrhythmias by direct operation. At present two syndromes account for the majority of cardiac operations performed with the specific intention of abolishing arrhythmias: the Wolff-Parkinson-White syndrome (one form of ventricular preexcitation) and recurrent, intractable ventricular tachycardia. Although unrelated in etiology and primary clinical manifestations, these two syndromes have in recent past come to share a common theme in regard to preoperative evaluation, intraoperative management, and characterization of the results of operative treatment. The unifying theme is the application of specific electrophysiologic study techniques, upon which current surgical approaches are based.

The following is a list of the arrhythmias that are amenable to surgical therapy:

1. Some ventricular tachycardias
2. Reentrant supraventricular tachycardia and rapid atrial fibrillation associated with the Wolff-Parkinson-White syndrome
3. Rapid atrial fibrillation associated with enhanced AV nodal conduction
4. Focal atrial tachycardia
5. AV nodal reentrant tachycardia

The objectives of electrophysiologic study in regard to these syndromes generally consist of documenting the sites of origin of the arrhythmia or anomalous pathways of conduction that are amenable to operative ablation preoperatively, followed by defining the same target abnormalities intraoperatively, with resolution of sufficient precision to guide an eradicative operative procedure without compromising the coronary circulation or specialized intracardiac structures (see Chapter 2). This chapter is keyed principally to the integrating role of electrophysiologic study, which rationalizes current surgical approaches to arrhythmias, giving a current "state of the art" summary. Limitations in understanding both the basic pathophysiology and technology, however, remain and emphasize the evolutionary nature of current experience. The advances already achieved promise even more definitive future surgical access to arrhythmias.

Of historical note, the earliest reported instance of a direct cardiac surgical procedure performed with the specific intention of abolishing ventricular arrhythmias occurred in 1956. In this case, as reported by Couch (1959), recurrent ventricular tachycardia followed myocardial infarction and left ventricular aneurysm formation. The justification for operative intervention was based on the long-recognized association between left ventricular aneurysm and recurrent ventricular tachycardia; aneurysmectomy was successful in abolishing further attacks. Many reports of empirical aneurysmectomy for recurrent ventricular tachycardia, with or without combined coronary artery bypass grafting, have followed this initial experience (Hunt, et al., 1969; Magidson, 1969; Ritter, 1969; Rolett, et al., 1969; Maloy, et al., 1971; Schlesinger, et al., 1971; Thind, et al., 1971; Wardekar, et al., 1972; Basta, et al., 1973; Graham, et al., 1973; Kenaan, et al., 1973; Welch, et al., 1973; Bett, et al., 1974; Buda, et al., 1979; Wald, et al., 1979). The results obtained, in terms of arrhythmia abolition, have been highly variable and unpredictable. Only recently have specific electrophysiologic study techniques been employed in the surgical management of patients with recurrent ventricular tachycardia associated with ischemic heart disease. Findings elucidated by intraoperative electrophysiologic studies have furnished at least a partial explanation for the unpredictability of outcome after empirical, blind, resectional procedures and have provided a rational foundation for current surgical treatment.

The modern era of electrophysiologically directed surgical intervention, however, grew out of experience with identification of accessory AV connections and operative division of such pathways, guided by intraoperative electrophysiologic mapping. It is, therefore, appropriate to consider first the evolution of experience with the Wolff-Parkinson-White syndrome.

THE WOLFF-PARKINSON-WHITE SYNDROME

The Wolff-Parkinson-White syndrome is the most commonly recognized and currently operable form of the preexcitation syndromes. The anatomic cause of the syndrome is an accessory pathway, classically referred to as the bundle of Kent (see Chapter 9). Such pathways are composed of working myocardium and originate from and insert into working myocardium across the AV valve rings (thereby providing an electrically excitable anomalous connection between atria and ventricles that is separate from the normal cardiac conduction system). Kent pathways are ordinarily quite small, with the widest dimension averaging slightly greater than 1 mm (Sealy, et al., 1978). The direction and depth of their course across the AV grooves are variable and unpredictable. They may be situated anywhere from an immediate subepicardial location in the AV sulcus to a position adjacent to, but not perforating, the annulus fibrosis of either AV valve (Sealy, et al., 1978). In surgically treated patients approximately 50% of accessory pathways have been found in the region of the free portion of the left AV junction, 20% in the right free-wall location, 20% in the posterior septal location, and 10% in the anterior septal region. In approximately 10% of surgically treated patients multiple pathways (usually two) have been present (Sealy, et al., 1978). Because of these considerations, it is clear that accurate localization of an accessory AV connection for purposes of surgical division requires intraoperative electrophysiologic mapping.

The pathophysiologic consequences of and implications for surgical treatment of patients with the Wolff-Parkinson-White syndrome derive from the presence of and differences in conduction properties of two AV conduction systems (normal and accessory pathways). The classical ECG abnormality seen during normal sinus rhythm consists of an abnormally short PR interval associated with a prolonged QRS complex with a slurred initial component, which is termed the delta wave. This ECG pattern is estimated to occur in 1-3 out of every 1000 patients (Gallagher, et al., 1978b). The absence of normal conduction delay in the accessory pathway is responsible for the abnormally short PR interval (preexcitation), as well as the abnormality of QRS morphology, which represents variable degrees of fusion of impulse propagation through the accessory and specialized pathways. In occasional patients ventricular preexcitation, although presumably potentially present since birth, may be delayed, and in other patients it may be intermittent, for reasons that are not understood. Moreover, the accessory pathway in some patients appears capable of only unidirectional conduction, either antegrade or retrograde.

Many patients with the Wolff-Parkinson-White syndrome exhibit tachyarrhythmias of some kind, but these arrhythmias are sufficiently severe, intractable, or dangerous to warrant surgical treatment in a minority of patients. The most common manifestation of the presence of dual AV conduction pathways is recurrent reentrant supraventricular tachycardia. Critically timed supraventricular or ventricular premature depolarizations initiate a sustained macroreentry tachycardia that usually utilizes the normal AV node in an antegrade fashion and the accessory connection in a retrograde direction. Because of the atypical responses of the accessory connection to antiarrhythmic agents, as compared to the AV node, and because of the complexities of interacting properties that are responsible for sustaining reciprocating tachycardia (e.g., the respective refractory periods and conduction velocities of the accessory pathways and involved portions of specialized conduction tissue), prevention of supraventricular tachycardia by pharmacologic means is often difficult. Frequent attacks may not only interfere seriously with the patient's lifestyle but may become truly disabling. Approximately 60% of reported operations in patients with the Wolff-Parkinson-White syndrome have been performed because of this indication (Sealy, et al., 1978).

Another type of arrhythmia sustained by patients with the Wolff-Parkinson-White syndrome is potentially fatal. This consists of atrial fibrillation (or, uncommonly, atrial flutter) with conduction to the ventricles through the accessory pathway. Because the refractory period of the accessory pathway may be short in some patients and because the accessory pathway does not exhibit decremental conduction, very rapid ventricular rates may result; this rhythm may then degenerate into ventricular fibrillation. Patients who are most susceptible to this complication usually present with a history of both atrial fibrillation and reciprocating tachycardia, tend to exhibit short refractory periods of the accessory pathway (as determined by electrophysiologic study and manifested clinically by very short RR intervals during atrial fibrillation), and may have multiple accessory pathways (Klein, et al., 1979). This manifestation of the Wolff-Parkinson-White syndrome constituted the primary indication for surgery in approximately 40% of patients in a Duke University study, which has been the largest series conducted to date (Sealy, et al., 1978).

Preoperative electrophysiologic evaluation of potential surgical patients is conducted to confirm the presence of preexcitation (this may occasionally be absent because of intermittent function or retrograde conduction only of the accessory pathway), clarify the nature of inducible tachyarrhythmias and confirm participation of the accessory pathway (or pathways), and localize the site of the accessory pathway to a region that is surgically accessible (left or right free-wall, posterior septal, anterior septal).

Identification of the region in which the accessory pathway is situated is usually achieved by careful examination of the retrograde activation pattern of the atria recorded during reciprocating tachycardia and/or ventricular pacing. Precise localization, upon which successful operation depends, requires direct intraoperative epicardial or, rarely, endocardial mapping.

Preoperative cardiac evaluation should also include screening by appropriate methods for disorders known to be associated with the Wolff-Parkinson-White syndrome. These associated disorders include Ebstein's anomaly of the tricuspid valve, prolapsing mitral valve, cardiomyopathy (congestive or hypertrophic), and, in older patients, coronary artery disease (Gallagher, et al., 1978b).

Intraoperative epicardial mapping studies can usually be performed before the institution of cardiopulmonary bypass. During sinus rhythm with preexcitation the ventricular side of the AV rings is explored in careful sequence to identify the site of earliest ventricular activation. Exploration of the atrial side of the AV grooves during reciprocating tachycardia or ventricular pacing (during which the atria are first activated by retrograde conduction over the accessory pathway) provides additional confirmation of the site of the accessory connection, which is neither visible nor palpable. Figures 11-1A and 11-1B illustrate electrophysiologic findings obtained during epicardial mapping in a patient undergoing operation for a left free-wall accessory pathway. Precise timing of ECG recordings obtained with the exploring electrode, relative to an appropriate reference signal from the left or right ventricle, allows exact localization of that portion of the AV groove containing the accessory connection.

The ability to ablate the accessory pathways responsible for the Wolff-Parkinson-White syndrome discretely was predicted by the study of Burchell and colleagues (1967), who identified a right free-wall connection by epicardial mapping in a patient undergoing repair of an atrial

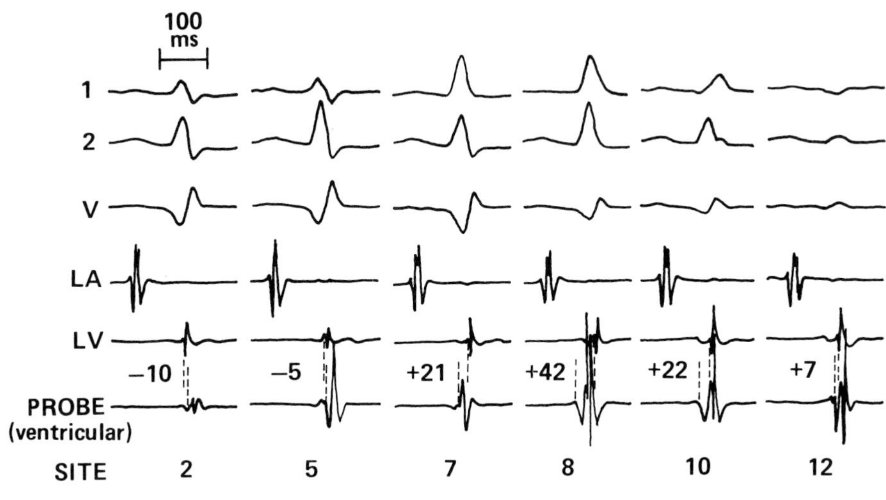

Figure 11-1A Intraoperative electrophysiologic recordings in a patient with a left-sided free-wall anomalous conduction pathway. Surface ECG leads 1, 2, and a V lead (V) positioned on the patient's back opposite the usual V_1 position are displayed on left atrial (LA), left ventricular (LV), and moving probe electrograms. Six single cardiac cycles during spontaneous supraventricular rhythm are shown. For each separate beat the probe-recording electrodes have been moved to new recording sites that are identified numerically. Sites 1-6 refer to the epicardial surface of the right AV groove from the infundibulum around to the crux of the heart, and numbers 7-12 refer to sites around the left AV groove from a position adjacent to the left anterior descending coronary artery around to the crux. The change in QRS configuration seen most prominently in the recordings from sites 8, 10, and 12 reflects the need to lift the heart to reach posterior left ventricular sites with the probe. The purpose of mapping in sinus rhythm is to find the location of earliest ventricular activation along the AV groove, which will identify the ventricular input site of the anomalous pathway. In this figure the timing in milliseconds from the onset of the left ventricular reference electrogram to onset of the initial major or rapid deflection on the moving probe electrogram is shown. Note that the earliest site of ventricular activation along the AV groove occurs at site 8 where the local electrogram precedes the left ventricular electrogram by 42 milliseconds.

septal defect. Temporary functional ablation of the pathway was produced by injection in situ of 1% procaine (Burchell, et al., 1967). In the following year direct surgical division of an accessory pathway, guided by intraoperative mapping, was achieved by researchers at Duke University (Sealy, et al., 1968 and 1969). The series subsequently developed by these investigators has provided a firm foundation for the current surgical approach (Gallagher, et al., 1978b; Sealy, et al., 1978).

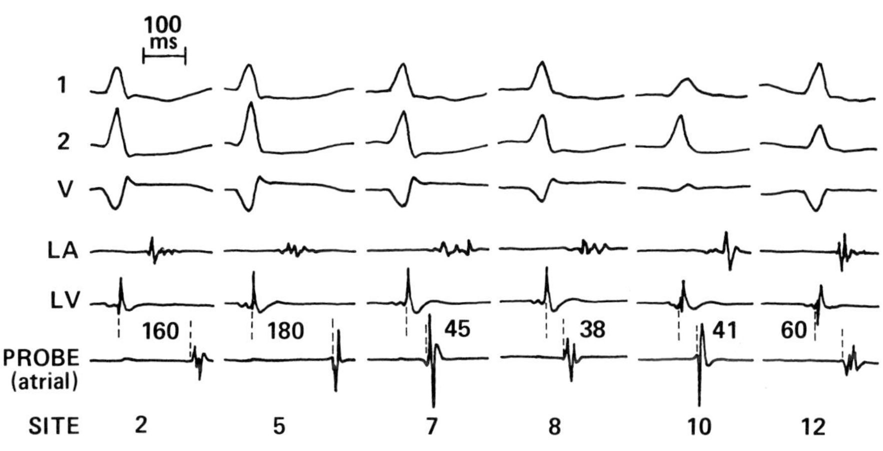

Figure 11-1B Intraoperative electrophysiologic recordings in a patient with the Wolff-Parkinson-White syndrome. This is the same patient shown in Figure 11-1A. In this series of mapping sites reentrant supraventricular tachycardia has been induced. During reentry the circuiting impulse returns to the atria by retrograde conduction from ventricle to atrium over the anomalous pathway. Thus, by locating the site of earliest atrial activation during supraventricular tachycardia the atrial input position of the anomalous pathway can be identified. The earliest atrial activity in this example was recorded when the probe electrodes were placed at site 8 on the atrial side of the AV groove. In this position the probe atrial electrogram occurred closest to the preceding left ventricular electrogram (LV probe interval was 38 milliseconds). Thus, as expected from the ventricular mapping during spontaneous sinus rhythm that was shown in Figure 11-1A, the atrial input location of the Kent fiber is at site 8, which corresponds to the lateral left AV groove.

The technical principle utilized most successfully for division of anomalous pathways is endocardial dissection of the AV grooves in the appropriate location. After institution of cardiopulmonary bypass by standard techniques and exposure of the pertinent AV valve, an endocardial incision is made 1-2 mm to the atrial side of the annulus in the area previously identified by mapping as containing the accessory pathway. The AV groove is then dissected downward along the crest of the ventricle to the level of reflection of the epicardium and upward to the point of reflection of epicardium on the external atrial surface. External epicardial dissection is combined with this maneuver for right-sided free wall pathways. In the paraseptal areas, both anterior and posterior, the dissection is more complex because of the proximity of the specialized cardiac conduction system and the convergence of several discrete portions of the cardiac fibrous skeleton. Nevertheless, refinements in the surgical technique in recent years now allow approach to these areas with success rates that are comparable to those obtained with free-wall connections (Sealy and Gallagher, 1980). An alternative technique to direct dissection is cryothermal ablation of the anomalous pathway with a specially designed freezing probe (Gallagher, et al., 1977). This procedure may be especially applicable to those connections defined by electrophysiologic mapping as occupying an immediate subepicardial location or to cases in which the safe period for duration of cardiopulmonary bypass appears to be limited because of associated disease. Experimental studies have shown that cryoablation techniques do not seriously jeopardize the functional integrity of the myocardial wall because of the resistance of collagenous elements to freezing injury, but coronary artery lesions consisting of mural fibrosis and intimal plaques do occur (Mikat, et al., 1977). This technique, therefore, should be applied judiciously with due consideration to the details of coronary artery anatomy in the region of intended cryoablation.

After interruption of the accessory pathway and cardiac resuscitation, repeat electrophysiologic study should be performed intraoperatively to confirm eradication of function of the accessory pathway. Repeat epicardial mapping on both sides of the AV grooves and attempts to induce reciprocating tachycardia by appropriately timed electrical stimulation provide data to confirm interruption of the accessory pathway. Occasionally, a secondary pathway may be unmasked by this maneuver, which requires additional dissection. At the completion of the operation the characteristic ECG abnormalities of the Wolff-Parkinson-White syndrome should no longer be present and, in the absence of additional cardiac disease, conversion of the ECG to normal can be expected. Preoperative and postoperative ECGs in the case of a left-sided free-wall pathway (type A) are illustrated in Figure 11-2. Prior to discharge a repeat, limited electrophysiologic study in the catheterization laboratory should be performed to confirm persistent ablation of accessory pathway function and to provide firm evidence for patient counseling. In rare cases evidence of preexcitation, which was abolished at operation, may return after variable periods (usually days), caused apparently by functional obtundation of an accessory pathway by operation but without anatomic division.

The results of surgical treatment in patients with the Wolff-Parkinson-White syndrome have steadily improved to the point that success may now be expected nearly routinely. The largest surgical study to date was conducted at Duke University (Gallagher, et al., 1978b; Sealy, et al., 1978). Cure rates now exceed 95%, regardless of the anatomic location of the accessory connection. Overall, the operative risk is very low, in the range of 1-2%, and is related primarily to associated cardiac disease. Barring the development and availability of new pharmacologic agents that are specifically effective for the electrophysiologic abnormalities encountered

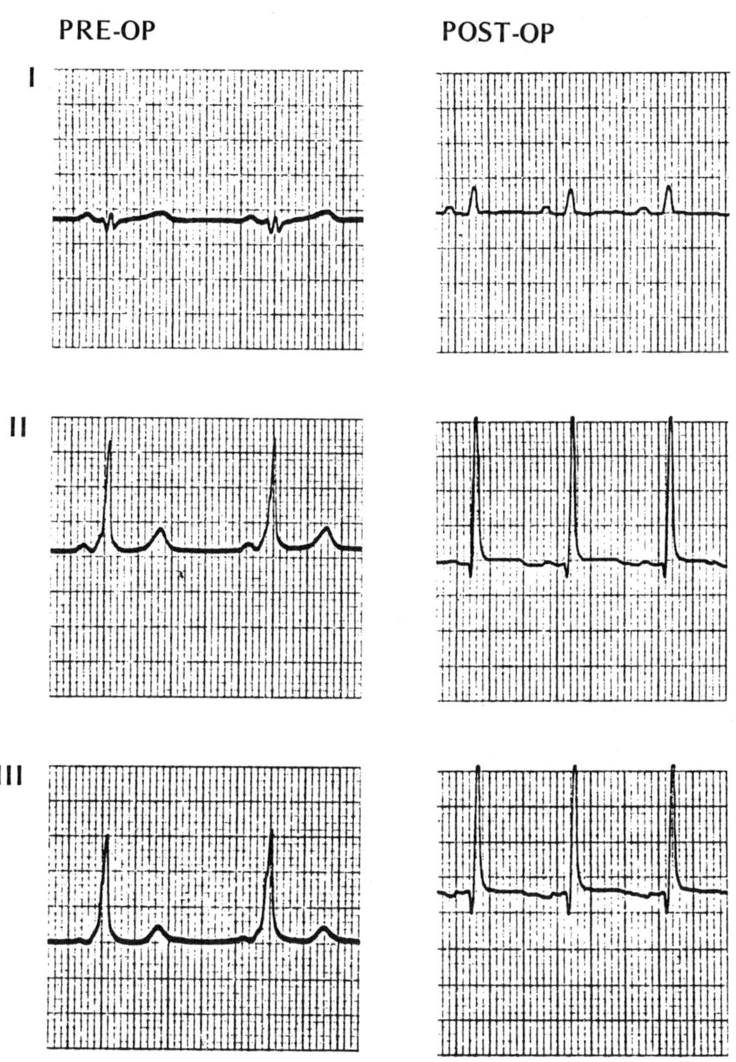

Figure 11-2 ECG recordings from a patient with the Wolff-Parkinson-White syndrome. Leads I, II, and III from a preoperative ECG in this patient show obvious delta waves that are directed inferiorly and to the right, which is consistent with a left free-wall bypass fiber. The same leads in the postoperative state show a dramatic change. The previously short PR interval now lasts 0.16 seconds. The delta waves have been eliminated and the total QRS duration shortened. Evidence no longer exists for preexcitation.

in the Wolff-Parkinson-White syndrome, the success rates now achieved with surgical treatment lend support to liberalizing the indications for operation. Needless to say, such a program of electrophysiologically directed surgical treatment should be pursued at institutions that have experienced electrophysiologic and cardiac surgical teams.

SURGICAL TREATMENT OF OTHER SUPRAVENTRICULAR TACHYCARDIAS

Several types of supraventricular tachycardias, other than those associated with the Wolff-Parkinson-White syndrome, may prove unresponsive to pharmacologic or pacemaker management. Such problems, if disabling, may justify consideration of surgical ablation of the AV node-His bundle, combined with pacemaker implantation. A variety of mechanisms may be responsible for such intractable supraventricular tachyarrhythmias, including paroxysmal atrial flutter or fibrillation with rapid ventricular rates that are not responsive to AV nodal depressant agents, reentrant mechanisms in the AV node or atria, ectopic atrial foci, or failed attempts at ablation of the accessory pathway in the Wolff-Parkinson-White syndrome. Direct surgical dissection with detachment of the AV node and proximal portion of the His bundle from the subjacent conduction system, as well as cryosurgical techniques, may be used (Sealy, et al., 1977; Klein, et al., 1980) and appear to be more successful than previous methods that employed suture ligation or electrocautery. Precise placement of the ablative lesion usually results in a residual intrinsic pacemaker site in the His system, but concomitant placement of a ventricular pacemaker is required because of potential instability of the residual junctional rhythm and the unpredictability of long-term electrophysiologic behavior. Pacemaker dependency is, therefore, a genuine consideration, and the treatment of supraventricular tachyarrhythmias by production of complete heart block remains controversial. A recently described catheter technique for ablating the AV conduction system may minimize the need for open-heart surgical procedures (Gallagher, et al., 1982). An alternative approach for ectopic atrial foci is electrical sequence mapping in the operating room to identify the location of the focus, followed by simple excision or electrical isolation from the rest of the atrium by an encircling incision (Wyndham, et al., 1980; Anderson, et al., 1982).

RECURRENT VENTRICULAR TACHYCARDIA

The majority of patients with life-threatening recurrent ventricular tachycardia that is refractory to control by pharmacologic or pacemaker treatment have ischemic heart disease. The remainder of patients constitute a heterogenous group in terms of disease etiology, clinical characteristics, and methods of surgical management. It is, therefore, appropriate to consider these two categories of patients separately.

Nearly all patients with recurrent ventricular tachycardia associated with ischemic heart disease have sustained prior myocardial infarction, with or without aneurysm formation. As noted earlier, it was the long-recognized association between left ventricular aneurysms and recurrent ventricular tachycardia that led to the development of left ventricular resection as empirical treatment for this disorder. The experience gained with mapping techniques for the precise surgical treatment of patients with the Wolff-Parkinson-White syndrome and several key observations in experimental myocardial infarction settings, however, have provided a foundation for the current guided approach to the operative treatment of ventricular tachycardia. The following is a list of the relevant experimental findings that have been confirmed in the clinical setting:

1. The ability to initiate ventricular tachycardia reproducibly by appropriately timed (programmed) electrical stimulation
2. The identification by activation sequence mapping in some cases of a discrete site (or sites) or origin of the arrhythmia on or near the endocardial surface, usually in the region of interface between infarcted and normal tissue
3. Directionally unpredictable spread of activation such that the earliest activity on the epicardial ventricular surface may be variably distant from a subendocardial focus
4. The ability to abolish inducible ventricular tachycardia by discrete ventricular resection guided by activation sequence mapping during the arrhythmia (Wittig and Bioneau, 1975; Josephson, et al., 1979).

These features rationalize, in part, the current operative approach to ablative surgical treatment of ventricular tachycardia, at least in patients with coronary artery disease and previous myocardial infarction. These features may also explain the unpredictable success rates achieved with empirical aneurysmectomy that leaves the margin between normal and infarcted myocardium intact to a variable degree to provide a fibrotic rim for secure suture placement. The basic cellular mechanisms responsible for the genesis of recurrent ventricular tachycardia, whatever the associated underlying myocardial disease process, remain controversial. A reentry mechanism, intermittently or continuously active in a relatively discrete and possibly protected region, has been accepted as a workable hypothesis by many investigators on the basis of the conditions necessary for initiation and termination of the arrhythmia by electrical stimulation; however, this surely does not represent the sole mechanism (Gallagher, et al., 1978a; Mason, et al., 1981).

The selection of patients for operative treatment of ventricular tachycardia is based at present on a set of criteria that may be expanded, reduced, or otherwise modified with future developments in pharmacologic therapy or improvements in surgical techniques. In general, ventricular tachycardia must be life-threatening, have occurred on more than one occasion, and have required active intervention (usually including cardioversion) to qualify for termination. The ventricular tachycardia should be documented to be resistant to control by both standard antiarrhythmic drugs and available investigational agents.

Complete electrophysiologic study should be performed preoperatively. Sustained, regular ventricular tachycardia should be inducible by programmed stimulation and should include the morphology (or morphologies) that are exhibited clinically and are responsible for the patient's symptoms. An example of sustained ventricular tachycardia initiated by programmed stimulation in a patient with ischemic heart disease is illustrated in Figure 11-3. In some cases catheter localization to regions of the left ventricle can be achieved (e.g., septum, lateral wall, apex) by virtue of identification of the site of earliest recorded endocardial activation during tachycardia (Josephson, et al., 1980). The site of earliest endocardial activation is presumed to be the site of origin in those cases that appear to be caused by a discrete focus of activity. Full hemodynamic and angiographic studies should also be performed to plan fully the surgical approach and to estimate the operative risk, which is determined principally by the state of left ventricular function.

Preoperative selection and evaluation of patients with intractable ventricular tachycardia of nonischemic etiology are conducted similarly, but heterogenous abnormalities may be identified. There may even be no apparent structural disorder. In contrast to patients with coronary artery disease, most of these patients have exhibited a tachycardia originating in the right ventricle. The arrhythmia may be attributable to cardiac involvement in a systemic disease (e.g., scleroderma) (Gallagher, et al., 1978), primary cardiomyopathy (Fontaine, et al., 1979a; Fontaine, et al., 1979b), a scar from previous ventriculotomy (Fontaine, et al., 1979b), Uhl's anomaly (Fontaine, et al., 1979a), or arrhythmogenic right ventricular dysplasia (Fontaine, et al., 1979a; Marcus, et al., 1982).

The sequence of intraoperative steps in the surgical treatment of ventricular tachycardia is straightforward, although this conceptually orderly procedure may be confounded by biologic variability and incomplete understanding of the electrophysiologic phenomena that are observed. The basic goals of surgery are to identify by direct mapping the cause of arrhythmia during induced tachycardia and to resect or otherwise functionally ablate cardiac tissue that is responsible or necessary for arrhythmia maintenance. Mapping is performed after institution of cardiopulmonary bypass. An epicardial map is first obtained according to a predetermined grid system for identification of the epicardial activation sequence. In the case of tachycardia of left ventricular origin this sequence may bear a variable anatomic relationship to the subendocardial

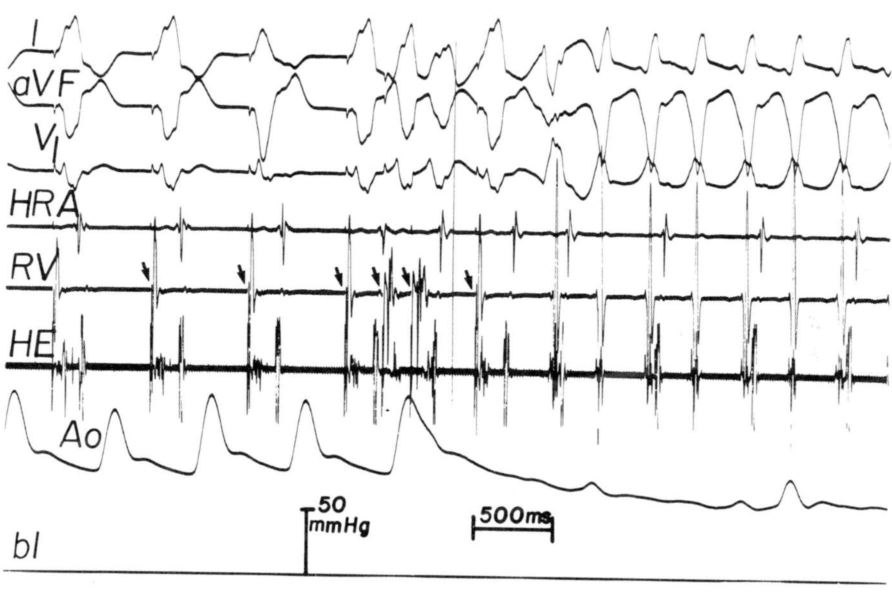

Figure 11-3A Ventricular tachycardia induction. Surface ECG leads 1, aVF, and V_1 are displayed with high right atrial (HRA), right ventricular (RV), and His (HE) electrograms. Aortic blood pressure (Ao) is also displayed above a zero pressure reference line (bl). Right ventricular pacing stimuli are indicated by the arrows. Three programmed extrastimuli were delivered to the ventricle during a period of right ventricular pacing at 100 beats/min. Sustained ventricular tachycardia with a right bundle branch block, left axis deviation pattern was induced with a resultant fall in the patient's blood pressure. Note the presence of 2:1 retrograde VA conduction during tachycardia. This tachycardia resembled perfectly the spontaneous rhythm disturbance in this patient, who eventually failed therapeutic attempts with all available antiarrhythmic agents. Intraoperative activation sequence mapping and myocardial resection were eventually required.

sequence. After incision through an aneurysm or infarct, if present, an endocardial map is derived to identify the mechanism of tachycardia. In some cases the earliest site of activation is considered to constitute the focus of arrhythmia genesis. In other cases macro-reentry is present (see Figure 1-9) or the arrhythmia mechanism cannot be identified with certainty (Mason, et al., 1981). In tachycardia of right ventricular origin epicardial recordings alone are usually enough to identify accurately the origin of the arrhythmia. Figure 11-4 is an example of endocardial electrograms defining the earliest site of activation during tachycardia in the region of border tissue between infarcted and normal myocardium.

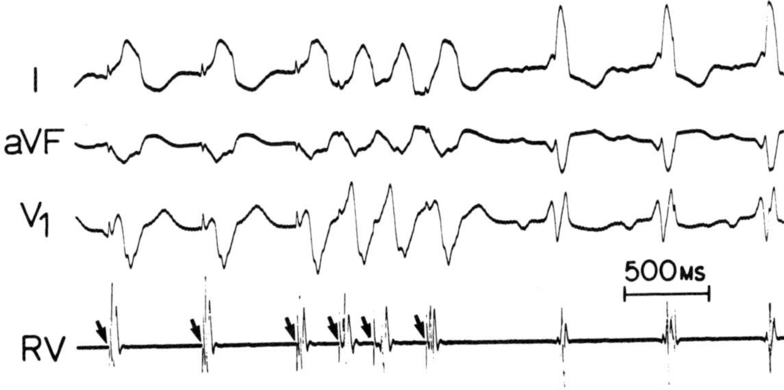

Figure 11-3B Postoperative ventricular tachycardia induction study. Two weeks after undergoing mapping and myocardial resection the patient, whose preoperative recordings were shown in Figure 11-3A, was subjected to repeat attempts at ventricular tachycardia induction. In this illustration surface ECG leads 1, aVF, and V_1 are displayed with a right ventricular electrogram recording (RV). An extrastimulation program similar to the one shown in Figure 11-3A (preoperative state) failed to initiate ventricular tachycardia in the postoperative state. This patient has had sustained relief from recurrent ventricular tachycardia paroxysms for 32 months.

After a site for ablation has been identified, the subendocardial region containing this site should be resected or a cryothermal lesion created. Repeat programmed stimulation should then be performed to reassess the inducibility of ventricular tachycardia. This sequence should be repeated, if necessary, until the arrhythmia can no longer be initiated. At this point hypothermic cardiac arrest should be produced, other procedures, such as coronary artery bypass grafting or mitral valve replacement, performed, and the ventriculotomy repaired. In patients with tachycardia of right ventricular origin simple ventriculotomy alone or very limited excision is usually sufficient to eradicate the origin of the arrhythmia. After cardiac resuscitation, programmed stimulation should be repeated once again to assess arrhythmia inducibility.

The postoperative care of such patients is routine for cardiac surgical patients, except that prolonged ECG monitoring and restudy in the electrophysiology laboratory are conducted prior to discharge. During this postoperative study inducibility of ventricular tachycardia should be ascertained once again. Currently, patients in whom tachycardia cannot be induced are discharged without antiarrhythmic medication. Those patients who have residual inducible arrhythmias receive pharmacologic therapy tailored according to the specific protective effects of drugs

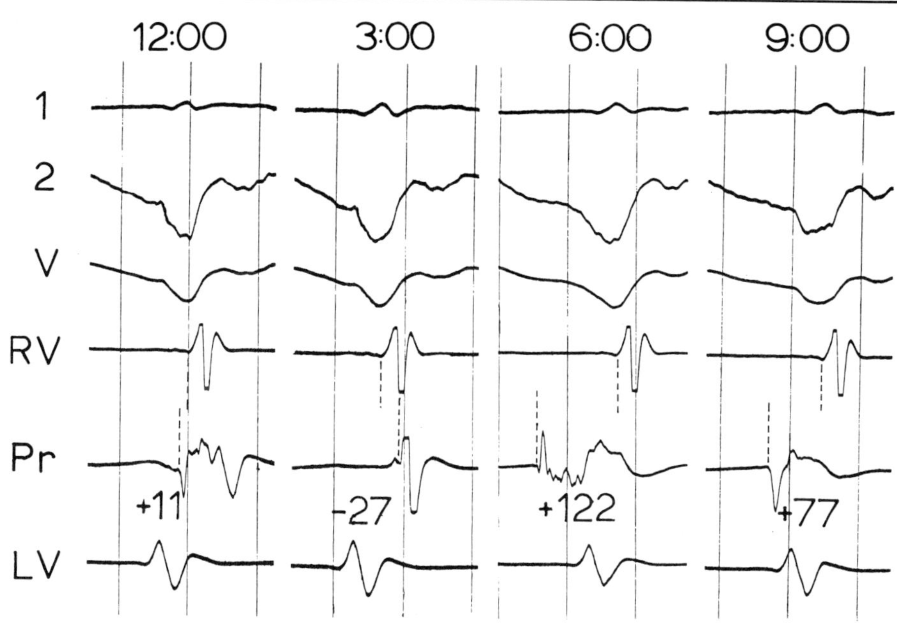

Figure 11-4 Intraoperative electrophysiologic recordings in a patient with recurrent ventricular tachycardia. Surface ECG leads 1, 2, and a precordial lead positioned on the patient's back (V) are displayed with right ventricular reference (RV), roving probe (PR), and left ventricular reference (LV) electrograms. Time lines of 100 milliseconds are shown. Mapping is carried out in the endocardial tissue at the border between normal and infarcted endocardium. Four different sites at 12:00, 3:00, 6:00, and 9:00, recorded with the mapping probe during sustained ventricular tachycardia, are shown. The clock-face format is used to identify recording positions within and around aneurysmal or akinetic scarred regions. In this example 12:00 corresponds to the cephalad extent of the aneurysm, 6:00 to its apical extent, 3:00 to its left ventricular free-wall extent, and 9:00 to the septal side of the aneurysm. Note that earliest electrical activity during ventricular tachycardia is recorded at 6:00. This electrogram occurs 123 milliseconds prior to the right ventricular reference electrogram, precedes the left ventricular reference electrogram, and also precedes by a few milliseconds the onset of the surface QRS complexes. In this patient recordings at 6:00 within the aneurysm and well into normal myocardium were also early but later than the electrogram recorded from the border tissue. Tissue at 6:00 in the border region was the putative arrhythmia focus in this case.

tested at this time. Figure 11-3B illustrates postoperative noninducibility of ventricular tachycardia, which was easily initiated by programmed stimulation preoperatively.

Overall, the risk of electrophysiologically guided surgery for recurrent ventricular tachycardia is dominated by the status of the patient's left ventricular function. According to the threshold criteria of acceptability for surgery, therefore, operative mortality rates vary from approximately 8% to 20%. Myocardial failure, especially in association with recent acute myocardial infarction, not residual tachycardia, is the commonest cause of operative death.

The success rate, in terms of arrhythmia control, is in the range of 70%-80% (Horowitz, et al., 1980; Mason, et al., 1982), which is higher than that obtained by empirical left ventricular resection in previously reported studies (Harken, et al., 1977; Mason, et al., 1982). The follow-up periods for guided operative resection are limited, however, and the time-related incidence of recrudescence of ventricular tachycardia in patients with extensive structural ventricular abnormalities cannot be well defined. Within the constraints of current follow-up intervals, though, this appears to be low.

ALTERNATIVE OPERATIVE PROCEDURES FOR VENTRICULAR TACHYCARDIA

Characterization by endocardial mapping of the usual anatomic location of the site of origin of ventricular tachycardia in patients with prior myocardial infarction lends some support for an innovative surgical technique that does not require intraoperative mapping: the encircling endocardial ventriculotomy (Guiraudon, et al., 1978). This procedure consists of an incision perpendicular to the endocardial surface, extended circumferentially at a variable depth around the limits of fibrosis that delineate aneurysm or akinetic infarct tissue. The theoretical justification for this surgical technique is interruption or isolation of assumed reentry circuits or foci of automaticity that originate in the border zone between infarcted and normal myocardium. The reported initial results of this technique appear encouraging, but the long-term outcome has not yet been defined. The scope of applicability of this procedure appears to be limited to patients with ischemic disease whose intracardiac pathology (i.e., regional endocardial fibrosis associated with infarction) can be visually delineated and in whom the encircling incision will not damage the papillary muscles. However, modifications of the technique in combination with selective subendocardial resection may be effective in a wider variety of patients when they are guided by intraoperative mapping data.

Myocardial revascularization by coronary artery bypass grafting has also been proposed as a principal or adjunctive method of treatment of ventricular tachycardia in patients with ischemic heart disease. Several previous reports, however, have indicated that bypass grafting, alone or in combination with ventricular resection, is often ineffective in the control of recurrent tachycardia (Ecker, et al., 1971; Lambert, et al., 1971; Bryson, et al., 1973; Mundth, et al., 1973; Nordstrom, et al., 1975; Tilkian, et al., 1976; Ricks, et al., 1977; Tabry, et al., 1978; Nakhjavan, et al., 1971; Mason, et al., 1982). One possible exception may be recurrent tachycardia that appears only in conjunction with documented acute ischemic episodes (Nordstrom, et al., 1975; Tabry, et al., 1978). Although coronary artery bypass grafting is often performed concomitantly with guided subendocardial resection, substantial evidence exists that myocardial revascularization does not play a substantial role in the control of recurrent tachycardia.

In some patients with the long QT interval syndrome recurrent ventricular tachycardia and even ventricular fibrillation may occur (see Chapter 10). In this syndrome an imbalance between right and left sympathetic nerve activity is presumed to exist, and left-sided cervicothoracic sympathectomy, including the stellate ganglion and the upper thoracic chain, has been reported to both normalize the QT interval and eliminate recurrent ventricular tachyarrhythmias (Moss and McDonald, 1971; Vincent, et al., 1974; Schwartz, et al., 1975; Crampton, 1979). Further experience is needed to define the mechanisms involved in this fascinating disorder more precisely.

Another innovative technique for surgical treatment of recurrent ventricular fibrillation has been described by Mirowski and colleagues (1978). This procedure consists of an implantable defibrillating unit that automatically monitors cardiac rhythm and delivers a defibrillating current when ventricular fibrillation is sensed (see Chapter 10). The two component electrodes consist of a transvenous catheter and a plaque that is sewn to the external pericardial surface of the left ventricular apex through a thoracotomy incision. The system has been validated experimentally and its efficacy has been described (Mirowski, et al., 1978); in the preliminary clinical experience with a small number of patients the initial results have been encouraging (Mirowski, et al., 1980 and 1981).

CONCLUSION

The efficacy of surgical treatment of various types of cardiac arrhythmias, both supraventricular and ventricular, has increased in recent years by virtue of both advanced understanding of basic mechanisms (although still far from complete) and refinement of the technology of cardiac surgery. The latter consideration includes improvements in surgical craftsmanship in the management of complications of coronary artery disease (e.g., excision of pathologic changes and ventricular reconstruction) and the development of new techniques for ablation or functional eradication of myocardial tissue identified by electrophysiologic study techniques as responsible for arrhythmia genesis or propagation. Progress has been achieved by the integrated efforts of specialized electrophysiologic and cardiac surgical teams.

Future evolution in the effectiveness and scope of applicability of surgical treatment will be linked to advances in basic understanding of the mechanisms of various arrhythmias and their anatomical causes. Increased precision in intraoperative identification of various portions of the specialized cardiac conduction system should allow selective ablation of any myocardial segment identified as essential to the genesis or propagation of otherwise unmanageable arrhythmias. Developments in this field over the past decade indicate that such expectations are not unreasonable.

REFERENCES

Anderson, K. P.; Stinson, E. B.; and Mason, J. W. 1982. Surgical exclusion of focal paroxysmal atrial tachycardia. *Am. J. Cardiol.* 49:869-873.

Basta, L. L.; Takeshita, A.; Theilen, E. O., et al. 1973. Aneurysmectomy in treatment of ventricular and supraventricular tachyarrhythmias in patients with postinfarction and traumatic ventricular aneurysms. *Am. J. Cardiol.* 32:693-699.

Bett, J. H. N.; Cooper, E.; Mushin, G., et al. 1974. Ventricular aneurysmectomy for recurrent tachyarrhythmias. *Aust. N.Z.J. Med.* 4(3):253-255.

Bryson, A. L.; Parisi, A. F.; Schechter, E., et al. 1973. Life-threatening ventricular arrhythmias induced by exercise: cessation after coronary bypass surgery. *Am. J. Cardiol.* 32:995-999.

Buda, A. J.; Stinson, E. B.; and Harrison, D. C. 1979. Surgery for life-threatening ventricular tachyarrhythmias. *Am. J. Cardiol.* 44:1171-1177.

Burchell, H. B.; Frye, R. L.; Anderson, M. W., et al. 1967. Atrioventricular and ventriculoatrial excitation in Wolff-Parkinson-White syndrome (type B): temporary ablation at surgery. *Circulation* 36:663-672.

Couch, O. A., Jr. 1959. Cardiac aneurysm with ventricular tachycardia and subsequent excision of aneurysm: case report. *Circulation* 20:251-253.

Crampton, R. 1979. Preeminence of the left stellate ganglion in the long Q-T syndrome. *Circulation* 59(4):769-778.

Ecker, R. R.; Mullins, C. B.; Grammer, J. C., et al. 1971. Control of intractable ventricular tachycardia by coronary revascularization. *Circulation* 44:666-670.

Fontaine, G.; Guiraudon, G.; and Frank, R. 1979a. Mechanism of ventricular tachycardia with and without associated chronic myocardial ischemia: surgical management based on epicardial mapping. In *Cardiac arrhythmias: electrophysiology, diagnosis, and management.* O. S. Narula, editor. Baltimore: Williams and Wilkins. pp. 516-545.

Fontaine G.; Guiraudon, G.; Frank, R., et al. 1979b. The surgical management of ventricular tachycardia. *Herz* 4:276-284.

Gallagher, J. J.; and Cox, J. L. 1979. Status of surgery for ventricular arrhythmias (editorial). *Circulation* 60(7):1440-1442.

Gallagher, J. J.; Sealy, W. C.; Anderson, R. W., et al. 1977. Cryosurgical ablation of accessory atrioventricular connections: a method for correction of the preexcitation syndrome. *Circulation* 55(3):471-479.

Gallagher, J. J.; Anderson, R. W.; Kasell, J., et al. 1978a. Cryoablation of drug-resistant ventricular tachycardia in a patient with a variant of scleroderma. *Circulation* 57:190-197.

Gallagher, J. J.; Pritchett, E. L. C.; Sealy, W. C., et al. 1978b. The preexcitation syndromes. *Prog. Cardiovasc. Dis.* 20(4):285-327.

Gallagher, J. J.; Svenson, R. H.; Kasell, J. H., et al. 1982. A catheter technique for closed-chest ablation of the atrioventricular conduction system. *N. Engl. J. Med.* 306:194-200.

Graham, A. F.; Miller, D. C.; Stinson, E. B., et al. 1973. Surgical treatment of refractory life-threatening ventricular tachycardia. *Am. J. Cardiol.* 32: 909-912.

Guiraudon, G.; Fontaine, G.; Frank, R., et al. 1978. Encircling endocardial ventriculotomy: a new surgical treatment for life-threatening ventricular tachycardias resistant to medical treatment following myocardial infarction. *Ann. Thoracic Surg.* 26:438-443.

Harken, A. H.; Josephson, M. E.; and Horowitz, L. N. 1977. Surgical endocardial resection for the treatment of malignant ventricular tachycardia. *Ann. Surg.* 190:456.

Horowitz, L. N.; Spear, J. F.; and Moore, E. N. 1976. Subendocardial origin of ventricular arrhythmias in 24-hour-old experimental myocardial infarction. *Circulation* 53:56-63.

Horowitz, L. N.; Harken, A. H.; Kastor, J. A., et al. 1980. Ventricular resection guided by epicardial and endocardial mapping for treatment of recurrent ventricular tachycardia. *N. Engl. J. Med.* 302(11):589-593.

Hunt, D.; Sloman, G.; and Westlake, G. 1969. Ventricular aneurysmectomy for recurrent tachycardia: case report. *Br. Heart J.* 31:264-266.

Josephson, M. E.; and Horowitz, L. N. 1979. Electrophysiologic approach to therapy of recurrent sustained ventricular tachycardia. *Am. J. Cardiol.* 43:631-641.

Josephson, M. E.; Horowitz, L. N.; Farshidi, A., et al. 1978a. Recurrent sustained ventricular tachycardia. 1. Mechanisms. *Circulation* 57:431-439.

Josephson, M. E.; Horowitz, L. N.; Farshidi, A., et al. 1978b. Recurrent sustained ventricular tachycardia. 2. Endocardial mapping. *Circulation* 57(3):440-447.

Josephson, M. E.; Horowitz, L. N.; and Farshidi, A. 1978c. Continuous local electrical activity: a mechanism of recurrent ventricular tachycardia. *Circulation* 57:659-665.

Josephson, M. E.; Horowitz, L. N.; Farshidi, A., et al. 1978d. Sustained ventricular tachycardia: evidence for protected localized reentry. *Am. J. Cardiol.* 42:416-424.

Josephson, M. E.; Horowtiz, L. N.; Farshidi, A., et al. 1979. Recurrent sustained ventricular tachycardia. 4. Pleomorphism. *Circulation* 59(3): 459-468.

Josephson, M. E.; Horowitz, L. N.; Spielman, S. R., et al. 1980. Comparison of endocardial catheter mapping with intraoperative mapping of ventricular tachycardia. *Circulation* 61(2):395-404.

Kenaan, G.; Mendez, A. M.; Zubiate, P., et al. 1973. Surgery for ventricular tachycardia unresponsive to medical treatment. *Chest* 64(5):574-578.

Klein, G. J.; Bashore, T. M.; Sellers, T. D., et al. 1979. Ventricular fibrillation in the Wolff-Parkinson-White syndrome. *N. Engl. J. Med.* 301(20): 1080-1085.

Klein, G. J.; Sealy, W. C.; Pritchett, E. L. C., et al. 1980. Cryosurgical ablation of the atrioventricular node-His bundle: long-term follow-up and properties of the junctional pacemaker. *Circulation* 61(1):8-15.

Lambert, C. J.; Adam, M.; Geisler, F. G., et al. 1971. Emergency myocardial revascularization for impending infarctions and arrhythmias. *J. Thoracic Cardiovasc. Surg.* 62:522-526.

Magidson, O. 1969. Resection of postmyocardial infarction ventricular aneurysms for cardiac arrhythmias. *Dis. Chest* 56:211-218.

Maloy, W. C.; Arrants, J. E.; Sowell, B. F., et al. 1971. Left ventricular aneurysm of uncertain etiology with recurrent ventricular arrhythmias. *N. Engl. J. Med.* 285:662-663.

Marcus, F. I.; Fontaine, G. H.; Guirauden, G., et al. 1982. Right ventricular dysplasia: a report of 24 cases. *Circulation* 65:384-398.

Mason, J. W.; Stinson, E. B.; Winkle, R. A., et al. 1981. Mechanisms of ventricular tachycardia: wide, complex ignorance. *Am. Heart J.* 102: 1083-1087.

Mason, J. W.; Stinson, E. B.; Winkle, R. A., et al. 1982. Surgery for ventricular tachycardia: efficacy of left ventricular aneurysm resection compared with operation guided by electrical activation mapping. *Circulation* 65:1148-1154.

Mikat, E. M.; Hackel, D. B.; Harrison, L., et al. 1977. Reaction of the myocardium and coronary arteries to cryosurgery. *Lab. Invest.* 37(6): 632-641.

Mirowski, M.; Mower, M. M.; Langer, A., et al. 1978. A chronically implanted system for automatic defibrillation in active conscious dogs: experimental model for treatment of sudden death from ventricular fibrillation. *Circulation* 58(1):90-94.

Mirowski, M.; Reid, P. R.; Mower, M. M., et al. 1980. Terminating malignant ventricular arrhythmias with an implanted automatic defibrillator in human beings. *N. Engl. J. Med.* 303:322-324.

Mirowski, M.; Reid, P. R.; Watkins, L., et al. 1981. Clinical treatment of life-threatening ventricular tachyarrhythmias with the automatic implantable defibrillator. *Am. Heart J.* 102:265-280.

Moss, A. J.; and McDonald, J. 1971. Unilateral cervicothoracic sympathetic ganglionectomy for the treatment of long QT interval syndrome. *N. Engl. J. Med.* 285(16):903-904.

Mundth, E. D.; Buckley, M. J.; DeSanctis, R. W., et al. 1973. Surgical treatment of ventricular irritability. *J. Thoracic Cardiovasc. Surg.* 66: 943-949.

Nakhjavan, F. K.; Morse, D. P.; Nichols, H. T., et al. 1971. Emergency aortocoronary bypass. Treatment of ventricular tachycardia due to ischemic heart disease. *J.A.M.A.* 216:2138-2140.

Nordstrom, L. A.; Lillehei, J. P.; Adicoff, A., et al. 1975. Coronary artery surgery for recurrent ventricular arrhythmias in patients with variant angina. *Am. Heart J.* 89(2):236-241.

Ricks, W. B.; Winkle, R. A.; Shumway, N. E., et al. 1977. Surgical management of life-threatening ventricular arrhythmias in patients with coronary artery disease. *Circulation* 56(1):38-42.

Ritter, E. R. 1969. Intractable ventricular tachycardia due to ventricular aneurysm with surgical cure. *Ann. Intern. Med.* 71:1155-1157.

Rolett, E.; Wessler, S.; and Avioli, L. V. 1969. Surgical management of ventricular aneurysm. *J.A.M.A.* 210(1):122-125.

Schlesinger, Z.; Lieberman, Y.; and Neufeld, H. N. 1971. Ventricular aneurysmectomy for severe rhythm disturbances. *J. Thoracic Cardiovasc. Surg.* 61:602-604.

Schwartz, P. J.; Periti, M.; and Malliani, A. 1975. The long Q-T syndrome. *Am. Heart J.* 89(3):378-390.

Sealy, W. C.; and Gallagher, J. J. 1980. The surgical approach to the septal area of the heart based on experiences with 45 patients with Kent bundles. *J. Thoracic Cardiovasc. Surg.* 79:542-551.

Sealy, W. C.; Boineau, J. P.; Wagner, G. S., et al. 1968. Successful surgical interruption of the bundle of Kent in a patient with Wolff-Parkinson-White syndrome. *Circulation* 38:1018-1028.

Sealy, W. C.; Hattler, B. G., Jr.; Blumenschein, S. D., et al. 1969. Surgical treatment of Wolff-Parkinson-White syndrome. *Ann. Thoracic Surg.* 8(1): 1-11.

Sealy, W. C.; Anderson, R. W.; and Gallagher, J. J. 1977. Surgical treatment of supraventricular tachyarrhythmias. *J. Thoracic Cardiovasc. Surg.* 73(4):511-522.

Sealy, W. C.; Gallagher, J. J.; and Pritchett, E. L. C. 1978. The surgical anatomy of Kent bundles based on electrophysiological mapping and surgical exploration. *J. Thoracic Cardiovasc. Surg.* 76(6):804-815.

Spielman, S. R.; Michelson, E. L.; Horowitz, L. N., et al. 1978. The limitations of epicardial mapping as a guide to the surgical therapy of ventricular tachycardia. *Circulation* 57:666-670.

Tabry, I. F.; Geha, A. S.; Hammond, G. I., et al. 1978. Effect of surgery on ventricular tachyarrhythmias associated with coronary arterial occlusive disease. *Circulation* (*Suppl.* I)58:I-166-170.

Thind, G. S.; Blakemore, W. S.; and Zinsser, H. F. 1971. Ventricular aneurysmectomy for the treatment of recurrent ventricular tachyarrhythmia. *Am. J. Cardiol.* 27:690-694.

Tilkian, A. G.; Pfeifer, J. F.; Barry, W. H., et al. 1976. The effect of coronary bypass surgery on exercise-induced ventricular arrhythmias. *Am. Heart J.* 92:707-714.

Vincent, G. M.; Abildskov, J. A.; and Burgess, M. J. 1974. Q-T interval syndromes. *Prog. Cardiovasc. Dis.* 16(6):523-530.

Wald, R. W.; Waxman, M. B.; Corey, P. N., et al. 1979. Management of intractable ventricular tachyarrhythmias after myocardial infarction. *Am. J. Cardiol.* 44:329-337.

Wardekar, A.; Son, B.; Gosaynie, C. D., et al. 1972. Recurrent ventricular tachycardia successfully treated by excision of ventricular aneurysm. *Chest* 62(4):505-508.

Welch, T. G.; Fontana, M. E.; and Vasko, J. S. 1973. Aneurysmectomy for recurrent ventricular tachyarrhythmia. *Am. Heart J.* 85:685-688.

Wellens, H. J. J. 1975. Pathophysiology of ventricular tachycardia in man. *Arch. Intern. Med.* 135:473-479.

Wellens, H. J. J.; Duren, D. R.; and Lie, K. I. 1976. Observations on mechanisms of ventricular tachycardia in man. *Circulation* 54:237-244.

Wittig, J. H.; and Bioneau, J. P. 1975. Surgical treatment of ventricular arrhythmias using epicardial, transmural, and endocardial mapping. *Ann. Thoracic Surg.* 20(2):117-125.

Wyndham, C. R. C.; Arnsdorf, M. R.; Levitsky, S., et al. 1980. Successful surgical excision of focal paroxysmal atrial tachycardia. *Circulation* 62: 1365-1372.

12 Arrhythmias Associated with Acute Myocardial Infarction

Ronald W. F. Campbell, M.D.

Honorary Consultant Cardiologist
The University of Newcastle-upon-Tyne
Newcastle-upon-Tyne, England

The association of cardiac arrhythmias with acute myocardial infarction has been recognized for many years; recently, however, fresh attention has been paid to this phenomenon. Although acute myocardial infarction is caused by a sudden reduction in coronary blood flow, the ensuing process of cell death is not instantaneous. Complex biochemical and metabolic events follow a distinct time course from the first instance of ischemia, and arrhythmias, which are an almost universal accompaniment of the process of infarction, are similarly time-dependent. Until recently the major source of information regarding the natural history of arrhythmias in acute myocardial infarction has been the visual observations of monitored ECGs of patients who are admitted to coronary care units. Currently, this knowledge has been expanded by data from mobile rescue squads and by continuous tape recording and analysis of ECGs. In the 1970s the increasing number of interventions and treatments that were recommended in various clinical situations of acute infarction and ischemia hampered the description of the natural history of arrhythmias.

The arrhythmias associated with acute myocardial infarction may occur for many reasons. Some, such as sinus bradycardia, can be a consequence of changes in autonomic tone. Ventricular ectopic beats and ventricular fibrillation are liable to occur in any patient with infarction, regardless of the site of origin, but AV block can often be ascribed to a particular anatomic area of damage. Finally, some arrhythmias, including atrial arrhythmias, may be related to hemodynamic changes.

ARRHYTHMIAS ASSOCIATED WITH AUTONOMIC UPSET

Sinus Bradycardia

Disturbances of autonomic tone are common in acute myocardial infarction, particularly in the earliest hours (Webb, et al., 1972). Sinus bradycardia and sinus tachycardia are the most commonly encountered manifestations of autonomic upset. Sinus bradycardia, especially, is associated with infarction of the inferior surface of the heart and, when present, may permit the appearance of ventricular escape rhythms or may result in marked hypotension. In this circumstance treatment should be directed at correcting the sinus bradycardia rather than the ventricular arrhythmia. Parenteral atropine (0.5-1.0 mg intravenously) is recommended. Isoproterenol infusion should be avoided because of its potential for extending the area of myocardial damage by increasing both contractility and rate.

Sinus Tachycardia

Sinus tachycardia is another common arrhythmia in acute myocardial infarction. Many factors may account for its presence, and relieving the patient's pain and anxiety is frequently enough to reduce the sinus rate to normal. Sinus tachycardia may also be a consequence of quite appropriate sympathetic drive in association with hypotension and cardiac failure. The treatment is generally directed at the underlying cause of the tachycardia.

AV Block

Disturbances of autonomic tone can also manifest as AV conduction disorders, particularly when inferior myocardial infarction has occurred. First-degree, second-degree, or complete heart block in this context can often be managed by atropine without recourse to endocardial pacing. Atropine administration in acute myocardial infarction is sometimes associated with the development of ventricular arrhythmias, and after it is administered, an increased propensity for ventricular arrhythmias to occur by mechanical stimulation appears to exist if an endocardial pacing electrode has to be inserted.

ARRHYTHMIAS ASSOCIATED WITH NONSPECIFIC MYOCARDIAL DAMAGE

In almost all patients the process of myocardial cell death is accompanied by electrical disturbances that produce ventricular arrhythmias. These phenomena are relatively independent of the anatomic location of the myocardial infarction; however, autonomic influences, infarct size, and previous myocardial damage are a few factors that play a role in the expression of these arrhythmias.

Ventricular Ectopic Complexes

Single ventricular ectopic complexes, multiform ventricular ectopic complexes, ventricular ectopic complex pairs, and R-on-T ventricular ectopic complexes are short isolated events, and, unless they occur in great numbers or are associated with prolonged postectopic pauses, do not usually have any hemodynamic significance and alone do not justify treatment. However, considerable controversy surrounds their importance as potential predictors of serious events (see the section on the anticipation of ventricular fibrillation in this chapter).

Ventricular Tachycardia

Ventricular tachycardia may have immediate significance for patients because, depending on its duration and rate, it can be of serious hemodynamic importance. It occurs in about 15% of patients in the first 48 hours after acute myocardial infarction (Bigger, et al., 1977), but significant hemodynamic deterioration occurs in only a few patients. Most events within the first 48 hours are self-terminating, but ventricular tachycardia occurring at a later period, particularly in the presence of shock, cardiac failure, or in association with a left ventricular aneurysm, may occur in long paroxysms. In situations of urgency a synchronized direct current shock should be used to abort an attack. The shock should coincide with the R wave of the ECG because inadvertent delivery in the area of the T wave may result in ventricular fibrillation. If this occurs, the defibrillator can be recharged and an unsynchronized shock can be applied.

A bolus and infusion of lidocaine are often indicated to prevent recurrences (see Chapter 3). Intravenous lidocaine can also be used to terminate the ventricular tachycardia when it is hemodynamically well tolerated and does not require immediate cardioversion. Other antiarrhythmic drugs may be useful if lidocaine fails. Intravenous procainamide is the most commonly used second-line agent because it can be administered intravenously over 20-30 minutes.

Ventricular tachycardia occurring in the first 48 hours after acute myocardial infarction is less likely to recur than when it appears in the later phase. Early ventricular tachycardia does not necessarily require long-term oral antiarrhythmic therapy. It is customary to prescribe oral therapy for at least 6-12 months when troublesome ventricular tachycardia occurs after the first 48 hours, although the efficacy of such therapy in preventing future morbidity or mortality is unknown.

Ventricular Fibrillation

This is the most feared arrhythmic complication of acute myocardial infarction. Rapid, uncoordinated electrical activity in the myocardium occurs and there is no organized myocardial contraction or effective cardiac output. Although the ECG manifestation of this arrhythmia is similar in most cases, several clinical factors do exist that allow ventricular fibrillation to be differentiated into the following types:

1. Primary ventricular fibrillation. Ventricular fibrillation occurring in the absence of shock or cardiac failure and generally considered to be within the first 24 hours of the onset of symptoms of acute myocardial infarction.
2. Late ventricular fibrillation. Ventricular fibrillation occurring in the absence of shock or cardiac failure and more than 24 hours after the onset of symptoms of acute myocardial infarction but in the absence of symptoms suggesting further infarction.
3. Secondary ventricular fibrillation. Ventricular fibrillation occurring in the presence of cardiac failure and/or shock.

4. Induced ventricular fibrillation. Ventricular fibrillation related to the use of drugs and/or mechanical intervention such as catheterization or temporary pacing.
5. Agonal ventricular fibrillation. Ventricular fibrillation occurring as part of the dying heart syndrome.
6. Ventricular fibrillation occurring in the absence of infarction.

The latter two categories will not be considered further.

The immediate management of ventricular fibrillation (see Chapter 14)
Speed is essential in the management of ventricular fibrillation. No cardiac output occurs during this arrhythmia and so, while specific measures to correct ventricular fibrillation are organized, the patient should be kept alive by cardiopulmonary resuscitation (CPR). Maintenance of cardiac output by continuous coughing in conscious patients has been reported (Criley, et al., 1976) but may require training the patient prior to the onset of the arrhythmia.

The primary goal of management is correction of ventricular fibrillation, and this can be accomplished in a few patients by thump version, which entails the delivery of a blow to the chest with a clenched fist (Gordon, 1972) and imparts considerable energy to the precordium. Thump version is only successful if used within seconds of the onset of the arrest. Transthoracic direct current defibrillation is the definitive management of ventricular fibrillation. The recommended energy content of the initial shock is controversial and varies from 100-400+ joules. The rhythm that occurs as a consequence of direct current shock in patients with out-of-hospital ventricular fibrillation has prognostic implications (Liberthson, et al., 1974) but data regarding the in-hospital population are lacking. In patients with prehospital ventricular fibrillation sinus rhythm and atrial fibrillation have a better long-term prognosis than junctional or idioventricular rhythms following successful direct current conversion.

If the initial direct current shock is unsuccessful, it should be repeated at a higher energy level up to the defibrillator's maximum. A significant acidosis, which usually develops during cardiac arrest, reduces the success rate of defibrillation but can be corrected by the administration of intravenous sodium bicarbonate. Antiarrhythmic drugs, particularly intravenous lidocaine, may also improve the success rate in this situation. Bretylium tosylate (see Chapter 3) is the drug of choice for patients who have ventricular fibrillation that is resistant to defibrillation. The dose of 5-10 mg/kg is given as a rapid intravenous bolus. In rare cases a spontaneous conversion to sinus rhythm may occur. In one series intravenous bretylium tosylate permitted successful defibrillation in 44% of patients (Holder, et al., 1977). Electrolyte upsets, especially potassium imbalances, are associated with difficulties in restoring sinus rhythm; however, correction of this factor is difficult unless it has been defined as a preexisting problem.

After successful conversion of ventricular fibrillation, measures should be taken to prevent its recurrence. The probability of recurrence and the methods of prophylaxis vary according to the clinical situation and will be discussed for each subtype of ventricular fibrillation.

Special aspects of ventricular fibrillation subtypes *Primary ventricular fibrillation* This serious arrhythmic complication of acute myocardial infarction is most frequent in the first minute after the infarction and declines in frequency thereafter (Adgey, et al., 1971). It is more common in association with large areas of myocardial damage but no clear relationship exists to age, sex, or the site of infarction (Mogensen, 1971). The occurrence of this type of ventricular fibrillation seems to confer little if any adverse prognostic risk for patients if it is treated quickly and successfully (Kushnir, et al., 1975). After direct current conversion, intravenous lidocaine should be given for at least 24 hours. It is probably not necessary to continue lidocaine therapy beyond this time because the initial arrhythmia reflects an acute electrical event in the myocardium, which undergoes evolutionary changes over the first 24 hours, and recurrences are uncommon.

Late ventricular fibrillation This type of ventricular fibrillation also occurs in the absence of shock or cardiac failure but presents more than 24 hours after the onset of symptoms of infarction. Unlike primary ventricular fibrillation, it is much more liable to recur after initial management, and, after 24 hours of intravenous lidocaine therapy, 6-12 months or more of oral antiarrhythmic therapy should be considered. When therapy is terminated, the arrhythmia may recur, and, although the value of inpatient monitoring or outpatient ambulatory ECG recording in this population is as yet unproven, a reasonable case can be made for reinstituting therapy in patients who show frequent ventricular arrhythmias.

In some patients late ventricular fibrillation may be related to a particular geometry of damage in the myocardium. Anteroseptal infarction, complicated by bundle branch block, has been reported in association with this form of ventricular fibrillation but the value of long-term prophylactic antiarrhythmic therapy is not yet known (Lie, et al., 1978a).

Secondary ventricular fibrillation This form of ventricular fibrillation, which occurs in the presence of shock or cardiac failure, has a poor prognosis. It reflects severe underlying myocardial damage and widespread electrical upset. It carries a high mortality because it is considerably more difficult to treat by direct current shock. After initial control, secondary ventricular fibrillation is liable to recur and prophylactic antiarrhythmic therapy should be used. Intravenous lidocaine has the advantage of a minimal negative inotropic effect, but in the management of secondary ventricular fibrillation it may be ineffective and second-line drugs may be required. Many of these second-line agents have potentially detrimental effects on left ventricular function. Intra-aortic balloon counter-pulsation pumping, which may be useful in improving the hemodynamic status of patients in shock or cardiac failure, may also stabilize this arrhythmia.

Long-term suppressive antiarrhythmic therapy is usually prescribed for 6-12 months for continued prophylaxis, but patients with this form of ventricular fibrillation have a poor prognosis despite such therapy. Amiodarone (Rosenbaum, et al., 1976), a promising new antiarrhythmic drug that has strong antifibrillatory effects and relatively little negative inotropic effect, may have particular application for this group of patients.

Drug-related ventricular fibrillation A wide variety of drugs, including atropine, sympathomimetics, and diuretics, and invasive procedures, including pacemaker insertion and cardiac catheterization for hemodynamic monitoring, may provoke ventricular fibrillation in patients with acute myocardial infarction. Antiarrhythmic drugs given to control ventricular arrhythmias can also, paradoxically, occasionally produce ventricular fibrillation. After correction of the precipitating event, no further prophylaxis for this arrhythmia is required, although in many institutions it is common to start a short course of intravenous lidocaine. Overdrive pacing at rates of 110-140 beats/min may have a special role in controlling drug-induced arrhythmias until the plasma drug levels decline.

Self-terminating ventricular fibrillation Almost all incidents of ventricular fibrillation are fatal unless they are electrically reversed. However, a few cases of self-terminating ventricular fibrillation have been described. The true incidence of this phenomenon is unknown. It is postulated that, in some circumstances, the patient, in falling to the ground, self-administers thump version but in other instances spontaneous termination in recumbent patients has occurred. In our own institution, from 1066 patients who had definite acute myocardial infarction, three cases of self-terminating ventricular fibrillation were known to have occurred. Ventricular fibrillation was of the primary type in one patient and self-terminated after 2 minutes; however, it recurred 4 hours later and direct current conversion was required. The other two cases were of the secondary type in patients who had combined severe shock and cardiac failure.

The mechanism of self-termination of ventricular fibrillation is unknown, but it is probable that only part of the myocardium is involved in the fibrillatory process, while the remainder of the myocardium stays in an organized rhythm or, at least, is not susceptible to fibrillation. After a period of time, the unaffected area becomes dominant and normal rhythm returns. This type of electrical dissociation within the myocardium has been described in the atria (Dietz, et al., 1957) and has been observed in the ventricles in experimental infarctions and during open-heart surgery.

Antiarrhythmic Strategy for Ventricular Arrhythmias in Acute Myocardial Infarction

The anticipation of ventricular fibrillation In the mid-1960s the advent of coronary care units and monitoring facilities for patients with acute myocardial infarction increased the knowledge of the ECG events occurring in this disease. Ventricular fibrillation was identified as the most serious arrhythmia, and it was shown to be amenable to therapy with a good outlook in many patients (Kushnir, et al., 1975). The initial management and prevention of recurrences of ventricular fibrillation were major aims of the coronary care unit. A classification of ventricular arrhythmias based on human-observer monitoring of the ECG was proposed (i.e., multiform, >5/min, R-on-T, and the occurrence of pairs and salvos) (Lown and Wolf, 1971), and such arrhythmias were considered to have predictive implications for the later occurrence of ventricular fibrillation (Julian, et al., 1964). Intravenous lidocaine was recommended for suppression of these so-called warning arrhythmias in the belief that ventricular fibrillation could be prevented (Lown, et al., 1967). However, subsequent reports suggested that ventricular fibrillation could occur in patients who had not demonstrated warning arrhythmias and in other patients ventricular fibrillation occurred despite lidocaine therapy (Lawrie, et al., 1968). Continuous tape recordings and computer analysis of ECGs revealed that human observations were inefficient and inaccurate and demonstrated that in acute myocardial infarction ventricular arrhythmias were occurring much more frequently than had been hitherto suspected (Romhilt, et al., 1973; Vetter and Julian, 1975). The concept of warning arrhythmias was reexamined using new monitoring technology, and warning arrhythmias were found as frequently in patients who did not develop ventricular fibrillation as in those who did (Lie, et al., 1975; El Sherif, et al., 1976). The result suggested that (from the monitored ECG) it was not possible to predict those patients who would develop ventricular fibrillation.

However, these studies encountered problems in comparing patients who had sustained ventricular fibrillation with patients who lacked this arrhythmia. The duration of the ECG available for the two groups of patients varied because, after the development of ventricular fibrillation, afflicted patients were ineligible for further analysis, while data from patients without ventricular fibrillation were collected for much longer periods. No account was taken of potential variations of arrhythmia frequency related to time from the onset of infarction. Finally, the drugs used in some of these studies may have altered the natural history of ventricular arrhythmias.

A further study of the natural history of ventricular fibrillation and ventricular arrhythmias in acute myocardial infarction has attempted to overcome these methodologic problems (Campbell, 1980). Its results suggest that R-on-T ventricular ectopic complex frequency may predict those patients who will develop primary ventricular fibrillation, but the sophisticated nature of this indicator renders it relatively impractical for use in coronary care unit monitoring.

Treating ventricular fibrillation as it arises The lack of a practical method of predicting those patients who will develop ventricular fibrillation has encouraged alternative management policies. In some coronary care units patients are particularly closely monitored with prompt correction of ventricular fibrillation on occurrence, but other ventricular arrhythmias (except those that are of hemodynamic significance) are ignored. This strategy has the advantage that antiarrhythmic therapy is administered only to patients who require it, but it demands a great deal of staff time and monitoring and resuscitation equipment. Although data suggest that primary ventricular fibrillation has little adverse prognostic significance in resuscitated patients (Kushnir, et al., 1975), the studies may have been too small to assess any influence of ventricular fibrillation on potential infarct size.

Drug prophylaxis of ventricular fibrillation This strategy demands that prophylactic therapy be given to all patients admitted with suspected acute myocardial infarction. In practice drugs will be administered to some patients who are later shown not to have sustained acute myocardial infarction and to other patients who may later develop serious consequences of acute myocardial infarction, including failure, shock, and heart block. The success of this approach depends on the availability of a drug that is highly effective in preventing ventricular fibrillation, is relatively nontoxic, has little or no effects on left ventricular function, sinus node function, and AV node conduction, and is easily administered. Intravenous lidocaine is the only drug that has so far been shown to reduce primary ventricular fibrillation significantly (Lie, et al., 1974). Unwanted effects, albeit minor, commonly occur at the recommended dosage level. Prophylactic intravenous lidocaine is now a widely accepted regimen in coronary care units, but intravenous administration of lidocaine can be expensive and the effects of the drug on infarction size and its safety in rare clinical situations are unclear. Little doubt exists that it can be used successfully to protect patients from ventricular fibrillation (Wyman and Hammersmith, 1974) but usually can only be administered in situations where a small portable defibrillator might be as effective in reducing mortality. Unfortunately, intramuscular administration of lidocaine appears to be ineffective (Lie, et al., 1978b). Other antiarrhythmic drugs have been evaluated as prophylactic agents but in each case too few episodes of ventricular fibrillation occurred for statistical analysis (Koch-Weser, et al., 1969; Jones, et al., 1974; Jennings, et al., 1976; Campbell, et al., 1979). In these studies other, more common ventricular arrhythmias were reduced significantly but this does not imply similar efficacy in preventing ventricular fibrillation. In many studies oral therapy was used, but it is unlikely that drugs administered by this route can be absorbed quickly enough to allow protection from ventricular fibrillation in the first hours after acute myocardial infarction (Prescott, 1978), which is the time when it is most required.

ARRHYTHMIAS ASSOCIATED WITH PARTICULAR INFARCTION ANATOMY

The appearance of AV conduction disorders in acute myocardial infarction is usually an indication of ischemia or infarction involving the AV node or the His-Purkinje system (see Chapter 6). The significance of first-degree, second-degree, or complete heart block depends on the type of associated infarction, but the immediate hemodynamic effect of these arrhythmias dictates their management. First-degree heart block does not itself require treatment but alerts the physician to the possibility of increasing degrees of AV block. Similarly, second-degree AV block is rarely of immediate hemodynamic significance, but it is particularly likely to progress to complete heart block. A significant reduction of heart rate and cardiac output occurs in complete heart block. Second-degree AV block and complete heart block are usually treated. Intravenous atropine may correct the problem, especially in the presence of inferior myocardial infarction. Intravenous isoproterenol may also be used but requires extremely careful administration because it may cause serious ventricular arrhythmias. Its routine use is not recommended. The treatment of choice for AV block in association with anterior infarction, and when atropine fails in patients with inferior myocardial infarction, is endocardial pacing. Placement of an endocardial pacing electrode following therapy with atropine or isoproterenol is associated with an increased risk of ventricular fibrillation and should be undertaken with care and with a defibrillator readily available.

Inferior Myocardial Infarction

AV conduction disorders are more common in inferior than in anterior infarction (Norris, 1969). As mentioned previously, AV block occurring in inferior infarction may be a consequence of vagal tone. It has been postulated that there are more vagal receptors in the right coronary artery than in the left, but the precise mechanism of this phenomenon is not understood. The inferior myocardial wall and the AV node receive their blood supply from the right coronary artery, but the His bundle is also supplied by branches from the left circumflex coronary artery, giving it relative protection from infarction. When complete heart block occurs in the context of an acute inferior infarction, the escape pacemaker is often relatively proximal in the His-Purkinje system, is relatively stable, and produces a reasonable ventricular rate with a narrow QRS complex (Norris and Croxson, 1970). (See also Chapter 6.)

Anterior Myocardial Infarction

AV conduction disorders associated with anterior myocardial infarction have a serious prognosis, usually reflecting severe myocardial damage involving the His-Purkinje system. The onset of AV conduction disorders is often sudden, and the escape pacemaker is distal in the His-Purkinje system, has a low rate, produces a broad QRS complex, and is frequently unstable (Norris and Croxson, 1970). Atropine is usually ineffective, and isoproterenol is often unreliable in improving cardiac output. Endocardial pacing is the treatment of choice, but the outlook is relatively poor because of the extent of underlying infarction.

Bundle branch block is also particularly associated with anterior myocardial infarction and carries an increased subsequent mortality (Scheinman and Brenman, 1972). It does not cause hemodynamic deterioration and, for this reason, does not require treatment. The relationship of bundle branch block to the development of complete heart block and asystole has stimulated interest in defining particular forms of bundle branch block for which prophylactic pacemaker electrode insertion is beneficial (see also Chapter 6). Right bundle branch block with left anterior fascicular block or left posterior fascicular block and PR prolongation with left anterior fascicular block or left posterior fascicular block, particularly with HV prolongation, are high-risk subtypes of bundle branch block (Scanlon, et al., 1970; Scheinman and Brenman, 1972). Unfortunately, the mortality of these patients is high despite endocardial pacing. Although there may be a small risk of producing ventricular fibrillation by placement of the electrode in the coronary care unit, it is often more convenient to anticipate the need for a pacemaker and insert it electively rather than in the presence of complete heart block or asystole.

Only a minority of patients who require endocardial pacemaking acutely during acute myocardial infarction require permanent generator implantations. The poor late prognosis of survivors of AV conduction disorders in anterior myocardial infarction has stimulated research into the value of prophylactic long-term pacemaking, but no firm conclusions are presently available. The recognition that some late mortality is caused by ventricular fibrillation rather than asystole (Lie, et al., 1978) introduces new therapeutic implications. (See also Chapter 6.)

OTHER ARRHYTHMIAS

Supraventricular Arrhythmias

Hemodynamically significant supraventricular arrhythmias are relatively uncommon in acute myocardial infarction but less severe forms are frequent. Many supraventricular arrhythmias are associated with cardiac failure and may be a consequence of altered cardiac hemodynamics and autonomic imbalance. In some cases they may be the result of atrial infarction. Most supraventricular arrhythmias can be ignored, but sustained arrhythmias such as atrial flutter or atrial fibrillation will require treatment to control the ventricular rates, and management differs little from their management in other settings (see Chapter 6).

Accelerated Idioventricular Rhythm

Considerable controversy surrounds the significance of this arrhythmia in acute myocardial infarction. It can occur as a normal escape mechanism when the sinus rate slows (Figure 12-1), but in some patients with

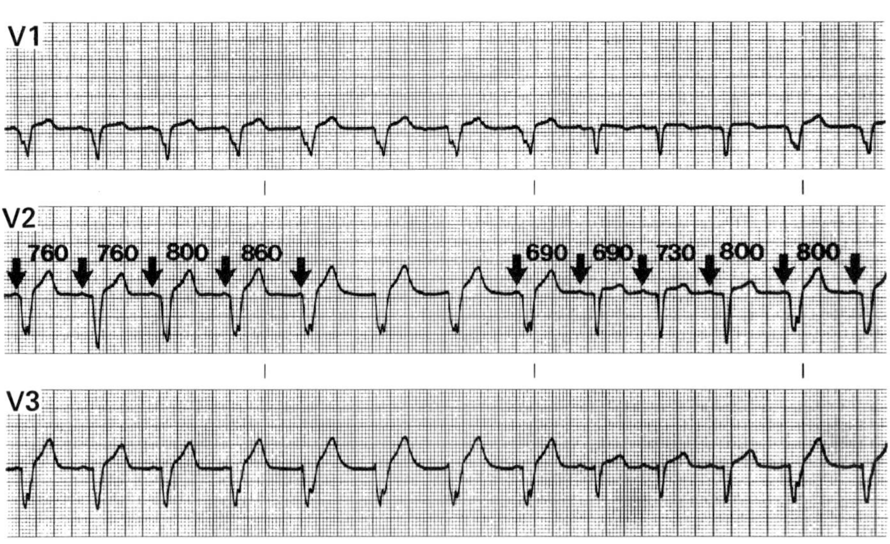

Figure 12-1 Example of accelerated idioventricular rhythm (AIVR) in a patient with an acute anterior infarction. Three simultaneous surface ECG leads are shown. The arrows show the discernible P waves and the numbers represent the sinus cycle length. Note that as the sinus cycle length increases (i.e., heart rate slows) the AIVR emerges, and as the cycle length shortens (i.e., faster heart rate) supraventricular capture beats (the narrow QRS complexes) occur.

accelerated idioventricular rhythm ventricular tachycardia at a rate arithmetically related to the rate of the accelerated idioventricular rhythm has been observed, suggesting a more serious significance of this arrhythmia (Lichstein, et al., 1975). In these circumstances a rapid ventricular focus may be subject to exit block and present as accelerated idioventricular rhythm on one occasion, but the block may later dissipate and rapid ventricular tachycardia may occur. At the present time therapy should be considered optional.

Asystole

Asystole is usually a consequence of severe myocardial damage. It carries a high immediate mortality. Treatment is by pacemaking or chronotropic drugs such as isoproterenol. The long-term outlook is grave, reflecting the extent of underlying disease.

REFERENCES

Adgey, A. A. J.; Allen, J. D.; Geddes, J. S., et al. 1971. Acute phase of myocardial infarction. *Lancet* 2:501-504.

Bigger, J. T., Jr.; Dresdale, R. J.; Heissenbuttel, R. H., et al. 1977. Ventricular arrhythmias in ischemic heart disease: mechanism, prevalence, significance, and management. *Prog. Cardiovasc. Dis.* 19:255-300.

Campbell, R. W. F. 1980. Relation of ventricular arrhythmias to primary ventricular fibrillation. *Br. Heart J.* 43:100.

Campbell, R. W. F.; Achuff, S. C.; Pottage, A., et al. 1979. Mexiletine in the prophylaxis of ventricular arrhythmias during acute myocardial infarction. *J. Cardiol. Pharm.* 1:43-52.

Criley, J. M.; Blaufuss, A. H.; and Kissel, G. L. 1976. Cough-induced cardiac compression. *J.A.M.A.* 236:1246-1250.

Dietz, G. W., III; Marriott, H. J. L.; Fletcher, E., et al. 1957. Atrial dissociation and uniatrial fibrillation. *Circulation* 15:883-888.

El Sherif, N.; Meyerburg, R. J.; Scherlag, B. T., et al. 1976. Electrocardiographic antecedents of primary ventricular fibrillation. *Br. Heart J.* 38:415.

Gordon, A. S. 1972. Technique of cardiopulmonary resuscitation (CPR) and pitfalls in performance. In *Coronary care.* L. E. Meltzer; and A. J. Dunning, editors. Amsterdam: Excerpta Medica. pp. 397-433.

Holder, D. A.; Sniderman, A. D.; Fraser, G., et al. 1977. Experience with bretylium tosylate by a hospital cardiac arrest team. *Circulation* 55:541-544.

Jennings, G.; Jones, M. B. S.; and Besterman, E. M. M. 1976. Oral disopyramide in prophylaxis of arrhythmias following myocardial infarction. *Lancet* 1:51-54.

Jones, D. T.; Kostuk, W. J.; and Gunton, R. W. 1974. Prophylactic quinidine in acute myocardial infarction. *Am. J. Cardiol.* 33:655-660.

Julian, D. G.; Valentine, P. A.; and Miller, G. G. 1964. Disturbance of rate rhythm and conduction in acute myocardial infarction. *Am. J. Med.* 37:915.

Koch-Weser, J.; Klein, S. W.; Foo-Canto, L. L., et al. 1969. Antiarrhythmic prophylaxis with procainamide in acute myocardial infarction. *N. Engl. J. Med.* 281:1253-1260.

Kushnir, B.; Fox, K. M.; Tomlinson, I. W., et al. 1975. Primary ventricular fibrillation and resumption of work, sexual activity, and driving after first acute myocardial infarction. *Br. Med. J.* 4:609.

Lawrie, D. M.; Higgins, M. R.; Godman, M. J., et al. 1968. Ventricular fibrillation complicating acute myocardial infarction. *Lancet* 2:523-528.

Liberthson, R. R.; Nagel, E. L.; Hirschman, J. C., et al. 1974. Prehospital ventricular defibrillation. *N. Engl. J. Med.* 7:317-321.

Lichstein, E.; Ribas-Meneclier, C.; Gupta, P. K., et al. 1975. Incidence and description of accelerated ventricular rhythm complicating acute myocardial infarction. *Am. J. Med.* 58:192-198.

Lie, K. I.; Wellens, H. J. J.; Von Capelle, F. J., et al. 1974. Lidocaine in the prevention of primary ventricular fibrillation. *N. Engl. J. Med.* 29: 1324-1326.

Lie, K. I.; Wellens, H. J.; Downar, E., et al. 1975. Observations on patients with primary ventricular fibrillation complicating acute myocardial infarction. *Circulation* 52:755-759.

Lie, K. I.; Liem, K. L.; Schuilenberg, R. M., et al. 1978a. Early identification of patients developing late in-hospital ventricular fibrillation after discharge from the coronary care unit. A 5½ year retrospective study of 1897 patients. *Am. J. Cardiol.* 41:674-677.

Lie, K. I.; Liem, K. L.; Louridtz, W. L., et al. 1978b. Efficiency of lidocaine in preventing ventricular fibrillation within 1 hour after a 300 mg intramuscular injection. A double-blind randomized study of 300 hospitalized patients with acute myocardial infarction. *Am. J. Cardiol.* 42: 486-488.

Lown, B.; and Wolf, M. 1971. Approaches to sudden death from coronary heart disease. *Circulation* 54:130-142.

Lown, B.; Fakhro, A. M.; and Hood, W. B. 1967. The coronary care unit. New perspectives and directions. *J.A.M.A.* 188:199.

Mogensen, L. 1971. A controlled trial of lidocaine prophylaxis in the prevention of ventricular tachyarrhythmias in acute myocardial infarction. *Acta Med. Scand.* 513:1-80.

Norris, R. M. 1969. Heart block in posterior and interior myocardial infarction. *Br. Heart J.* 31:352-356.

Norris, R. M.; and Croxson, M. S. 1970. Bundle branch block in acute myocardial infarction. *Am. Heart J.* 79:728-733.

Prescott, L. F. 1978. Pharmacokinetic abnormalities in myocardial infarction. In *Management of ventricular tachycardia—role of mexiletine.* Amsterdam: Excerpta Medica. pp. 465-471.

Romhilt, D. W.; Bloomfield, S. S.; Chou, T., et al. 1973. Unreliability of conventional electrocardiographic monitoring for arrhythmia detection in coronary care units. *Am. J. Cardiol.* 31:457-461.

Rosenbaum, M. B.; Chiale, P. A.; Halpern, M. S., et al. 1976. Clinical efficacy of amiodarone as an antiarrhythmic agent. *Am. J. Cardiol.* 38: 934-944.

Scanlon, P. J.; Pryor, R.; and Blount, S. G. 1970. Right bundle branch block associated with left superior or inferior intraventricular block associated with acute myocardial infarction. *Circulation* 42:1135-1142.

Scheinman, M. M.; and Brenman, B. A. 1972. Clinical and anatomical implications of intraventricular conduction block in acute myocardial infarction. *Circulation* 46:753-760.

Vetter, N. J.; and Julian, D. G. 1975. Comparison of arrhythmia computer and conventional monitoring in coronary care unit. *Lancet* 1:1151-1154.

Webb, S. W.; Adgey, A. A. J.; and Pantridge, J. F. 1972. Autonomic disturbances at onset of acute myocardial infarction. *Br. Med. J.* 3:89-92.

Wyman, M. G.; and Hammersmith, L. 1974. Comprehensive treatment plan for the prevention of primary ventricular fibrillation in acute myocardial infarction. *Am. J. Cardiol.* 33:661-667.

13 Digitalis Toxicity

Roger J. Hall, M.D., M.R.C.P.

Consultant Cardiologist and Physician
Royal Victoria Infirmary
Queen Victoria Road
Newcastle-upon-Tyne, England

When William Withering (1785) used digitalis preparations to treat cardiac failure, he realized that a therapeutic effect was often followed quickly by toxicity, usually in the form of vomiting. This side-effect was so common that its onset was often used as an indication that an adequate dosage of the drug had been given. After 200 years, side-effects remain a major problem of digitalis therapy, occurring in between 10% and 20% of patients receiving the drug (Beller, et al., 1971; Evered and Chapman, 1971; Carruthers, et al., 1974). Arrhythmias occur in more than 80% of these patients. Although the extracardiac effects of digitalis toxicity can be unpleasant, cardiac arrhythmias are the major problem and may prove fatal in as many as 5%-10% of cases of intoxication (Rodensky and Wasserman, 1961; Beller, et al., 1971). The enormous size of this problem can be appreciated when it is realized that digoxin is the fourth most commonly prescribed drug in the United States (Schick and Scheuer, 1974).

DIGITALIS AND THE MANAGEMENT OF HEART FAILURE

Despite their toxicity, digitalis glycosides remain a mainstay of antiarrhythmic treatment because of their unique ability to slow conduction through the AV node in atrial fibrillation without depressing cardiac contractility and their effectiveness in treating many supraventricular arrhythmias. The other common use of digitalis is in patients with sinus rhythm and cardiac failure. Because this use contributes significantly to the incidence of toxicity and is controversial, it is worth examining the evidence supporting the use of chronic oral digitalization in patients with cardiac failure who are in sinus rhythm.

1. *Does an inotropic effect occur, and is it sustained during chronic administration?* This was a controversial area for many years. However, recent research, using a variety of techniques to assess cardiac function both at rest and on exercise, has established a definite, if modest, sustained inotropic effect in patients with heart failure who are in sinus rhythm (Braunwald, et al., 1961; Crawford, et al., 1976; Dobbs, et al., 1977; Kleiman, et al., 1978; Arnold, et al., 1980; Griffiths, et al., 1982; Lee, et al., 1982; Murray, et al., 1982).
2. *Are such changes in measured cardiac function clinically beneficial?* There are several difficult problems in interpreting all studies of digitalis glycosides in sinus rhythm. First, patients frequently have cardiac failure resulting from many causes, but they are grouped together in the assumption that they will all behave in the same way. Second, nearly all studies have only examined the effects on resting cardiac output, when the major problem for such patients is often an inability to increase cardiac output adequately with exercise. Recent studies

have shed light on the situation. Dobbs and colleagues (1977), in a double-blind trial, substituted a placebo for digoxin and found that 30% of their patients deteriorated when this substitution was made. Salt and water retention was the usual mode of deterioration. The studies of Hull and MacIntosh (1977) and McHaffie and colleagues (1978) suggest that in many patients adjustments of diuretics when digoxin is withdrawn will prevent such deterioration. Because digitalis toxicity is both prevalent and dangerous, a reasonable approach to patients with congestive heart failure is to attempt to control the patient initially with diuretics alone. If the maximum effect of a reasonable dose of diuretics provides inadequate response, digitalis can be added in an attempt to obtain a further improvement. If no improvement occurs, the digitalis glycoside can be withdrawn (Figure 13-1).

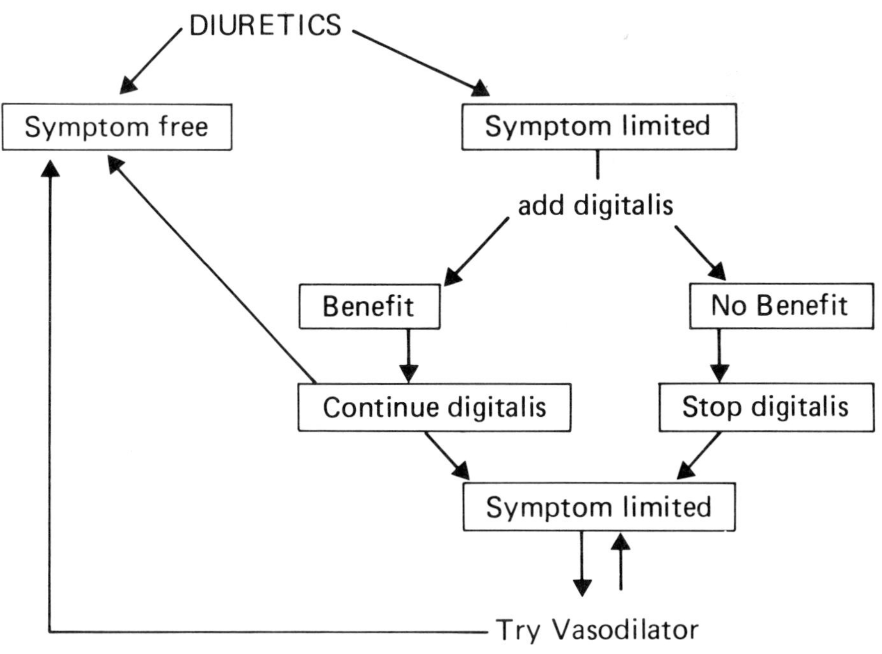

Figure 13-1 Scheme for the use of digitalis for the treatment of cardiac failure in patients with sinus rhythm.

MECHANISM OF THE THERAPEUTIC AND TOXIC ACTIONS OF DIGITALIS

The cardiovascular actions of digitalis glycosides are particularly complex because the drug acts at different but interrelated levels in the circulation. It has direct effects on the myocardium and peripheral vasculature and is also a potent neuroexcitatory drug, producing autonomic effects on the heart and circulation. Its actions are frequently modified in clinical practice by alterations in plasma electrolytes, pH and PaO_2 levels, the patient's age, concurrent therapy, and the severity and type of heart disease.

Digitalis is a potent inhibitor of sodium and potassium transport across the cell membrane (Schatzmann, 1953), and this inhibition of ionic transport results from digitalis blocking a specific enzyme system, Na^+, K^+–ATPase (Skou, 1957). The attractive idea of a specific enzyme receptor for the actions of digitalis has led to an enormous amount of work to establish whether the enzyme is the digitalis receptor and whether inhibition of the enzyme can explain both the inotropic and toxic actions of digitalis.

Inotropic Effects

Good evidence exists that the inotropic actions of digitalis are a direct cardiac effect and not mediated by alterations in autonomic tone (Spann, et al., 1966; Ezrailson, et al., 1977) and occur at an extracellular site (Okarma, et al., 1972). There are several attractive hypotheses for the mechanism by which digoxin produces its inotropic effects, all of which depend on a final step of providing more available intracellular calcium to stimulate the interaction of the contractile proteins. Several hypotheses postulate that alteration of Na^+, K^+–ATPase activity produces changes in ionic movements that result in increased calcium availability (Langer, 1972; Nayler, 1975). However, explanations based on a modification of sodium pumping have been seriously challenged (Okita, et al., 1973).

It is possible that the link between digitalis binding to Na^+, K^+–ATPase and the onset of inotropy is more indirect than a simple inhibition of ion transport. A recent hypothesis (Gervais, et al., 1975) suggests that the binding of digitalis to Na^+, K^+–ATPase produces a conformational change in the cell membrane, which in turn alters sarcolemmal calcium affinity and, hence, makes more calcium available to the contractile protein.

Toxicity

As with the hypotheses put forward to explain inotropy, controversy exists as to whether Na^+, K^+–ATPase inhibition and the toxic effects of digitalis are linked. However, most investigators feel that Na^+, K^+–ATPase inhibition and the changes in intracellular electrolytes that occur as a result of this are important factors in digitalis toxicity. Although intracellular electrolyte changes are absent or slight when therapeutic doses of digitalis are given, larger and toxic doses reduce intracellular potassium and increase intracellular calcium and sodium levels, and these electrolyte changes can be related to the occurrence of arrhythmias (Okita, et al., 1973).

Unlike the inotropic effects, which appear to be independent of the autonomic system, the toxic effects of digitalis glycosides are by no means confined to their direct action on the heart. Indirect cardiac effects mediated by the autonomic system have an important additive and modifying effect on the direct toxic effects of digitalis. Although a tendency exists to regard the therapeutic and toxic effects of digitalis as separate entities with separate mechanisms, the difference is often one of degree. For example, moderate impairment of AV conduction in atrial fibrillation produces a clinically beneficial slowing of the rate of atrial fibrillation, but an excessive impairment of AV conduction can produce a dangerous bradyarrhythmia.

Autonomic Effects of Digitalis

At normal therapeutic dosage digitalis produces only minor direct alterations in cardiac electrophysiology, and the autonomic effects produce most of the observed changes in heart rate and rhythm. These autonomic effects may, if excessive, also cause some of the toxic effects of digitalis. At normal therapeutic dosage the most important effect is vagotonia, produced by the parasympathetic nervous system; however, as toxic levels are reached, less well-recognized sympathetic stimulation also becomes important.

Vagotonic effects The vagotonic effects of digitalis occur in the following three ways (Gillis, et al., 1975; Rosen, et al., 1975):

1. Potentiation of the afferent limb of the carotid and aortic baroreceptor reflexes so that at any given level of blood pressure the digitalized patient develops more afferent traffic to the medullary vasomotor center with a subsequent increase in vagal outflow and a reduction in sympathetic outflow.
2. Direct stimulation of the parasympathetic medullary control centers.
3. Potentiation of the action of the vagal discharge at the level of the cardiac parasympathetic receptors.

This vagotonic action has only modest effects on the sinus node in humans and may occasionally lead to some slowing of the sinus rate. It has far more important effects on the rest of the atrium, where it enhances conduction, shortens the effective refractory period, and reduces the automaticity of ectopic pacemakers. The best known and perhaps the single most important therapeutic effect of digitalis results from its vagotonic action, which slows the conduction of impulses from the atria to the ventricles. This slowing of AV conduction occurs entirely in the AV node (Przybyla, et al., 1974).

Reduction of sympathetic activity Under normal circumstances digitalis causes withdrawal of sympathetic tone both by its alteration of the baroreceptor reflexes and by alleviating cardiac failure. Digitalis also has a direct effect on supraventricular pacemakers, decreasing their sensitivity to sympathetic influences (Nadeau and James, 1963).

Increased sympathetic outflow The most recently recognized and controversial autonomic effect of digoxin is its ability, in toxic doses, to excite the central nervous system and enhance sympathetic outflow in cardiac, phrenic, and peripheral sympathetic nerves (Gillis, et al., 1972). Recent animal experiments (Somberg and Smith, 1979) suggest that the central arrhythmogenic effects of digitalis glycosides are mediated by the area *postrema* in the hind brain. The chemoreceptor trigger zone through which the common noncardiac side-effect of vomiting is mediated is also located in this area. The area *postrema* lacks a blood/brain barrier, which explains why polar glycosides (e.g., digoxin) that do not cross the blood/brain barrier and nonpolar glycosides (e.g., digitoxin) that do are equally effective in producing centrally mediated toxic effects. Toxic doses may also excite the sympathetic nervous system peripherally, producing increased activity in pre- and postganglionic nerves and sympathetic ganglia.

Other effects Suggestions have been made of a serotonergic mechanism of digitalis action, both centrally and peripherally. The evidence for a central serotonergic mechanism in digitalis toxicity is poor (Helke, et al., 1978b), but experiments in the cat have suggested that peripheral blockade of serotonin with, for example, methysergide or cyproheptadine reduces digitalis-induced arrhythmias (Helke, et al., 1978a). The effect of serotonin blockers in digitalis toxicity in humans is unknown.

ARRHYTHMOGENIC EFFECTS

As toxic digitalis levels are reached, the direct electrophysiologic effects of digitalis become important and combine with the autonomic effects to produce arrhythmias.

Increased Automaticity

Enhanced diastolic depolarization As the level of digitalis increases, diastolic (phase 4) depolarization (Figure 13-2) becomes more rapid in

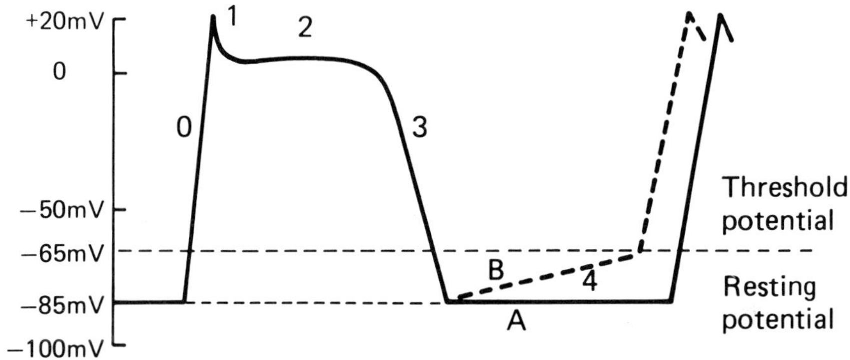

PHASE 0 — upstroke
1 — early rapid depolarisation
2 — plateau phase
3 — repolarisation
4 — (A) Resting potential maintained in non-pacemaking cells
(B) 'Phase 4' pacemaker depolarisation in potential pacemaker cells

Figure 13-2 The normal cardiac action potential in nonpacemaker and pacemaker cells. The extent of membrane polarization is shown on the left. Phase 4 differs depending on whether the cell is a nonpacemaker (A) or pacemaker cell (B).

cells in the His-Purkinje system. This enhanced diastolic depolarization means that a cell that does not normally act as the dominant pacemaker may reach threshold before it is depolarized by the next impulse from the normal pacemaker, producing a premature depolarization. This may occur as a result of altered sodium pumping and cation conductance and is exacerbated by reduced potassium levels (Ito, et al., 1970). Recent work suggests that a slow inward calcium current, rather like that occurring during the plateau phase of the normal action potential, occurs during phase 4 of the action potential in digitalis toxicity and speeds diastolic (phase 4) depolarization (Tse and Han, 1975). Even if this accelerated phase 4 depolarization does not reach threshold, another subthreshold stimulus may combine with this higher than normal membrane potential and produce a premature depolarization. Phase 4 depolarization is also stimulated by the increased sympathetic outflow to the heart that is produced by digitalis toxicity; thus, both direct and autonomic effects combine to create enhanced automaticity. This combined effect is most likely to occur below the AV node, where there is no opposing vagal influence. Exceptions to this may occur in some patients with heart disease. Such patients often have impaired vagal function (Eckberg, et al., 1971), and this may partly explain the observation that patients with heart disease tend to develop increased automaticity, particularly in the form of ventricular premature contractions and atrial ectopic rhythms, as a manifestation of digitalis toxicity, whereas in patients with normal hearts the vagotonic actions of digitalis predominate.

Late after-depolarizations Recently, attention has been focused on late after-depolarizations occurring in the His-Purkinje system as an important electrophysiologic mechanism underlying tachyarrhythmias, particularly in digitalis toxicity (Rosen, et al., 1975; Cranefield, 1977) (see Chapter 1). Following a normal depolarization, in the presence of digitalis toxicity, the membrane potential falls below normal (hyperpolarizes) and then rises again rapidly to a higher-than-normal level, producing the late after-depolarization (Figure 13-3), which may reach threshold and trigger a premature depolarization. This premature depolarization may itself be followed by the same chain of events, thereby setting up a repetitive arrhythmia. Repetitive arrhythmias are especially likely to occur because late after-depolarizations are more common following a premature depolarization. This phenomenon is potentiated by sympathetic stimulation and hypokalemia. The mechanism underlying the late after-depolarization appears to be calcium-dependent and may result from alterations in intracellular calcium occurring as a result of the interaction between digitalis and Na^+, K^+–ATPase (Tsien and Carpenter, 1978).

Reduced resting membrane potential The most easily understood, directly mediated toxic effect of digitalis is the reduction of the resting membrane potential that occurs in atrial and ventricular muscle and the His-Purkinje system. The resting membrane potential depends almost exclusively on the ratio of intracellular to extracellular potassium. If intracellular potassium is reduced by inhibition of Na^+, K^+–ATPase, the value of this ratio falls and results in a fall in the resting membrane potential. A reduced resting membrane potential brings the cell nearer to threshold and, hence, increases automaticity.

Decreased Conduction

Autonomic effects The vagotonic actions of digitalis have their most important therapeutic effect in slowing conduction through the AV node. If this effect becomes excessive, either because of toxic drug levels or because normal levels have an excessive effect on conduction that was impaired before digitalis therapy, heart block may occur and escape rhythms below the level of the block may take over.

Reduced resting membrane potential Reduction of the resting membrane potential may cause increased automaticity as described above, but it also

A **Normal action potential**

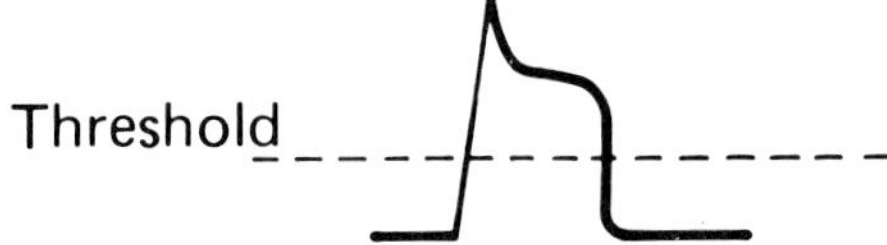

B **Late afterdepolarisation I**

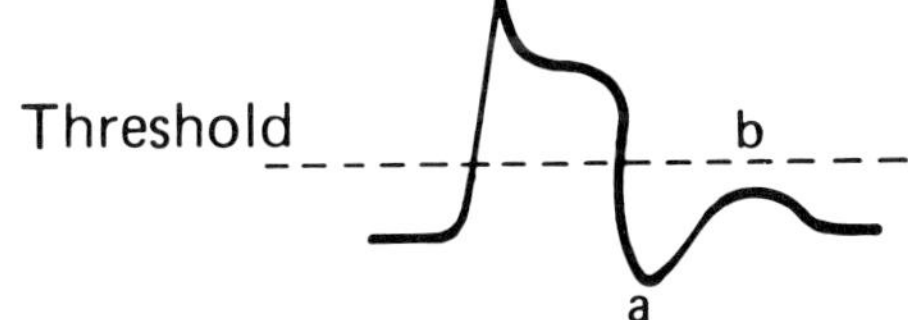

a = early afterhyperpolarisation
b = late afterdepolarisation

C **Late afterdepolarisation II**

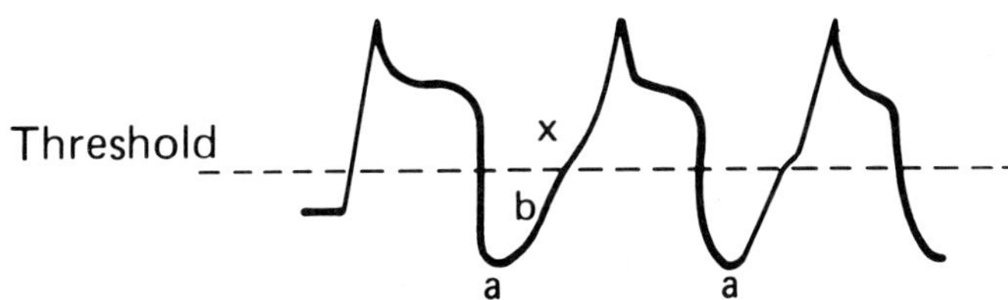

The late afterdepolarisation reached threshold at x

Figure 13-3 Late after-depolarizations in digitalis toxicity. A (top part of the figure) shows a normal action potential. In B the action potential is followed by an early hyperpolarization (a) and a late after-depolarization (b) that does not reach threshold. In C the late after-depolarization reaches threshold at x and triggers another action potential, which is itself followed by an after-depolarization that triggers another response. Note that the upstroke of the action potential is slower in the responses triggered by the late after-depolarization and, hence, conduction will be slower.

affects conduction. The lower the resting membrane potential is when a cell is depolarized (i.e., the nearer it is to threshold potential), the slower is the upstroke (phase 0) of the potential. Slowing the rate of rise of the upstroke of the action potential directly reduces the rate of conduction in excitable tissue. Such slow conduction may set up the conditions required to allow reentry to occur.

FACTORS PREDISPOSING TO TOXICITY

A number of extrinsic factors can alter myocardial sensitivity to digitalis, either directly or by altering digitalis blood levels by changing metabolism or renal clearance. A patient who is well controlled on a maintenance dosage of digitalis is not at great risk from toxicity unless some other change occurs (either as a result of progression of heart disease, alterations in other therapy, or intercurrent disease) that unbalances the situation.

Electrolytes

Hypokalemia Hypokalemia is the single most important precipitating cause of digitalis toxicity. Hypokalemia frequently results from diuretic-induced potassium loss, but it is also exacerbated by poor dietary intake by anorectic patients with cardiac failure and by secondary hyperaldosteronism, which is a normal physiologic response to the reduced cardiac output that occurs in cardiac failure. The well-known, but anecdotal, potentiation of digitalis toxicity by hypokalemia in clinical practice has recently been demonstrated more scientifically. Shapiro (1978) found that in hypokalemic patients digitalis-induced arrhythmias occur at lower serum digoxin levels than in normokalemic patients, and Steiness and Olesen (1976) produced digitalis toxicity in a group of patients by withdrawing potassium supplements while maintaining the same dose of digoxin. The mean serum potassium level in the group fell from 4.37 to 3.41 mmol/L and 50% of the patients developed arrhythmias ascribed to digoxin, which disappeared when potassium was reintroduced.

Alterations of intracellular electrolytes, particularly a fall in intracellular potassium and an increase in intracellular sodium and calcium levels, are important in producing digitalis toxicity. Because hypokalemia and digitalis both alter the activity of Na^+, K^+–ATPase, the potentiating effect of hypokalemia may be mediated by this enzyme. Experimental evidence (Allen and Schwartz, 1970; Goldman, et al., 1975) suggests that extracellular potassium and cardiac glycosides compete for a membrane receptor site, probably Na^+, K^+–ATPase. If this is so, hypokalemia would be expected to promote the binding of cardiac glycosides to Na^+, K^+–ATPase and, hence, the inhibition of this enzyme. Most studies (Binnion and Morgan, 1970; Hall, et al., 1977) suggest that this is the case, although one research team (Francis, et al., 1973) was unable to show this effect. Hypokalemia alone inhibits Na^+, K^+–ATPase activity and might combine with any digitalis-induced inhibition. Although hypokalemia does increase digitalis binding, this effect only explains part of the potentiation of toxicity (Hall, et al., 1977). The additional potentiation is independent of digitalis binding and Na^+, K^+–ATPase inhibition and may be caused by the direct effects of hypokalemia on membrane excitability.

Magnesium deficiency Magnesium deficiency is rarely recognized clinically, although it may often be produced by prolonged use of diuretics (Lim and Jacob, 1972; Sheehan and White, 1982). Experimental studies in animals (Seller, et al., 1970) and observation of patients (Beller, et al., 1970) suggest that hypomagnesemia potentiates digitalis toxicity. The mechanism underlying this potentiation is, as yet, unclear.

Other electrolytes Alterations in plasma calcium levels can alter the sensitivity of the heart to digitalis under experimental conditions, but it is doubtful whether fluctuations of serum calcium seen under normal clinical conditions are important; however, digitalis toxicity may be enhanced in patients with pathologically high levels of calcium. The effects of hyponatremia on digitalis toxicity have not been assessed in enough detail to allow any useful conclusions.

Acid-Base Changes

The effects of acid-base changes on digitalis toxicity are complex. Both acidosis and alkalosis may precipitate cardiac arrhythmias in the absence of digitalis and, hence, would be expected to exacerbate arrhythmias caused by digitalis toxicity. In addition, acid-base changes may alter autonomic activity and have effects on intracellular and extracellular potassium levels. Although the effect of altered pH on potassium movement is complex and varies from tissue to tissue, the extracellular potassium level generally rises during acidosis and falls during extracellular alkalosis. Rapid falls in serum potassium levels may occur during correction of an acidosis and, therefore, particular care should be taken in this situation with the digitalized patient.

Hypoxia

There is a clinical impression that cardiac glycoside toxicity is more common in patients with pulmonary disease. The role of hypoxia is difficult to define, but it appears from experimental studies that acute changes in the arterial oxygen tension tend to promote digitalis toxicity more than chronic changes (Beller, et al., 1975).

Age

With advancing years, patients become less tolerant to digitalis and more likely to develop toxicity. This may be related to declining renal function (Chamberlain, et al., 1970), but the volume of drug distribution also tends to fall as body composition changes with age. There may also be a genuine change in myocardial sensitivity (Grahame-Smith, 1978). At the other end of the age range, after the first few months of life, during which time renal excretion of glycosides is relatively poor, the opposite situation occurs. Children need much larger maintenance doses of digitalis glycosides (for example, up to the age of 2 years nearly three times as much digoxin is needed in children as in adults). Animal experiments suggest that this is caused by an increased volume of distribution. These large maintenance doses produce plasma glycoside levels in children that are similar to those seen in adults receiving a smaller maintenance dose (Cree, et al., 1975).

Renal Function

The fate of cardiac glycosides within the body varies. Digoxin and other polar glycosides, such as cedilanid and medigoxin (4β-methyldigoxin), are highly dependent on renal excretion, whereas the relatively nonpolar long-acting glycoside digitoxin is mainly metabolized. Some 34% of the body's store of digoxin is eliminated daily if renal function is normal, but only 14% is lost per day if the patient is anuric (Aronson and Grahame-Smith, 1976a). Decreased renal function can precipitate digitalis toxicity, especially when the most commonly used glycoside, digoxin, is involved, and, therefore, renal function must be assessed before starting digitalis therapy. Reduced elimination means that smaller maintenance doses are required. The volume of distribution is also reduced to about half in renal failure (Aronson and Grahame-Smith, 1976b), thus, the loading (digitalizing) dose of any glycoside must be halved. Digitoxin elimination is only slightly altered in renal failure (Vohringer, et al., 1976), and, therefore, it has been suggested that this is the most suitable drug to use in this situation. However, many physicians are so much more familiar with the use of digoxin that they prefer to use a reduced maintenance dose rather than a very long-acting drug with which they are unfamiliar.

Thyroid Function

Alterations in thyroid function change the sensitivity of the heart to digitalis glycosides. Patients with hypothyroidism are particularly susceptible to digitalis toxicity. Although this increased susceptibility has not been completely explained, reduced renal clearance, reduced distribution volume (Grahame-Smith, 1978), reduced biliary secretion of glycosides (Aronson and Grahame-Smith, 1976a), and altered myocardial uptake (Bakoulas, et al., 1976) may all be important. In addition, the slow resting heart rate may be a predisposing factor to the bradycardic effects of digitalis.

Other Drugs

Although some agents, such as dicoumarol anticoagulants, sulfonylureas, sulfonamides, and clofibrate, displace cardiac glycosides from the serum proteins to which they bind, this effect does not significantly promote toxicity even with highly protein-bound drugs such as digitoxin.

Recent studies have suggested that anti-inflammatory agents, such as indomethacin, aspirin, and ibuprofen, which are inhibitors of prostaglandin synthesis, decrease the dose of digitalis needed to produce toxicity in animals. Although this has been shown in animal experiments (Wilkerson, et al., 1980), no clinical evidence exists to suggest that these agents promote digitalis toxicity; however, further studies are needed to clarify this point. This effect may be mediated by catecholamine release because prior depletion of cardiac catecholamines with guanethidine prevents this potentiating effect (Wilkerson and Glenn, 1977). Certain other drugs modify the metabolism of digitoxin. Phenobarbitone (phenobarbital), phenytoin, and phenylbutazone all induce hepatic enzymes and, hence, may increase digitoxin metabolism and maintenance requirements. Digitoxin requirements may also be increased by agents, such as cholestyramine, that bind digitoxin undergoing enterohepatic circulation, so that it is excreted in the feces rather than reabsorbed. Drugs, such as digoxin, that are mainly eliminated by renal excretion and undergo little enterohepatic circulation are not affected to any significant degree by these agents.

Drugs that have a molecular structure similar to digitalis, such as the canrenoates and spironolactone, competitively block the renal tubular excretion of digitalis glycosides. They may also displace glycosides from cardiac receptors to a minor degree, and it has been suggested that these drugs can combat toxicity in this way (de Guzman and Yeh, 1975). Other researchers have suggested that any beneficial effect produced by displacing digitalis from cardiac receptors is more than outweighed by the ability of these drugs to raise serum digitalis levels by blocking renal excretion.

A recent report (Lindenbaum, et al., 1981) has drawn attention to the microbial metabolism of digoxin that takes place in the gut of some individuals. In about 10% of patients who are given oral digoxin the gut flora metabolize nearly half the drug to inactive compounds. When antibiotics (e.g., tetracycline or erythromycin) (Lindenbaum, et al., 1981) are given to these individuals, the gut flora are altered and digoxin breakdown is decreased. This results in an increase in plasma glycoside levels, which may be doubled in susceptible individuals. At present, there is no easy way to identify the patients in whom this will occur, and it is not yet clear whether digitalis dosage should be reduced in all patients receiving antibiotics so as to avoid possible digitalis toxicity.

Digoxin/Quinidine Interaction

One of the most effective drug combinations used over the years to treat arrhythmias has been a combination of digitalis and quinidine. Recently, a great deal of attention has been focused on the interaction between these two agents since the discovery that quinidine administration can have a very significant effect on serum digoxin levels (see Chapter 3). Doering (1979) has shown that serum digoxin levels at least double during quinidine administration. This effect of quinidine is dose-dependent and is not seen at doses below 500 mg/day. Quinidine elevates serum digoxin levels by reducing renal clearance and also by reducing the volume of distribution (Doering, 1979; Hager, et al., 1979; Risler, et al., 1980). Quinidine may also reduce digitalis binding to tissue Na^+, K^+–ATPase (Straub, et al., 1978). Therefore, the effects of quinidine on the toxic and therapeutic manifestations of digoxin therapy are difficult to predict. Clinical evidence suggests that quinidine does increase the incidence of both cardiac and noncardiac toxicity produced by coincident digoxin administration (Cohen, et al., 1977; Leahey, et al., 1978). Some other antiarrhythmic drugs, including procainamide and disopyramide (which have many electrophysiologic actions in common with quinidine), do not alter digitalis levels (Doering, 1979). Amiodarone, a powerful antiarrhythmic drug that is only available in the United Kingdom and Europe, increases serum digoxin levels by an unknown mechanism and can lead to clinical toxicity (Moysey, et al., 1981). The calcium antagonists, verapamil and nifedipine, consistently increase serum digoxin levels in healthy volunteers (Belz, et al., 1981). Although clinical toxicity has not been reported as a result of this interaction, caution is necessary when prescribing these drugs in combination with digitalis.

Chronic Lung Disease

Epidemiologic evidence exists that patients with chronic lung disease have an increased incidence of digitalis-induced arrhythmias. It is not clear whether this is caused by chronic hypoxia or other factors such as acute fluctuations in arterial oxygen saturation, excessive dosages of digitalis, hypokalemia caused by diuretics, and sympathomimetic bronchodilator agents.

THE EFFECT OF CARDIAC DISEASE ON THE ACTIONS OF DIGITALIS

The type of underlying cardiac disease present in a patient receiving digitalis may significantly modify the effects of digitalis. Experimental work in vitro has shown that stretched and damaged fibers are more likely to develop electrophysiologic abnormalities in the face of excess levels of digitalis. The clinical counterpart of this observation is that patients with significant underlying heart disease tend to develop tachyarrhythmias as a result of digitalis toxicity, whereas patients with normal underlying hearts show predominantly the vagal effects and develop bradyarrhythmias.

Unwanted Inotropic Effects

In acute myocardial infarction digitalis, like any inotropic agent, has the potential for increasing myocardial necrosis (Maroko, et al., 1971) and should be avoided unless specifically indicated. Mild degrees of heart failure in patients with acute myocardial infarction can usually be managed with diuretics alone. Despite the theoretical hazard of increasing the size of a myocardial infarct, digitalis is often the most appropriate agent for control of a rapid tachyarrhythmia, particularly in a patient who has compromised left ventricular function. In these circumstances slowing the heart rate may be important in limiting infarct size, and the possible deleterious effects of increased inotropy as a result of digitalis should be ignored. There is no convincing evidence that digitalis toxicity is more common in the setting of acute ischemia, although impaired renal clearance of cardiac glycosides may occur, which can be countered by careful dose adjustment (Sharpe, et al., 1975). However, there is no evidence to the contrary, and, therefore, digitalis is best avoided in this setting unless definitely indicated. The other clinical situation in which the inotropic effect of digoxin is undesirable is in hypertropic cardiomyopathy. Like all inotropic agents, digoxin exacerbates the hemodynamic and symptomatic disturbances by increasing left ventricular outflow obstruction. When atrial fibrillation occurs in this condition, it can often be controlled by beta blockade. Should beta blockade fail, digitalis can be tried cautiously and is sometimes successful.

Effects on Impulse Formation and Conduction

In the sick sinus syndrome supraventricular arrhythmias, such as supraventricular tachycardia and atrial fibrillation, which respond to digitalis, often occur. Although recent reports (Vera, et al., 1978) suggest that digitalis does not have a deleterious effect on sinus node function or on the heart rate as assessed by ambulatory ECG monitoring, both clinical experience and the wide variety of conduction disturbances that can occur in this syndrome dictate that digoxin be used with great care.

Digitalis is likely to exacerbate both first- and second-degree heart block, unless it is of the Mobitz type II variety, and should generally be avoided unless the patient is paced. If the disturbance in conduction is simply one of isolated left or right bundle branch block, digitalis is generally safe. Although there is no evidence that digitalis causes serious conduction disturbance below the AV node, caution is necessary if there is a complicated conduction disturbance such as bifascicular or trifascicular block because such patients often have significant disturbances in AV node conduction, which cannot be detected from the surface ECG. Digitalis rarely produces complete heart block, as a toxic manifestation, in patients who have previously normal AV conduction. Fortunately, when digitalis does produce complete heart block in patients with previously compromised AV conduction, which may not have been recognized clinically, the diverse nature of the toxic effects of digoxin offers some margin of safety because escape rhythms are usually, but not always, accelerated (Fisch, et al., 1964). Digitalis should not, however, be used to speed the ventricular rate in complete heart block because pacemaker acceleration is definitely a toxic effect and may be quickly followed by other serious arrhythmias.

Wolff-Parkinson-White Syndrome

Some patients with the Wolff-Parkinson-White syndrome develop atrial fibrillation, and when this occurs conduction from the atrium to the ventricle is generally via the bypass tract (see Chapters 2, 8, and 9). The resulting ventricular rate depends on the conduction properties of the bypass and may be very rapid. If the shortest RR interval is less than 220 milliseconds when the patient has atrial fibrillation, there is a definite risk of ventricular fibrillation occurring because of the very rapid bombardment of the ventricle with impulses from above. In about one-third of patients with the Wolff-Parkinson-White syndrome digitalis, in therapeutic doses, accelerates conduction via the bypass, and this may increase the risk of ventricular fibrillation (Sellers, et al., 1977). The patients at risk for this serious complication cannot be recognized with certainty from the surface ECG and, therefore, digitalis should be avoided in patients with the Wolff-Parkinson-White syndrome unless electrophysiologic studies have shown that digitalis administration is safe.

DIAGNOSIS OF DIGITALIS TOXICITY

Digitalis toxicity is so frequent and the consequences may be so serious that unexplained arrhythmias and new symptoms in a patient receiving digitalis should always be considered to be caused by digitalis toxicity until proven otherwise. This approach inevitably leads to overdiagnosis, particularly with regard to nonspecific, noncardiac symptoms. Some 20% of patients taking digitalis who are not intoxicated complain of symptoms such as nausea and anorexia (Doering and König, 1978).

Laboratory Investigations

Plasma potassium level A low plasma potassium level significantly increases the chances that any arrhythmia is digitalis-induced in a patient receiving digitalis. The plasma potassium level is not generally altered in patients with toxicity resulting from therapeutic usage; however, hyperkalemia is often a prominent feature of massive digitalis ingestion (Smith, et al., 1982).

Plasma glycoside levels When accurate, rapid assay systems to measure plasma levels of cardiac glycosides became available, they were greeted with enthusiasm as an accurate method for controlling digitalis dosage and diagnosing toxicity. Experience with these techniques has led to some disenchantment. Ingelfinger and Goldman (1976) concluded that measurement of plasma glycoside levels was no more useful than knowledge of the dosage received, renal function, and plasma potassium levels. Other researchers have suggested that plasma levels of digoxin below 1 ng/mL are generally subtherapeutic and those above 3 ng/mL are usually toxic (Dobbs, et al., 1976). The confusion and dispute over the value of estimating plasma glycoside levels result from the multiple factors that modify the actions of cardiac glycosides. Shapiro (1978) critically reviewed the same question in a large series of patients with digitalis toxicity and made the following conclusions:

1. In normokalemic patients toxicity is rarely seen if the plasma digoxin level is less than 2 ng/mL.
2. In hypokalemic patients toxicity frequently occurs with plasma levels of less than 2 ng/mL and can occur occasionally even when the level is below 0.5 ng/mL.
3. Serious underlying heart disease may predispose the patient to toxicity even with plasma levels less than 2 ng/mL.

If these reservations are kept in mind, an estimation of plasma glycoside levels provides some useful information when considered with all the other clinical information available. The diagnosis of toxicity cannot be made simply by measuring the plasma glycoside level.

Patient noncompliance to prescribed dosages is so frequent (Johnstone, et al., 1978) that measurement of plasma levels will occasionally show that the patient was not taking the digitalis at all. Similarly, very high plasma levels (>5 ng/mL) make toxicity very likely.

Pharmacologic Testing

Several pharmacologic tests designed to enhance or reduce digitalis toxicity have been devised, but, to date, all tests have proved to be inconclusive or have major dangers. Administration of the short-acting glycoside acetylstrophanthidin to briefly increase toxicity has been advocated but is too dangerous for general use. Edrophonium chloride administration may increase AV block transiently in digitalized patients if the dosage is not maximal, but the results are often difficult to interpret or are inconclusive. Calcium chelating agents may transiently reverse toxicity, but again the results are often inconclusive and the agents themselves may be toxic.

Carotid Sinus Massage

Supraventricular tachyarrhythmias caused by digitalis toxicity are not usually terminated by carotid sinus massage, and several researchers have suggested that carotid sinus massage may very occasionally cause ventricular fibrillation in patients who are suffering from digitalis toxicity. This risk is probably very low if massage is attempted for less than 5 seconds. Other investigators (Lown and Levine, 1961) have suggested that carotid sinus massage may reveal digitalis toxicity by producing AV block, premature ventricular contractions with fixed coupling, or junctional rhythms. The results of this procedure are unpredictable and potentially dangerous. They do not help in making clinical decisions because, if digitalis toxicity is suspected, administration of the glycoside should be stopped regardless of the results of the test. Therefore, carotid sinus massage does not have an important place in the diagnosis of digitalis toxicity.

CLINICAL FEATURES

Clinically, digitalis toxicity is similar regardless of the glycoside that is administered, although minor differences may occur from drug to drug. Cardiac and extracardiac manifestations of toxicity may occur at the same time in the same patient but either may precede the other.

Extracardiac Manifestations

Gastrointestinal disturbances Anorexia, nausea, and vomiting, sometimes accompanied by diarrhea, are the most frequently recognized extracardiac manifestations of digitalis toxicity, although minor lassitude and weakness may be very frequent and are often overlooked (Lely and Van Enter, 1970). Occasionally, nausea and vomiting are caused by gastric irritation and do not denote generalized toxicity; in these situations changing the patient to another glycoside (e.g., from digoxin to lantoside-C or digitoxin) may remedy the situation. More frequently, the gastrointestinal upset results from the glycoside directly stimulating the chemoreceptor trigger zone (Borison and Wang, 1953), which is closely related to the vagal nuclei in the medulla. The vagotonic effects of digitalis also produce gastrointestinal disturbance by altering motility. This effect may result in poor tolerance to digitalis in patients with chronic gastrointestinal disease such as peptic ulceration or ulcerative colitis. The effect of digitalis on appetite may occasionally be so severe and insidious that it leads to chronic anorexia and severe weight loss.

Visual disturbances The visual disturbances of digitalis toxicity are relatively uncommon, compared to the gastrointestinal effects. They usually consist of disturbances of color vision, with objects taking on a yellow or green hue (xanthopsia), and the appearance of flashing lights and visual scotomata (Robertson, et al., 1966). These effects seem to be produced by the direct action of digitalis on the visual cortex.

Other clinical features The digitalis glycosides have a structural similarity to estrogens and can induce gynecomastia in men. Patients on long-term therapy have raised serum estrogen levels and decreased levels of luteinizing hormone. Under these circumstances digitalis has been postulated to act as a substrate from which estrogen is produced (Stoffer, et al., 1973). In rare cases headaches, confusion, and even psychosis have been attributed to digitalis toxicity.

Cardiac Manifestations

Digitalis administration produces changes in the resting ECG that are often characteristic. The most common features are a slight prolongation of the PR interval, shortening of the QT interval, and changes in the ST segment. These changes may occasionally be atypical, and, because of this, it is very difficult to interpret changes in the ST segment in patients receiving digoxin. Furthermore, ST changes caused by digitalis may increase dramatically on exercise and prevent or obscure the diagnosis of myocardial ischemia. Unfortunately, changes in the ECG do not give a precise guide to the degree of digitalization or provide an early warning that cardiac toxicity may occur. Joubert and colleagues (1975) devised an index incorporating T-wave amplitude and QT and PR intervals, from which they suggest that the degree of digitalization and the risk of toxicity can be computed. This has yet to be confirmed by other researchers.

The Arrhythmias of Digitalis Toxicity

Although almost any rhythm disturbance can result from digitalis toxicity, certain disturbances are much more common than others (Table 13-1). The incidence of these disturbances varies from report to report, probably because of differences in the patient populations studied. Multiple rhythm disturbances in the same patient are extremely common.

Sinus node Minor toxicity often causes sinus arrhythmia and/or sinus bradycardia, and, in this situation, a further increase in toxicity leads to sinus arrest or sinoatrial (SA) exit block with or without the Wenckebach phenomenon. Although sinus tachycardia has been described as a toxic manifestation (Lown, et al., 1960), the bradycardic effects are usually much more common.

Table 13-1 Relative frequency of digitalis-induced arrhythmias

Frequency	Type of arrhythmia
Very common	Ventricular premature contractions (75%) First- or second-degree AV block (30%)
Common (10%-20%)	AV dissociation Junctional rhythms Atrial tachycardia (usually with block)
Less common (<10%)	Atrial fibrillation and atrial flutter Premature atrial and junctional ectopic beats Ventricular tachycardia Ventricular fibrillation Asystole and complete heart block
? Never	Parasystole Mobitz type II heart block Paroxysmal junctional tachycardia

Atrial arrhythmias Atrial tachycardia with AV block is commonly, although not always (Storstein, et al., 1977), caused by glycoside toxicity. Sir Thomas Lewis first described this arrhythmia in 1906, and within 5 years Sir James MacKenzie had attributed it to digitalis toxicity. This is an area in which confusion of terminology has occurred. Any tachycardia with block tends to be called "paroxysmal atrial tachycardia with block," even though the arrhythmia of digitalis toxicity is often sustained, and, therefore, should not be called paroxysmal. It is not necessarily a stable arrhythmia and may show evolution as toxicity progresses, so that the atrial rate in the early stages of toxicity may be between 100 and 150 beats/min and later increase to 150-250 beats/min. When the atrial rate is above 140 beats/min, some form of AV block is usually present. The ventricular response is determined by the degree of AV block and may be either regular, with the block fixed at 2:1 or 3:1, or irregular, with varying degrees of block and Wenckebach phenomenon. Occasionally, the P waves may be so inconspicuous and the ventricular response so irregular that distinguishing atrial tachycardia with AV block from atrial fibrillation becomes difficult or impossible. This is a particularly dangerous situation because the digitalis dosage may be mistakenly increased further. This arrhythmia commonly occurs in patients who were originally in sinus rhythm but may also occur in the presence of atrial fibrillation. The P waves may be very small and are often best seen in ECG lead V_1. The PP interval is often regular but may be irregular, and P-wave morphology may vary considerably, giving rise to the so-called multifocal atrial tachycardia, or chaotic atrial rhythm (see Chapter 8). Occasionally, especially when there is left atrial hypertrophy (e.g., in mitral valve disease), the P waves are broad and distinction from atrial flutter may be difficult or impossible.

Atrial fibrillation and, less commonly, atrial flutter occasionally occur as a toxic manifestation of cardiac glycosides. These arrhythmias usually develop in patients who previously had sinus rhythm. Digitalis toxicity may sometimes cause speeding-up of the ventricular responses in patients with established atrial fibrillation. If this phenomenon is seen, the clinician should always suspect digitalis toxicity and resist the temptation to increase the digitalis dosage further.

Atrial premature contractions also occur as a result of digitalis toxicity, and, because AV conduction is often compromised, the conduction of these ectopic beats to the ventricles may be blocked.

Junctional dysrhythmias Junctional dysrhythmias, as a manifestation of digitalis toxicity, are particularly common in patients in whom atrial fibrillation is the basic rhythm, although they may also occur in patients who are in sinus rhythm. The dual effects of impaired AV conduction (either in a retrograde direction alone or in an antegrade direction as well) and increased automaticity of nodal pacemakers result in interesting and often complex dysrhythmias. The rate of the junctional pacemaker is quite variable. In sinus rhythm a frequent situation is that of a junctional rhythm that is just faster than the sinus rate. Retrograde block allows the sinus node to keep control of the atria, while the faster junctional focus controls the ventricles most of the time. The majority of the sinus impulses arrive at the AV node when it is refractory because of depolarization from below by the faster nodal pacemaker, but sinus impulses occasionally reach the AV node when it is not refractory and conduct to the ventricle, producing a capture beat. In atrial fibrillation impaired antegrade conduction allows a junctional pacemaker, speeded by digitalis, to take over the ventricle as a slow nodal rhythm or a nodal tachycardia, depending on the extent to which nodal automaticity is enhanced. If the ventricular response becomes regular in a patient who is receiving digitalis for atrial fibrillation, this often means that a junctional rhythm has taken over, which is a sign of toxicity. It is also an indication that the digitalis dosage should be reduced. As toxicity progresses the arrhythmias may become more complex. In some instances exit block from the junctional pacemaker, with or without the Wenckebach phenomenon, may slow the ventricular rate and make it irregular. In other instances the rhythm may accelerate and varying exit block from the pacemaker may make the ventricular response fast and irregular. When either of these situations occur, and particularly when the ventricular response is fast, differentiation from atrial fibrillation may become extremely difficult or impossible, although a careful analysis of the ECG may reveal regularly repeated sequences of beats. AV junctional rhythms with retrograde block often coexist with atrial tachycardia, and, depending on whether antegrade conduction is possible, capture beats may or may not occur. Other complicated junctional dysrhythmias include double nodal tachycardias, where two nodal pacemakers at different rates control the atria and ventricles, and bidirectional junctional tachycardias. Although the latter is rare, it is almost invariably caused by digitalis toxicity (Stock, 1970). The ECG shows a regular tachyarrhythmia with a narrow QRS interval, in which alternate beats are written in opposite directions except in leads V_1 and AVR. This may result from alternating block of conduction in the anterior and posterior fascicles of the left bundle. This is a particularly serious arrhythmia, and four of the 10 patients described by Stock (1970) died.

Ventricular arrhythmias Premature ventricular contractions (PVCs) are the most common arrhythmia produced by digitalis toxicity and are particularly frequent when the patient has serious heart disease. PVCs rarely affect cardiac function adversely, and their significance is as a forerunner of more serious problems. PVCs are common in heart disease, but when they first occur during digitalis therapy, toxicity should be suspected, especially if the PVCs are multiform, bigeminal, or occur as pairs of opposite directions. Ventricular tachyarrhythmias are uncommon, but when they do occur, they carry a mortality quoted by various researchers as between 68% and 100%. As with any arrhythmia, the prognosis depends on how exhaustive the search has been for that arrhythmia. In many of the reported studies with high mortalities these arrhythmias were detected by ECG monitoring or on standard ECGs in patients who were already hospitalized for digitalis toxicity. Modern monitoring techniques are much more efficient in detecting the true incidence of dysrhythmias, and the mortality of patients with ventricular tachycardia detected in this way would be expected to be substantially lower. Ventricular tachycardia produced by digitalis toxicity is occasionally bidirectional, that is, the QRS morphology alternates in direction. The RR interval may be regular, suggesting a single focus with regularly alternating conduction, or it may alternate in duration (suggesting two foci or two reentry pathways of different length or conduction velocity). Ventricular tachycardia can coexist with nodal or atrial tachyarrhythmias and AV block.

AV conduction arrhythmias Slight prolongation of the PR interval is common with digitalis administration. This prolongation does not usually bring the PR interval outside normal limits but may occasionally cause first-degree heart block. When second-degree heart block occurs, it is usually of the Wenckebach variety (Mobitz type I). Complete heart block is relatively uncommon as a manifestation of digitalis toxicity unless there is preexisting conduction disease. Because toxic doses of digitalis usually increase automaticity, the escape ventricular response is often relatively rapid (50-60 beats/min) when complete heart block is the result of digitalis toxicity. Because of this, Stokes-Adams attacks are rare.

Arrhythmias Rarely Caused by Digitalis

A few arrhythmias are infrequently, if ever, caused by digitalis (Chung, 1977). These include parasystole, Mobitz type II second-degree heart block, paroxysmal AV junctional tachycardia, and the type of accelerated ventricular rhythm commonly seen in association with myocardial infarction.

TREATMENT OF DIGITALIS TOXICITY

As in every clinical situation, the relative risks of an active or conservative approach to the problem must be carefully considered before therapeutic enthusiasm is allowed to triumph over caution and inactivity. There are essentially three different clinical situations that are encountered in patients with digitalis toxicity, as follows:

1. The patient with arrhythmias that are thought to be the result of digitalis toxicity in whom these arrhythmias do not cause any hemodynamic embarrassment or suggest likely progression to more serious, life-threatening arrhythmias.
2. The patient on digitalis therapy in whom arrhythmias compromise cardiac performance or are thought to be a forerunner of more serious and life-threatening disturbances.
3. The patient with digitalis toxicity as the result of a single massive dose of a glycoside, taken either accidentally or as a suicide attempt.

The Hemodynamically Stable Patient

This situation is relatively common. Frequent PVCs are often an early sign of toxicity and usually do not produce hemodynamic disturbance. Similarly, nonparoxysmal AV junctional dysrhythmias (another frequent manifestation) often have a relatively slow rate (60-120 beats/min) and are usually well tolerated. In these patients the plasma potassium level must be checked immediately and, if reduced, restored to normal by intravenous infusion and then maintained with oral supplements. If the level is at or below the lower normal range, it should be restored to the upper normal range (4-4.5 mEq/L in most institutions) by intravenous infusion. If the plasma potassium level is already in this range, infusion of potassium chloride with frequent checks on the plasma level may reduce arrhythmias without raising the plasma potassium level, possibly because an undetected intracellular depletion is corrected. Extreme care is necessary because hyperkalemia may exacerbate conduction disturbances (Bashour, et al., 1975).

Intravenous potassium can be given at rates of between 20 and 40 mEq/hr. If given via peripheral veins, concentrations of above 40 mEq/L should be avoided because more concentrated solutions produce considerable pain at the infusion site and also need very precise control to prevent serious hyperkalemia. The disadvantage of this method is that large fluid volumes may be needed to adequately replace potassium in patients who cannot tolerate the fluid load because of their hemodynamic problems. An easier way to give potassium in this situation is to use an accurate infusion pump and administer more concentrated solutions via a central venous catheter (e.g., 1 mEq/mL). It is wise to take blood samples to estimate the magnesium level at an early stage because these tests are often not routine, and, consequently, there may be some delay in obtaining the result. If magnesium deficiency is demonstrated, the plasma magnesium level should be returned to normal. Magnesium can be given as 10-20 mL of 20% $MgSO_4$ solution given intravenously over 10-20 minutes, followed by 500 mL of 2% $MgSO_4$ over the next 6 hours.

An estimation of serum glycoside concentration is also useful because, although it has limited value in diagnosis, serial levels taken in the same patient during an episode of intoxication may give information that will be helpful in the future when used to guide digitalis dosage. Beyond these simple measures, the best therapeutic policy in this situation is one of inactivity, withholding digitalis until all signs of toxicity disappear, because relatively innocent arrhythmias, which will disappear with time, may need large doses of potentially toxic antiarrhythmic agents to be suppressed.

The Hemodynamically Disturbed Patient or the Dangerous Arrhythmia

In this situation a more aggressive therapeutic approach is necessary. The dual toxic effects of digitalis (increased automaticity and impaired AV conduction) must both be considered when selecting a therapeutic agent. Hemodynamic deterioration is frequently caused by tachyarrhythmias and less often by bradyarrhythmias; however, rapid tachyarrhythmias and significant bradyarrhythmias may often occur in the same patient within a short space of time. Although this transition often occurs spontaneously, it is particularly likely to occur when antiarrhythmic drugs, which have a depressant effect on AV conduction, are used. For this reason, the ideal drug for treating digitalis-induced dysrhythmias would be one that reduces automaticity reliably and has minimal effects on AV conduction. The degree and duration of the patient's cardiovascular decompensation is also important. If the patient has had a serious dysrhythmia for a short period of time, the restoration of a more advantageous rhythm will usually produce immediate clinical improvement, but if the dysrhythmia has been present for hours or days, cardiac failure and pulmonary edema may be present, and hypoxia, acidosis, and high sympathetic tone may exacerbate and potentiate the dysrhythmia, requiring urgent attention. The arterial pH level should be carefully monitored because changes in pH may exacerbate digitalis toxicity, either directly or by altering potassium levels. Acidosis elevates the plasma potassium level because of shifts of potassium from the intracellular to the extracellular compartments, and, if corrected rapidly by bicarbonate infusion, the plasma potassium level may fall precipitously and exacerbate dysrhythmias unless extra potassium is given at the same time.

Coincident cardiac failure should also be treated, with opiates, vasodilators, and intravenous diuretics, as appropriate. Inotropic catecholamines should be avoided if possible because they potentiate the increased automaticity produced by digitalis toxicity and may lead to serious tachyarrhythmias. If intravenous diuretics are needed, the additional potassium loss must be adequately replaced.

A clinical impression exists that PVCs that are multifocal or occur as pairs or triplets or short runs of ventricular tachycardia are likely to precede more prolonged ventricular tachycardia or ventricular fibrillation. Because of the relative infrequency of ventricular tachycardia and ventricular fibrillation as manifestations of digitalis toxicity, it is unlikely that this clinical impression will ever be tested scientifically, and, therefore, clinical caution dictates that an active approach be taken to these arrhythmias. This is particularly sensible because direct current cardioversion of ventricular tachycardia or ventricular fibrillation resulting from digitalis toxicity has a lower success rate than in other situations and may be accompanied by serious complications (see the section on direct current cardioversion in this chapter).

Specific Measures

Adequate potassium replacement, possibly with magnesium replacement, and treatment of cardiac failure often terminate the arrhythmias so that no other antiarrhythmic treatment is needed. However, other specific measures are occasionally required (see Table 13-2).

Antiarrhythmic agents *Lidocaine* Lidocaine is often effective in patients with ventricular arrhythmias resulting from digitalis toxicity and has little or no depressant effect on AV conduction. Because it is in frequent use in other clinical situations and the dosage schedules are generally well known by the medical and nursing staff, it is the agent of first choice in this situation. Lidocaine has little or no place in the treatment of supraventricular disturbances. Its action is purely on membrane excitability and does not seem to depend on any alterations in digitalis binding.

Table 13-2 Treatment of digitalis-induced arrhythmia

Type of arrhythmia	Treatment
All arrhythmias	1. Potassium infusion to produce normal plasma potassium level 2. Potassium infusion in normokalemic patients 3. Glycoside-specific Fab fragments*
Ventricular arrhythmias	1. First-line treatment: lidocaine or phenytoin 2. Second-line treatment: procainamide; disopyramide; beta blockers plus standby pacing; magnesium infusion; special pacing techniques; direct current cardioversion with prior lidocaine or phenytoin administration
Atrial or junctional tachycardias	1. First-line treatment: phenytoin (often ineffective, but safe); procainamide; beta blockers plus standby pacing 2. Second-line treatment: disopyramide; magnesium infusion; direct current cardioversion with prior lidocaine or phenytoin administration
Bradycardia and AV block	1. Atropine (occasionally effective) 2. Pacing 3. Avoid catecholamines

*Not generally available yet.

Diphenylhydantoin (phenytoin) Although phenytoin is only weakly or moderately effective when used against nondigitalis-induced arrhythmias, it appears to have a powerful, specific antidysrhythmic effect in digitalis toxicity (Wit, et al., 1975). Phenytoin does not impair AV conduction and has an advantage over lidocaine in that it often suppresses both atrial and ventricular arrhythmias caused by digitalis. Its mechanism of action in digitalis toxicity is poorly understood. At low plasma potassium levels it may reverse the digitalis-induced changes in resting membrane potential and the slowing of the upstroke of the action potential, theoretically improving conduction and eliminating reentry. At normal potassium levels it may reduce the late after-depolarizations and speeded-up phase 4 depolarizations that are produced by digitalis. Some, if not all, of phenytoin's antiarrhythmic effect may be mediated centrally by reducing the increased autonomic outflow occurring in digitalis toxicity (Evans and Gillis, 1974). Although the drug is effective in suppressing atrial tachycardia with block, ventricular dysrhythmias, and, sometimes, reversing digitalis-induced atrial fibrillation and flutter, it is not particularly effective in junctional tachyarrhythmias. Although there is some evidence that phenytoin may even improve AV conduction, its use is not contraindicated in atrial fibrillation because it does not seem to produce a significant increase in ventricular response.

Quinidine Although quinidine will suppress some of the ventricular and supraventricular arrhythmias produced by digitalis toxicity, it should be avoided if at all possible because of the growing evidence that it may potentiate digitalis toxicity.

Procainamide Procainamide may depress AV conduction, especially in high doses, and produce hypotension when given intravenously, but it does not have quinidine's disadvantage of potentiating digitalis toxicity. Procainamide is often effective in treating ventricular arrhythmias and, less frequently, in managing supraventricular arrhythmias that are associated with digitalis toxicity.

Beta blockers Beta blockers (e.g., propranolol, metoprolol, or nadolol, which are available in the United States, and many other agents that are available in Europe) suppress both supraventricular and ventricular arrhythmias caused by digitalis toxicity effectively (Gibson and Sowton, 1969). However, these drugs have some potentially serious disadvantages when used in this situation because they exacerbate preexisting AV conduction disturbances and may also exert significant negative inotropic effects in patients with already severely compromised cardiac function. Some of these agents, such as propranolol, have quinidine-like membrane-stabilizing properties, and in the past it was thought that this feature was important in countering digitalis toxicity. Recently, with the development of other beta blockers lacking this action (such as practolol and metoprolol), opinion has changed because these agents are also effective. It now appears that the effectiveness of beta blockers in digitalis toxicity depends on their ability to block beta-sympathetic effects. This may be a particularly important property in digitalis toxicity because of the arrhythmogenic effects of increased sympathetic outflow as a result of central stimulation by digitalis. Because of the risk of serious impairment of AV conduction, it is sensible to insert a temporary pacing wire before beginning treatment with beta blockers.

Disopyramide Disopyramide's antiarrhythmic properties are very similar to those of quinidine, but it does not have the disadvantage of altering plasma digoxin levels in the same way as quinidine (Doering, 1979). Clinical experience and experimental animal studies suggest that the drug is effective in controlling both supraventricular and ventricular arrhythmias resulting from digitalis toxicity. Its effects on AV conduction are not significant because the direct inhibition of conduction is offset in clinical practice by disopyramide's powerful anticholinergic, vagolytic effects. The drug has a powerful negative inotropic effect and must be avoided in patients with left ventricular dysfunction.

Other antiarrhythmic agents There are several new lidocaine-like agents (mexiletine and tocainide) under development in the United States or in use in Europe that are active both orally and intravenously and may prove to be useful in the treatment of digitalis-induced ventricular arrhythmias. In general, they all share the properties of lidocaine, especially of being effective in suppressing ventricular arrhythmias with minimal depressant effects on AV conduction. Ajmaline is a rauwolfia alkaloid with powerful quinidine-like effects. Conflicting evidence exists about its effects on AV conduction, and it may produce profound bradycardia in digitalized patients with atrial fibrillation. Although some researchers (Obayashi, et al., 1976) have recommended its use in digitalis toxicity, the uncertainty about its effects means that caution is required, and it cannot be recommended for use in this context at present. Ajmaline is not on the market either in the United Kingdom or the United States but has been available in Europe for many years. Verapamil, which is an effective agent for terminating supraventricular arrhythmias in other circumstances, is also best avoided in the complex situation of digitalis intoxication. The canrenoates and spironolactone have steroid nuclei that are similar to digitalis and compete with digitalis for its membrane-binding sites. Toxicity might be reduced by displacement of digoxin from these sites, and there is some evidence that potassium canrenoate, marketed as a diuretic (Soldactone), effectively diminishes digitalis-induced tachyarrhythmias in both dogs (de Guzman and Yeh, 1975) and humans (Yeh, et al., 1976) but is ineffective against other types of dysrhythmia. Because it does not seem to affect left ventricular function or AV conduction, its use in this situation seems worth pursuing. At present its use cannot be generally recommended until further clinical trials have been carried out. Spironolactone may have a similar, weak effect on myocardial digitalis binding, but in digitalis toxicity this is substantially outweighed by its more prominent effect of reducing digoxin clearance by the kidney, and it should, therefore, be avoided in this situation (Waldorff, et al., 1978).

Cholestyramine binds digitalis glycosides in the gastrointestinal tract. This is not important with agents such as digoxin, which are excreted principally by the kidneys, but it may significantly increase the clearance of digitoxin, which undergoes enterohepatic circulation. This is a useful adjunct to therapy in digitoxin toxicity because this agent has a long half-life, and toxicity may take a long time to disappear after drug administration is stopped.

Magnesium controls all types of digitalis-induced arrhythmias effectively (Szekely and Wynne, 1951; Singh, et al., 1976) and may also suppress arrhythmias that are not the result of digitalis toxicity (Iseri, et al., 1975). If magnesium salts are given to patients with normal serum magnesium levels in the doses recommended for the replacement of magnesium in deficient patients, toxic effects are likely. The possible mechanisms of action have already been discussed. Unfortunately, the ECG is not altered predictably with rising plasma magnesium levels, and, hence, great care is required. As blood levels rise to 6 mEq/L the deep tendon reflexes disappear, and this clinical sign can be used to predict impending toxicity. If plasma magnesium levels rise even higher (10 mEq/L), paralysis and respiratory depression occur. Magnesium is simple to use and well worth considering in patients with life-threatening arrhythmias in whom maximal doses of the first-line drugs, such as lidocaine or phenytoin, have failed.

When serious dysrhythmias are encountered, early insertion of a temporary transvenous pacing electrode may be helpful. This may be direct therapy for many bradyarrhythmias caused by digitalis toxicity, and when drugs other than lidocaine or phenytoin are used, the risk of serious impairment of AV conduction can be countered by having temporary pacing immediately available. Digitalis-induced tachyarrhythmias may be rate-dependent, and altering the heart rate by pacing may produce dysrhythmias occasionally. Mechanical stimulation of the myocardium while positioning the pacing wire may also, on occasions, result in serious dysrhythmias such as ventricular fibrillation (Bismuth, et al., 1977; Bremner, et al., 1977). This risk can be minimized by giving lidocaine intravenously before inserting the pacing wire.

The recent introduction of specific glycoside antibodies is an exciting development in the treatment of digitalis toxicity. Experimental digitalis intoxication can be reversed both by the whole IgG molecule and even more rapidly by the Fab fragment (Lloyd and Smith, 1978). Successful treatment of massive suicidal ingestion of digoxin and clinical intoxication by the same agent (Smith, et al., 1976; Smith, et al., 1982) and of clinical "toxicity" caused by lantoside-C (Hess, et al., 1979) with digoxin-specific Fab antibody fragments has been reported. The antibody rapidly clears the glycoside from the circulation, and beneficial clinical effects soon follow, although there is some delay, presumably because digitalis is released more slowly from the myocardial binding sites than it is cleared from the circulation. Modern methods of protein purification and the use of only the Fab fragment minimize the chances of adverse reactions to the foreign protein, which is usually prepared in sheep. The rapid clearance of the Fab fragment from the circulation by glomerular filtration appears to be one reason why adverse reactions to the Fab fragment are rare. Although the antibody is not yet commercially available other than as an investigational agent, early experiments and clinical studies suggest that this will prove to be the most effective and specific means of therapy available for serious toxicity and poisoning.

Direct current cardioversion As direct current cardioversion became a routine procedure in the early 1960s, reports of occasional ventricular fibrillation or ventricular tachycardia as a complication of this treatment began to appear. This complication usually occurred in patients in whom there was clinical evidence of digitalis toxicity (Graff and Etkins, 1964; Rabbino, et al., 1964). The larger the initial shock, the higher the chance of serious dysrhythmia. If there is any clinical suspicion of digitalis toxicity, there is a 50% chance of some form of ventricular ectopy developing (Kleiger and Lown, 1966). Castellanos and colleagues (1967) described the occurrence of PVCs with low energy shocks as a warning that digitalis toxicity might be present. This led to the policy of starting with low energy shocks in patients with possible digitalis toxicity. Hagemeijer and Van Houwe (1975) reported the safety of using titrated energy. They used an initial setting of 12.5 watt-seconds and subsequently doubled the energy until the patient's arrhythmia reverted. The risk of serious dysrhythmias can be reduced by pretreatment with intravenous lidocaine or phenytoin (Kleiger and Lown, 1966). On the basis of this experimental and clinical information several guidelines for the use of direct current cardioversion can be made as follows:

1. The plasma potassium level, if possible, should be normal.
2. Direct current cardioversion should not be regarded as an immediate treatment of choice for any dysrhythmia thought to be caused by digitalis toxicity, except ventricular fibrillation.
3. If all reasonable pharmacologic approaches have failed to correct a serious tachyarrhythmia thought to be caused by digitalis or a lack of adequate cerebral perfusion precludes extensive trials of drug therapy, the patient should be pretreated with lidocaine or phenytoin and synchronized direct current cardioversion attempted. The lowest possible energy setting should be used initially (usually 5-10 watt-seconds) and the energy setting subsequently doubled with each shock. If conversion does not occur, but significant ectopy follows a shock, further lidocaine or phenytoin should be given before proceeding.
4. Digitalis should always be discontinued for an appropriate period before elective cardioversion. Digoxin should be stopped 48 hours prior to conversion, and longer-acting agents should be stopped for a longer period of time (e.g., 4 days for digitoxin). If there is any doubt about the patient's digitalis status, the procedure should be deferred until the correct situation is established. There is no place for prophylactic antiarrhythmic agents in elective cardioversion; it is much safer (even though more inconvenient) to wait.
5. If a patient undergoing elective direct current conversion has recently been taking digitalis, the titrated energy method should be used, and if dysrhythmias, particularly premature ventricular contractions, occur

without arrhythmia conversion, the procedure should be abandoned until a later date.

Massive Digitalis Ingestion

Massive digitalis ingestion usually occurs as an unexpected disaster in a preschool child or as one of the more successful ways of committing suicide. The overall mortality for massive digitalis ingestion is approximately 20% (Bismuth, et al., 1977). Hyperventilation, drowsiness, severe vomiting, and diarrhea are often clinical features. In younger patients and those without severe heart disease the vagal effects of digitalis usually predominate, causing bradyarrhythmias and heart block, although supraventricular and ventricular tachyarrhythmias may also occur. In older patients the vagal effects also occur, but supraventricular and ventricular tachyarrhythmias are more common than in younger patients (Smith and Willerson, 1971; Bremner, et al., 1977). Hyperkalemia may be prominent, especially when a very large amount of glycoside has been ingested (Smith and Willerson, 1971). This rise in the plasma potassium level probably results from the release of intracellular potassium because of the widespread blockade of Na^+, K^+–ATPase but may be absent even when plasma glycoside levels are very high (Bremner, et al., 1977). As in toxicity occurring during the therapeutic use of digitalis, correction of potassium and magnesium levels, maintenance of fluid balance and arterial pH, and appropriate treatment of arrhythmias are the mainstays of treatment. Certain other procedures may be beneficial, and the following points are worth noting:

1. *Gastric lavage.* This may remove some unabsorbed tablets, although usually the severe vomiting induced by digitalis toxicity will have already emptied the stomach effectively.
2. *Oral cholestyramine.* Instillation of cholestyramine and activated charcoal via the lavage tube may capture some of the glycoside that has been ingested and not as yet absorbed. In the case of digitoxin overdosage cholestyramine can be given on a regular basis orally because it will capture some of the drug as it undergoes enterohepatic circulation.
3. *Digitalis elimination.* Digitalis elimination cannot be increased usefully by forced diuresis or by dialysis, but there have been some encouraging reports of removal of digitalis from the circulation by hemoperfusion through activated charcoal (Gilfrich, et al., 1978). Other reports are not so encouraging (Warren and Fanestil, 1979), and a recent review of published cases concluded that hemoperfusion might be beneficial in severe digoxin intoxication, but more experience is required before it can be recommended as routine therapy (Gibson, 1980).

4. *Glycoside-specific antibodies.* Glycoside-specific antibodies have been shown to be life-saving but are not yet generally available.
5. *Electrolyte imbalance.* Electrolyte imbalance and pH abnormalities are frequent because of the violent vomiting and diarrhea that often accompany massive overdosage, and it is essential that these conditions be carefully corrected.
6. *Prophylactic pacing.* A pacing electrode should be inserted into the right ventricle as soon as possible, and, because there is a risk of inducing dysrhythmias while doing this, the procedure should be covered with intravenous phenytoin or lidocaine.
7. *Other therapy.* Dysrhythmias should be treated as they occur using the principles already outlined in the previous section.

Despite all efforts, the mortality associated with the ingestion of large amounts of a cardiac glycoside, either accidentally or on purpose, remains extremely high. It is hoped that the more widespread use of glycoside-specific antibodies will change this situation.

REFERENCES

Allen, J. C.; and Schwartz, A. 1970. Effects of potassium, temperature, and time on ouabain interaction with the cardiac Na^+, K^+–ATPase: further evidence supporting an allosteric site. *J. Mol. Cell. Cardiol.* 1:39-45.

Arnold, S. B.; Byrd, R. C.; Meister, W., et al. 1980. Long-term digitalis therapy improves left ventricular function in heart failure. *N. Engl. J. Med.* 303:1443-1448.

Aronson, J. K.; and Grahame-Smith, D. G. 1976a. Digoxin therapy: textbooks, theory, and practice. *Br. J. Clin. Pharm.* 3:639-648.

Aronson, J. K.; and Grahame-Smith, D. G. 1976b. Altered distribution of digoxin in renal failure—a cause of digoxin toxicity? *Br. J. Clin. Pharm.* 3:1045-1051.

Bakoulas, G.; Voridis, E. M.; Tsiala-Parashos, E., et al. 1976. Study of myocardial and serum concentrations of ^{3}H-digoxin in disturbed thyroid function. *Abstract 7th Eur. Cong. Cardiol.* p. 328.

Bashour, T.; Hsu, I.; Gorfinkel, H. J., et al. 1975. Atrioventricular and intraventricular conduction in hyperkalemia. *Am. J. Cardiol.* 35:199-203.

Beller, G. A.; Hood, W. B.; Smith, T. W., et al. 1970. Prevalence of hypomagnesemia in a prospective clinical study of digitalis intoxication (abstract). *Am. J. Cardiol.* 26:625.

Beller, G. A.; Smith, T. W.; Abelmann, W. H., et al. 1971. Digitalis intoxication: a prospective clinical study with serum level correlations. *N. Engl. J. Med.* 284:989-997.

Beller, G. A.; Giamber, S. R.; Salz, S. B., et al. 1975. Cardiac and respiratory effects of digitalis during chronic hypoxia in intact conscious dogs. *Am. J. Physiol.* 229:270-274.

Belz, G. G.; Aust, P. E.; and Munkes, R. 1981. Digoxin plasma concentrations and nifedipine. *Lancet* 1:844-845.

Binnion, P. F.; and Morgan, L. M. 1970. Effect of acute hyper- and hypokalemia on left ventricular myocardial ^{3}H-digoxin uptake. *Irish J. Med. Sci.* 3:191-193.

Bismuth, C.; Motte, G.; Conso, F., et al. 1977. Acute digitoxin intoxication treated by intracardiac pacemaker: experience in sixty-eight patients. *Clin. Toxicol.* 10:443-456.

Borison, H. L.; and Wang, S. C. 1953. Physiology and pharmacology of vomiting. *Pharmacol. Rev.* 5:193-230.

Braunwald, W.; Bloodwell, R. D.; Goldberg, L. I., et al. 1961. Studies on digitalis. IV. Observations in man on the effects of digitalis preparations on the contractility of the non-failing heart and on total vascular resistance. *J. Clin. Invest.* 40:52-59.

Bremner, W. F.; Third, J. L. H. C.; and Lawrie, T. D. V. 1977. Massive digoxin ingestion. Report of a case and review of currently available therapies. *Br. Heart J.* 39:688-692.

Carruthers, S. G.; Kelly, J. G.; and McDevitt, D. G. 1974. Plasma digoxin concentrations in patients on admission to hospital. *Br. Heart J.* 36:707-712.

Castellanos, A.; Lemburg, L.; Brown, J. P., et al. 1967. An electrical digitalis tolerance test. *Am. J. Med. Sci.* 254:717-725.

Chamberlain, D. A.; White, R. T.; Howard, M. R., et al. 1970. Plasma digoxin concentrations in patients with atrial fibrillation. *Br. Med. J.* 3:429-432.

Chung, E. K. 1977. *Principles of cardiac arrhythmias.* Second ed. Baltimore: Williams and Wilkins Co. pp. 639-641.

Cohen, I. S.; Jick, H.; and Cohen, S. I. 1977. Adverse reactions to quinidine in hospitalized patients: findings based on data from the Boston Collaborative Drug Surveillance Program. *Prog. Cardiovasc. Dis.* 20:151-163.

Crawford, M. H.; Karliner, J. S.; O'Rourke, R. A., et al. 1976. Favorable effects of oral maintenance digoxin therapy on left ventricular performance in normal subjects: echocardiographic study. *Am. J. Cardiol.* 38:843-847.

Cranefield, P. F. 1977. Action potentials, afterpotentials, and arrhythmias. *Circ. Res.* 41:415-423.

Cree, J. E.; Coltart, D. J.; and Howard, M. R. 1975. Plasma digoxin concentration in children with heart failure. *Br. Med. J.* 1:443-446.

de Guzman, N. T.; and Yeh, B. K. 1975. Sodium canrenoate in the treatment of long-term digoxin-induced arrhythmias in conscious dogs. *Am. J. Cardiol.* 35:413-420.

Dobbs, S. M.; Rodgers, E. M.; Mawaer, G. E., et al. 1976. Serum digoxin concentrations. *Br. J. Clin. Pharmacol.* 3:674.

Dobbs, S. M.; Kenyon, W. I.; and Dobbs, R. J. 1977. Maintenance digoxin after an episode of heart failure: placebo-controlled trial in outpatients. *Br. Med. J.* i:749-752.

Doering, W. 1979. Quinidine-digoxin interaction. Pharmacokinetics, underlying mechanism, and clinical implications. *N. Engl. J. Med.* 301: 400-404.

Doering, W.; and König, E. 1978. *Digitalis intoxication: specificity of clinical and electrocardiographic signs. Cardiac glycosides.* G. Bodem; and H. J. Dengler, editors. New York: Springer-Verlag. pp. 358-363.

Eckberg, D. L.; Drabinsky, M.; and Braunwald, E. 1971. Defective parasympathetic control in patients with heart disease. *N. Engl. J. Med.* 285: 877-891.

Evans, D. E.; and Gillis, R. A. 1974. Effect of diphenylhydantoin and lidocaine on cardiac arrhythmias induced by hypothalamic stimulation. *J. Pharmacol. Exp. Ther.* 191:506-517.

Evered, D. C.; and Chapman, C. 1971. Plasma digoxin concentrations and digoxin toxicity in hospital patients. *Br. Heart J.* 33:540-545.

Ezrailson, E. G.; Potter, J. D.; Michael, L., et al. 1977. Positive inotropy induced by ouabain, by increased frequency, by X537A (R02-2985), by calcium, and by isoproterenol, the lack of correlation with phosphorylation Tn I. *J. Mol. Cell. Cardiol.* 9:693-698.

Fisch, C.; Greenspan, K.; Knoebel, S. B., et al. 1964. Effect of digitalis on conduction of the heart. *Prog. Cardiovasc. Dis.* 6:343-365.

Francis, D. J.; Gearoff, M. E.; Jackson, B., et al. 1973. The effect of insulin and glucose on the myocardial and skeletal muscle uptake of tritiated digoxin in acutely hypokalemic and normokalemic dogs. *J. Pharmacol. Exp. Ther.* 188:564-574.

Gervais, A.; Lindenmayer, G.; Entman, M. C., et al. 1975. A mechanism for ouabain action involving calcium-Na^+, K^+–ATPase interaction. *Circulation* 51 and 52 (*Suppl.* II):25.

Gibson, D. G.; and Sowton, E. 1969. The use of beta-adrenergic receptor blocking drugs in dysrhythmias. *Prog. Cardiovasc. Dis.* 12:16-39.

Gibson, T. P. 1980. Hemoperfusion of digoxin intoxication. *Clin. Toxicol.* 17:501-513.

Gilfrich, H. J.; Okonch, S.; Manns, M., et al. 1978. Digoxin and digitoxin elimination in man by charcoal hemoperfusion. *Klin. Wochensehr.* 56: 1179-1183.

Gillis, R. A.; Raines, A.; Sohn, Y., et al. 1972. Neuroexcitatory effects of digitalis and their role in cardiac arrhythmias. *J. Pharmacol. Exp. Ther.* 183:154-168.

Gillis, R. A.; Pearle, D. L.; and Levitt, B. 1975. Digitalis: a neuroexcitatory drug. *Circulation* 52:739-742.

Goldman, R. H.; Coltart, D. J.; Schweizer, E., et al. 1975. Dose response in vivo to digoxin in normo- and hyperkalemia: associated biochemical changes. *Cardiovasc. Res.* 9:515-523.

Graff, W. S.; and Etkins, J. P. 1964. Ventricular tachycardia after synchronized direct current countershock. *J.A.M.A.* 190:470-474.

Grahame-Smith, D. G. 1978. Some aspects of the clinical pharmacology of digoxin. In *Developments in cardiovascular medicine.* C. J. Dickinson; and J. Marks, editors. London: MTP Press Ltd. pp. 235-254.

Griffiths, B. E.; Penny, W. J.; Lewis, M. J., et al. 1982. Maintenance of the inotropic effect of digoxin on long-term treatment. *Br. Med. J.* 284: 1819-1822.

Hagemeijer, F.; and Van Houwe, E. V. 1975. Titrated energy cardioversion of patients on digitalis. *Br. Heart J.* 37:1303-1357.

Hager, W. D.; Fenster, P.; Mayersohn, M., et al. 1979. Digoxin-quinidine interaction. Pharmacokinetic evaluation. *N. Engl. J. Med.* 300:1238-1241.

Hall, R. J.; Gelbart, A.; Silverman, M., et al. 1977. Studies on digitalis-induced arrhythmias in glucose and insulin-induced hypokalemia. *J. Pharmacol. Exp. Ther.* 201:711-722.

Helke, C. J.; Quest, J. A.; and Gillis, R. A. 1978a. Effects of serotonin antagonist on digitalis-induced ventricular arrhythmias. *Eur. J. Pharmacol.* 47:443-449.

Helke, C. J.; Souza, J. D.; Hamilton, B., et al. 1978b. No evidence for a central serotonergic mechanism in arrhythmogenic effects of deslanoside. *Nature* 274:925.

Hess, T.; Stucki, P.; Barandun, S., et al. 1979. Treatment of a case of lantoside-C intoxication with digoxin-specific F $(ab')_2$ antibody fragments. *Am. Heart J.* 98:767-769.

Hull, S. M.; and MacIntosh, A. 1977. Discontinuation of maintenance digoxin therapy in general practice. *Lancet* ii:1251-1254.

Ingelfinger, J. A.; and Goldman, P. 1976. The serum digitalis concentration—does it diagnose digitalis toxicity? *N. Engl. J. Med.* 294:867-870.

Iseri, L. T.; Freed, J.; and Bures, A. R. 1975. Magnesium deficiency and cardiac disorders. *Am. J. Med.* 58:837-846.

Ito, M.; Hollander, P. B.; Marks, B. A., et al. 1970. The effects of six cardiac glycosides on transmembrane potential and contractile characteristics of the right ventricle of guinea pigs. *J. Pharmacol. Exp. Ther.* 172: 188-195.

Johnstone, G. D.; Kelly, J. G.; and McDevitt, D. G. 1978. Do patients take digoxin? *Br. Heart J.* 40:1-7.

Joubert, D. H.; Müller, F. O.; Pansegrouw, P. F., et al. 1975. A correlative study of serum digoxin levels and electrocardiographic measurements. *S. Afr. Med. J.* 49:1177-1181.

Kleiger, R.; and Lown, B. 1966. Cardioversion and digitalis. II. Clinical studies. *Circulation* 33:878-887.

Kleiman, J. H.; Ingels, W. B.; Daughters, G., et al. 1978. Left ventricular dynamics during long-term digoxin treatment in patients with stable coronary artery disease. *Am. J. Cardiol.* 41:937-942.

Langer, G. A. 1972. Effects of digitalis on myocardial ionic exchange. *Circulation* 46:180-187.

Leahey, E. B.; Reiffel, J. A.; Drusin, R. E., et al. 1978. Interactions between quinidine and digoxin. *J.A.M.A.* 240:533-534.

Lee, D. C-S.; Johnson, R. A.; Bingham, J. B., et al. 1982. Heart failure in outpatients. A randomized trial of digoxin versus placebo. *New Engl. J. Med.* 306:699-705.

Lely, A. H.; and Van Enter, C. H. J. 1970. Large-scale digitoxin intoxication. *Br. Med. J.* 3:737-740.

Lim, P.; and Jacob, P. 1972. Magnesium deficiency in patients on long-term diuretic therapy for heart failure. *Br. Med. J.* 3:620-622.

Lindenbaum, J.; Rund, D. G.; Butler, V. P., et al. 1981. Inactivation of digoxin by gut flora: reversal by antibiotic therapy. *New Engl. J. Med.* 305:789-794.

Lloyd, B. L.; and Smith, T. W. 1978. Contrasting rates of reversal of digoxin toxicity by digoxin-specific IgG and Fab fragments. *Circulation* 58:280-283.

Lown, B., and Levine, S. A. 1961. The carotid sinus. Clinical value of its stimulation. *Circulation* 23:766-789.

Lown, B.; Block, H.; and Moore, F. D. 1960. Digitalis, electrolytes, and the surgical patient. *Am. J. Cardiol.* 6:309-337.

McHaffie, D. J.; Purcell, H.; Mitchell-Heggs, P., et al. 1978. The clinical value of digoxin in patients with heart failure and sinus rhythm. *Q. J. Med.* 188:47, 401-419.

Maroko, P. R.; Kjekhus, J. K.; Sobel, B. G., et al. 1971. Factors influencing infarct size following experimental coronary artery occlusions. *Circulation* 43:67-82.

Moysey, J. O.; Jaggaro, N. S. U.; Grundy, E. N., et al. 1981. Amiodarone increases plasma digoxin concentrations. *Br. Med. J.* 282:272.

Murray, R. G.; Tweddel, A. C.; Martin, W., et al. 1982. Evaluation of digitalis in cardiac failure. *Br. Med. J.* 284:1526-1528.

Nadeau, R. A.; and James, T. N. 1963. Antagonistic effects on the sinus node of acetylstrophanthidin and adrenergic stimulation. *Circ. Res.* 13: 388-391.

Nayler, W. G. 1975. Ionic basis of contractility, relaxation, and cardiac failure. In *Modern trends in cardiology*. M. F. Oliver, editor. London: Butterworths. pp. 154.

Obayashi, K.; Nagasawa, K.; Mandel, W. J., et al. 1976. Cardiovascular effects of ajmaline. *Am. Heart J.* 92:487-496.

Okarma, T. B.; Tramell, P.; and Kalman, S. M. 1972. The surface interaction between digoxin and cultured heart cells. *J. Pharmacol. Exp. Ther.* 183:559-573.

Okita, G. T.; Richardson, F.; and Roth-Schechter, B. F. 1973. Dissociation of the positive inotropic action of digitalis from the inhibition of sodium- and potassium-activated adenosine triphosphatase. *J. Pharmacol. Exp. Ther.* 185:1-11.

Przybyla, A. C.; Paulay, K. L.; Stein, E., et al. 1974. Effects of digoxin on atrioventricular conduction patterns in man. *Am. J. Cardiol.* 33:344-350.

Rabbino, W.; Likoff, W.; and Dreifus, L. S. 1964. Complications and limitations of direct current counter-shock. *J.A.M.A.* 190:417-420.

Risler, T.; Peters, U.; Grabensee, B., et al. 1980. Quinidine-digoxin interaction (letter). *N. Engl. J. Med.* 302:175.

Robertson, D. M.; Hollenhorst, R. W.; and Callahan, J. A. 1966. Ocular manifestations of digitalis toxicity: discussion and report of three cases of central scotomas. *Arch. Ophthalmol.* (Chicago) 76:640-645.

Rodensky, P. L.; and Wasserman, F. 1961. Observations on digitalis intoxication. *Arch. Intern. Med.* 108:171-188.

Rosen, M. R.; Witt, A. L.; and Hoffman, B. F. 1975. Electrophysiology and pharmacology of cardiac arrhythmias. IV. Cardiac antiarrhythmic and toxic effects of digitalis. *Am. Heart J.* 89:391-399.

Schatzmann, J. J. 1953. Herzglykoside als Hemmstoffe für den aktiven Kalium—und Natriumtransport durch die Erythrocytenmembran. *Helv. Physiol. Pharmacol. Acta* 11:346-354.

Schick, D.; and Scheuer, J. 1974. Current concepts of therapy with digitalis glycosides. Part I. *Am. Heart J.* 87:253-258.

Seller, R. H.; Cangiano, J.; Kim, K. E., et al. 1970. Digitalis toxicity and hypomagnesemia. *Am. Heart J.* 79:57-68.

Sellers, T. D.; Bashore, T. M.; and Gallagher, J. J. 1977. Digitalis in the preexcitation syndrome. Analysis during atrial fibrillation. *Circulation* 56: 260-267.

Shapiro, W. 1978. Correlative studies of serum digitalis levels and the arrhythmias of digitalis intoxication. *Am. J. Cardiol.* 41:852-859.

Sharpe, D. N.; Norris, R. M.; and White, B. 1975. Serum digoxin levels after myocardial infarction. *Br. Heart J.* 37:530-533.

Sheehan, J.; and White, A. 1982. Diuretic-associated hypomagnesaemia. *Br. Med. J.* 285:1157-1159.

Singh, R. B.; Dube, K. P.; and Srivastau, P. K. 1976. Hypomagnesemia in relation to digoxin intoxication in children. *Am. Heart J.* 92:144-147.

Skou, J. C. 1957. The influence of some cations on an ATPase from peripheral nerves. *Biochem. Biophys. Acta* 23:394-401.

Smith, T. W.; and Willerson, J. T. 1971. Suicidal and accidental digoxin ingestion. *Circulation* 44:29-36.

Smith, T. W.; Haber, E.; Yeatman, L., et al. 1976. Reversal of advanced digoxin intoxication with Fab fragments of digoxin-specific antibodies. *N. Engl. J. Med.* 294:797-800.

Smith, T. W.; Butler, V. P.; Haber, E., et al. 1982. Treatment of life-threatening digitalis intoxication with digoxin-specific Fab antibody fragments. *New Engl. J. Med.* 307:1357-1362.

Somberg, J. C.; and Smith, T. W. 1979. Localization of the neurally mediated arrhythmogenic properties of digitalis. *Science* 204:321-323.

Spann, J. R., Jr.; Sonnenblick, E. H.; Cooper, T., et al. 1966. Studies on digitalis XIV. Influence of cardiac epinephrine stores on the response of isolated heart muscle to digitalis. *Circ. Res.* 19:326-331.

Steiness, E.; and Olesen, K. H. 1976. Cardiac arrhythmias induced by hypokalaemia and potassium loss during maintenance digoxin therapy. *Br. Heart J.* 38:167-172.

Stock, J. P. P. 1970. *Diagnosis and treatment of cardiac arrhythmias.* Second ed. London: Butterworths. pp. 226.

Stoffer, S. S.; Hynes, K. M.; Jiang, N. S., et al. 1973. Digoxin and abnormal serum hormone levels. *J.A.M.A.* 225:1643-1644.

Storstein, O.; Hansteen, V.; Hatle, L., et al. 1977. Studies on digitalis XIII. A prospective study of 649 patients on maintenance treatment with digitoxin. *Am. Heart J.* 93:434-443.

Straub, K. D.; Kane, J. J.; Bissett, J. K., et al. 1978. Alteration of digitalis binding by quinidine: a mechanism of digitalis-quinidine interaction. *Circulation* 57 and 58 (*Suppl.* II):II-58.

Szekely, P.; and Wynne, N. A. 1951. The effect of magnesium on cardiac arrhythmias caused by digitalis. *Clin. Sci.* 10:241-253.

Tse, W. W.; and Han, J. 1975. Effect of manganese chloride and verapamil on automaticity of digitalized Purkinje fibers. *Am. J. Cardiol.* 36:50-55.

Tsien, R. W.; and Carpenter, D. O. 1978. Ionic mechanisms of pacemaker activity in cardiac Purkinje fibers. *Fed. Proc.* 37:2127-2131.

Vera, Z.; Miller, R. R.; McMillin, D., et al. 1978. Effects of digitalis on sinus nodal function in patients with sick sinus syndrome. *Am. J. Cardiol.* 41:318-323.

Vohringer, H. F.; Rietbrock, N.; Spurny, P., et al. 1976. Disposition of digitoxin in renal failure. *Clin. Pharmacol. Ther.* 19:387-395.

Waldorff, S.; Andersen, J. D.; Heebøll-Nielsen, N., et al. 1978. Spironolactone-induced changes in digoxin kinetics. *Clin. Pharm. Ther.* 24: 162-167.

Warren, S. E.; and Fanestil, D. D. 1979. Digoxin overdose. Limitations of hemoperfusion hemodialysis treatment. *J.A.M.A.* 242:2100-2101.

Wilkerson, R. D.; and Glenn, T. M. 1977. Influence of nonsteroidal anti-inflammatory drugs on ouabain toxicity. *Am. Heart J.* 94:454-459.

Wilkerson, R. D.; Mockridge, P. B.; and Massing, G. K. 1980. The effects of selected drugs on serum digoxin concentrations in dogs. *Am. J. Cardiol.* 45:1201-1210.

Wit, A. L.; Rosen, M. R.; and Hoffman, B. F. 1975. Electrophysiology and pharmacology of cardiac arrhythmias: VIII. Cardiac effects of diphenylhydantoin. A and B. *Am. Heart J.* 90:265-272.

Withering, W. 1785. An account of the foxglove, and some of its medical uses: with practical remarks on dropsy, and other diseases. Birmingham, England: M. Swinney.

Yeh, B. K.; Chiang, B. N.; and Sung, P. K. 1976. Antiarrhythmic activity of potassium canrenoate in man. *Am. Heart J.* 92:308-314.

14 Cardiac Arrest

Michael Eliastam, M.D., M.D.P.
Assistant Professor of Medicine and Surgery
Director, Emergency Services
Stanford University Medical Center
Stanford, California

GENERAL COMMENTS

The Process of Resuscitation

The evaluation and treatment of cardiac arrest are unusual in medicine because treatment must begin almost immediately with only an initial preliminary evaluation. Subsequently, evaluation and treatment must be done in parallel, with evaluation focusing on both excluding unusual causes of cardiac arrest and assessing the impact of the resuscitation efforts. These procedures must be repeated throughout the resuscitation until either the patient is successfully resuscitated or the clinician decides to stop the cardiopulmonary resuscitation (CPR) efforts.

Leadership and the Team

Resuscitation should be carried out by a team with an identified leader to whom all pertinent clinical information should go and from whom all major clinical orders should come. The leader may delegate a function to a colleague (e.g., airway management to the anesthesiologist), but it is mandatory that the leader be aware continually of all drugs administered and all procedures performed by others. This is essential to avoid confusion among the team members and adverse effects on the patient. The cardiac arrest team should be familiar with its equipment and drugs and should practice resuscitation routines regularly. After a resuscitation, the team should review its performance and correct any identified deficiencies. A useful technique is to assign an uninvolved member of the hospital staff (a physician, nurse, or inhalation therapist) to observe the process and evaluate it against predetermined criteria. This procedure may be developed as part of the hospital's quality care audit program.

When to Stop CPR

It is clear that certain patients should not be resuscitated. Obvious examples include those patients in whom cardiac arrest brings a merciful end to a terminal illness or who have sustained a major injury that has resulted in extensive brain damage. Such patients should have "do not resuscitate" orders written in accordance with hospital policy to avoid inappropriate resuscitation efforts being initiated.

With the specific exceptions of hypothermia, drowning, and exsanguination from major trauma in young people, unsuccessful resuscitation may be halted when the following criteria have been met (Eliastam, et al., 1977):

1. Apnea and pulselessness are known to have exceeded 10 minutes.
2. No response after more than 30 minutes of advanced cardiac life support (ACLS) (including ACLS administered in the field).
3. No ventricular ECG activity after more than 10 minutes of ACLS.

For the exceptions resuscitation should be aggressive and pursued for longer periods of time. The team leader, in consultation with the patient's primary care physician, should be the one to decide when and if to terminate the resuscitation efforts.

In patients with hypothermia cardiac arrest occurs at a core temperature of about 25 C (Conn, 1979). Body temperature below 30 C affects the central nervous system, resulting in decreased mentation, dilated pupils, and hyporeflexia. These findings, along with an impalpable pulse caused by hypotension, may cause the patient to appear dead. However, because patients have been resuscitated successfully with core temperatures as low as 17 C, resuscitation of hypothermic patients must not cease until rewarming to a core temperature near normal has been achieved and evidence of cerebral and cardiac death is obvious (Reuler, 1978). For all hypothermic cardiac arrest patients, including drowning victims, CPR should begin immediately in the field. However, rewarming should be initiated outside the hospital only in those patients who have a core temperature below 30 C (Conn, 1979). A number of rewarming techniques are available for use in the hospital setting and should be implemented immediately while continuing aggressive resuscitation (Reuler, 1978). In patients with hypothermia the heart is relatively unresponsive to atropine, electrical pacing, and countershock. However, defibrillation should be attempted if ventricular fibrillation occurs. Rewarming accompanied by correction of hypoxia and acidosis will usually abolish the arrhythmias, and medications should be used judiciously because of the potential for adverse effects caused by the delayed metabolism of these drugs (Reuler, 1978).

Noncardiac Causes of Cardiac Arrest

Not all cardiac arrests are primarily the result of cardiac causes. Cardiac arrest is the final common pathway for a number of fatal illnesses and injuries, and a search should be made for less common primary causes that may have specific therapies. Examples of these are opiate overdose requiring naloxone, beta blocking drug overdose requiring isoproterenol or glucagon, tricyclic antidepressant drug abuse requiring physostigmine, and pneumothorax in a patient with obstructive pulmonary disease requiring chest tube insertion.

Chest X-Rays

Throughout the resuscitation efforts, repeated evaluation and reevaluation are necessary. As soon as a perfusing cardiac rhythm is obtained, a chest x-ray (portable) should be obtained if the adequacy of ventilation is questioned or if unexplained hypoxia and/or acidosis exists. The placement of central lines via neck or subclavian routes should be followed by a chest x-ray performed to exclude the possibility of a pneumothorax and to check the location of the intravenous line.

EVALUATION AND TREATMENT

The initial evaluation of any apparently dead patient is similar whether it is done by a lay person, paramedic, nurse, or physician. Basic life support (CPR) must be instituted immediately and maintained as long as necessary. The principles of advanced life support (ALS) are generally the same whether the ALS is delivered in the prehospital care phase or after admission to the hospital. However, paramedic emergency ambulance units often have a limited range of drugs, and the personnel may not be allowed to perform specific skills that are commonplace in the hospital setting such as tracheal intubation and central intravenous line placement.

Basic Life Support

The following ABC'S should be performed for basic life support:

1. *A = Airway.* The airway should be opened by hyperextending the neck, except in patients with head or neck injuries for whom the best method is the jaw thrust (Figure 14-1). The victim's mouth should be checked for loose dentures, foreign bodies, or excessive secretions.
2. *B = Breathing.* The victim's breathing should be checked by looking at the chest, listening over the mouth, and feeling air rushing out of the mouth against the examiner's ear. If the victim is not breathing, four quick breaths should be given and the chest observed to be certain that is is being inflated by these breaths. If no chest movement occurs, obstructed airway maneuvers should be initiated. The victim should be rolled toward the examiner and given four back blows between the shoulder blades. If this is unsuccessful, four abdominal thrusts should be administered by kneeling close to the hips of a supine victim or kneeling astride the victim. For very obese or pregnant victims four chest thrusts are the preferred maneuver. If repeated evaluation of the mouth for a foreign body using the finger sweep and repeated attempts at ventilation are unsuccessful, the above sequence should be repeated.
3. *C = Circulation.* The victim's carotid pulse should be checked. If it is absent, cardiac compression, at a rate of 80 beats/min in adults, should be initiated. The CPR should be continued, interspersing two ventilation breaths after every 15 cardiac compressions in one-person CPR. In two-person CPR ventilation should be given once for every five cardiac compressions without interrupting the cardiac compression. The cardiac compression rate is 60 beats/min in two-person CPR. Although it was initially felt that the mechanism of blood flow during closed-chest CPR was compression of the heart between the sternum and the spine, recent studies indicate that in most patients the blood flow probably occurs because of the increase in intrathoracic pressure. This pressure increase is transmitted unequally to the extrathoracic vessels with a resultant peripheral arteriovenous pressure gradient and forward flow

of blood (Rudikoff, et al., 1980). Thoracotomy for open-chest cardiac massage, with or without cross-clamping of the aorta, should be considered if closed cardiac compression appears to be ineffective.

4. *S = Spine and stop bleeding.* Whenever trauma is a possible cause of the cardiac arrest, movement of the victim's neck should be minimized to avoid spinal cord damage. Any major bleeding should be stopped by direct pressure.

Advanced Life Support

Airway management As soon as possible, a trained person should assume responsibility for managing the patient's airway. It is not necessary to intubate the trachea at this point. Adequate ventilation can be achieved with an oropharyngeal airway and a bag-valve mask. Although this arrangement does not protect the patient against aspiration of stomach contents, it does allow the patient to be rapidly oxygenated in a relatively simple manner. The esophageal obturator airway can also be used. While this instrument reduces the risk of aspiration, it does require additional personnel to obtain a good seal of the mask against the patient's chin, nose, and cheeks. Once the patient is well ventilated using the bag-valve mask or esophageal airway, tracheal intubation should be done by a person trained in airway management. A maximum of 15 seconds should be allowed for each attempt at intubation, and failed attempts should be followed by 30-40 seconds of adequate bag-valve mask ventilation before intubation is reattempted. Careful attention should be paid to the length of the endotracheal tube to avoid right mainstem bronchus intubation.

Intravenous line placement and other routes of drug administration Peripheral venous lines are adequate for the initial resuscitation of most cardiac arrest victims. Only those patients requiring large fluid volume replacement, those needing an immediate evaluation of central venous pressure, or those in whom it is impossible to find an accessible peripheral vein require central lines. For many of these patients the femoral vein will provide adequate access, although this vein is often difficult to find during cardiac arrest because of poor landmarks in the absence of a palpable femoral pulse. Subclavian lines are easier to insert but interfere with cardiac compression and carry a relatively high risk of incidental

Figure 14-1 Top panel: the most common cause of airway obstruction in the unconscious victim is the tongue. Middle panel: as long as there is enough tone in the muscles of the jaw, tilting the head back will cause the lower jaw to move forward and open the airway. Bottom panel: because the tongue is attached to the lower jaw, moving the lower jaw forward lifts the tongue away from the back of the throat and opens the airway.

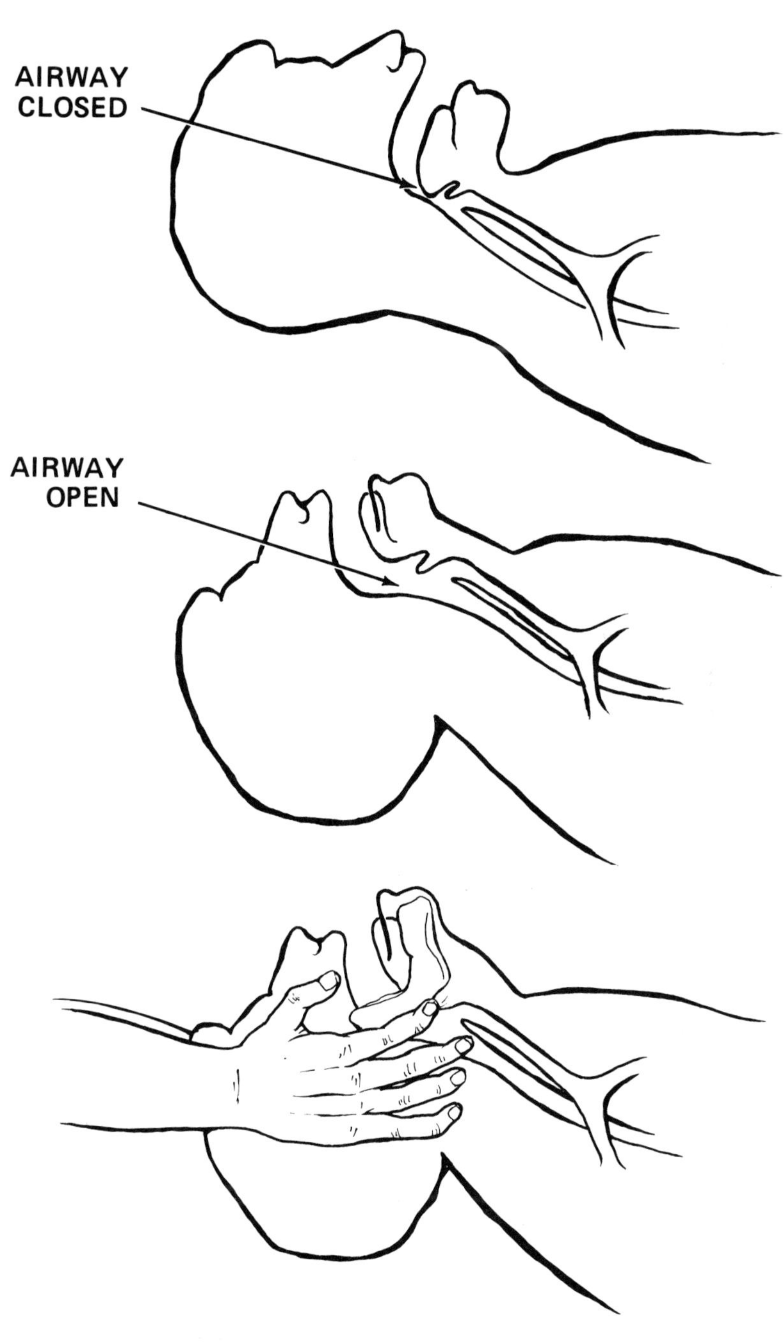
AIRWAY
CLOSED
AIRWAY
OPEN

pneumothorax. Internal jugular vein lines carry less risk of complication. However, during the early phase of resuscitation there is no place for jugular vein cannulation until the airway is secure and ventilation is satisfactory. In hypovolemic patients normal saline or lactated Ringer's solution should be infused initially, while D5W should be used in all other patients. Trauma patients need large volumes of fluids, especially blood.

Intracardiac drug administration should be used sparingly because of the potential for coronary artery damage and injection of drugs into the myocardium itself, which may produce intractable arrhythmias. The endotracheal tube has been investigated recently as a route for drug administration and is very useful (Greenberg, et al., 1979). Epinephrine, lidocaine, and atropine can be given safely via this route, and initial dosages are similar to parenteral doses, but repeat doses need adjustment down because the duration of effect appears to be longer. Drugs may be diluted in saline, although water appears to be better, and instilled into the endotracheal tube. Vigorous ventilation after instillation promotes movement of the drug into the alveoli, which facilitates absorption. Consideration should be given to using the sublingual route, which is a very vascular area with easy access. Strong evidence exists supporting the efficacy of naloxone and epinephrine through this route, and administration of 5 mL of lidocaine sublingually without adverse effect has been reported (Pomeroy and Loehr, 1977).

Arrhythmia management In the cardiac arrest situation cardiac output is usually zero or inadequate to produce a palpable femoral or carotid pulse. The most important aspects of this management phase, in addition to the drug therapy that is outlined below, are the presence of adequate ventilation and oxygenation, uninterrupted cardiac compression, and the correction of acid-base imbalances. Ventricular fibrillation is the most common cardiac arrest arrhythmia (occurring in about 60% of patients), but the exact frequency of its occurrence depends on the time from onset of the arrhythmia to discovery of the arrested patient. Ventricular fibrillation may degenerate into ventricular asystole over a variable period of time. In the field about 25% of cardiac arrest patients present in asystole and an additional 10% of patients present with other bradyarrhythmias (Eisenberg, et al., 1979).

The following is a list of the common cardiac arrest arrhythmias:

1. Ventricular asystole
2. Ventricular fibrillation or sustained ventricular tachycardia
3. Electromechanical dissociation
4. Pulseless idioventricular rhythm

The therapy for each of these arrhythmias is described below.

Ventricular asystole This arrhythmia has a very poor prognosis and may result from either total cardiac standstill or complete heart block with no ventricular escape rhythm. The drug therapy is as follows:

1. Epinephrine: 0.5-1.0 mg in 10 mL as a 1:10,000 solution given intravenously and rapidly. If difficulty inserting an intravenous line is encountered, the initial dose of epinephrine can be instilled intratracheally, followed by vigorous ventilation to distribute the drug as far into the bronchial tree as possible.
2. Sodium bicarbonate: the initial amount of this agent given should be based on an estimate of the time the patient spent without adequate ventilation and perfusion. If more than 5 minutes has elapsed, about 1.0-1.5 mEq/kg should be given as the initial bolus. The next dose should be based on the results of arterial blood gas determination and clinical review carried out every 5-10 minutes, and should take into account the adequacy of ventilation and perfusion and the patient's response to drugs. Generally, cardiac arrests occurring inside the hospital require much less sodium bicarbonate than those that occur outside the hospital and are brought to the emergency department.
3. Atropine: recently, it has been suggested that cardiac arrest caused by total cardiac standstill may be caused or aggravated by profound vagal tone. Therefore, atropine may be given in cardiac arrests caused either by complete heart block or total cardiac standstill. Dosage recommendations vary from 0.5-4.0 mg, given intravenously. Atropine should be accompanied by 0.5 mg of epinephrine every 10 minutes for three doses. While only a few published reports are available regarding the value of atropine in cardiac arrests, the grave prognosis for this subgroup of patients makes its use reasonable and potentially worthwhile (Brown, et al., 1979). Because atropine produces mydriasis, this clinical sign should be interpreted cautiously in cardiac arrest patients receiving this drug.
4. Isoproterenol: isoproterenol may be given in a dose of 2 mg in 250 mL of D5W administered by intravenous infusion. Because this drug is a potential cause of serious arrhythmias, its use must be monitored carefully once a response has been obtained.
5. Calcium chloride: this drug should be given intravenously, 500-1000 mg as a 10% solution. Data on the absorption of calcium chloride via the tracheal route are not available. Unavailability of an intravenous line may necessitate the administration by the intracardiac route.
6. Pacemakers: temporary pacemakers are generally of little use in treating cardiac arrest. It is possible that future research will identify a role for pacemakers in a subset of patients with bradysystolic cardiac arrest, but such evidence is lacking at present.

Ventricular fibrillation or sustained ventricular tachycardia Cardiac arrest patients with these arrhythmias have the best prognosis. Survival is often directly related to the time that elapsed before defibrillation was begun.

Defibrillation must be carried out as soon as possible after the diagnosis of ventricular fibrillation is made. While it is now widely accepted that direct current defibrillation is far superior to that of alternating current, considerable controversy exists regarding the optimal defibrillation dose for the individual patient (Bander, 1979). The most relevant study on the subject is by Weaver and colleagues (1982) and shows no difference in the rate of reversion to an organized rhythm or survival of out-of-hospital cardiac arrest victims randomized to either 175 or 320 joules for the first two defibrillations. The controversy is further complicated by confusion resulting from the disparity between the energy level selected on the defibrillator meter by the physician and the actual amount of energy delivered at the paddle surface. Studies have shown a wide variation in delivered energy (ranging from 155 to 400 joules, or watt-seconds) for a meter setting of 400 joules. Therefore, it is important to be aware of the energy delivered by the particular defibrillator being used in the resuscitation efforts at a given meter setting. Most newer defibrillators have meters that read delivered energy rather than stored energy.

Significant argument exists over whether heavier adults (i.e., those weighing more than 80 kg) require significantly larger amounts of energy for rapid defibrillation to occur. The proponents of this view recommend delivered energy levels of 5 joules/kg for patients weighing more than 100 kg and 4 joules/kg for those weighing 50-100 kg. The opponents recommend repeated defibrillation shocks using not more than 2 joules/kg each time, being certain that impedance is minimized by using the correct electrode surface area, careful electrode placement, and choice of the most effective interface material. While the potential for myocardial damage from high-energy machines is evident, actual documented evidence of this effect is sparse, especially where energy levels up to 400 joules have been used. For pediatric patients the defibrillation dose has been firmly established at 1-2 joules/kg (Gutgesell, et al., 1976).

While the defibrillator is being charged and the paddle contact surface prepared, effective CPR must be maintained to minimize hypoxia and acidosis. Special attention should be paid to ensuring that the skin contact is firm, that arcing does not occur between the two paddles, and that no personnel are in contact with the patient or bed when the shock is given. Paddles should be placed over the apical impulse area and to the right of the sternum. Immediately after the defibrillation shock is administered, CPR should be resumed and femoral pulses looked for. The time during which the CPR is stopped to check the ECG rhythm and feel for femoral pulses should be limited to no more than 10 seconds at any one time.

An unsuccessful defibrillation attempt should be followed by a second attempt as soon as possible because skin resistance is reduced following the first shock. If a second shock is unsuccessful, 50-100 mEq of sodium bicarbonate should be administered by an intravenous push. Adequate ventilation should be confirmed and femoral pulses felt for to ensure that cardiac compression is effective. After 1-2 minutes of effective CPR, the defibrillation should be repeated as above. If defibrillation is repeatedly unsuccessful, consideration should be given to using a high-energy defibrillator or anteroposterior paddles if they are available.

When ventricular fibrillation is resistant to defibrillation despite correction of acidosis and the presence of adequate oxygenation, pharmacologic agents should be given.

Epinephrine, 0.5-1.0 mg (5-10 mL of 1:10,000 solution), may be given intravenously or, if an intravenous line is unavailable, via the endotracheal tube. A less desirable alternative is to use the intracardiac route. Epinephrine is reputed to coarsen fine ventricular fibrillation and make the arrhythmia more responsive to defibrillation.

Lidocaine, 1-2 mg/kg, may be given by rapid intravenous bolus. In this setting it is postulated that defibrillation may occur immediately after the shock is administered, but fibrillation recurs immediately. The lidocaine is given to prevent this refibrillation. If the drug is successful, an additional bolus should be given 5-10 minutes later and an intravenous infusion to run at 2-4 mg/mL initiated immediately.

Bretylium sulfate, 5-10 mg/kg by rapid intravenous bolus, has on rare occasions been documented to pharmacologically reverse intractable ventricular fibrillation. In most patients administration of bretylium appears to facilitate successful electrical defibrillation. In one study bretylium administration following 30 minutes of unsuccessful comprehensive resuscitation resulted in 44% of the patients being successfully defibrillated and discharged alive from the hospital (Holder, et al., 1977). In another study randomization of cardiac arrest patients to either lidocaine or bretylium showed no difference in terms of immediate or long-term outcome (Haynes, et al., 1981).

Procainamide, 100 mg over 1 minute followed by 200 mg over 5 minutes up to a total loading dose of 1 g by intravenous infusion, may permit conversion of intractable ventricular fibrillation.

Propranolol, 1-5 mg by intravenous bolus, given as 1 mg/min, may be successful occasionally in this setting but is generally avoided because of its myocardial depressant actions.

Calcium chloride, 0.5-1.0 g by intravenous push, is occasionally useful in this setting. Its exact action is unknown.

Electromechanical dissociation This arrhythmia has a grave prognosis and is characterized by nearly normal ECG complexes and an absent pulse. The heart lacks mechanical action and cardiac output is negligible, despite the apparently adequate ECG activity. While this rhythm is most often caused by left ventricular power failure, severe hypovolemia, massive pulmonary embolus, and cardiac rupture or tamponade must be considered depending on the clinical setting. Specific therapeutic interventions, such as pericardiocentesis or pulmonary embolectomy, may be life-saving.

Pharmacologic therapy is limited to administering calcium and cardiac stimulants, such as epinephrine and isoproterenol, in addition to maintaining adequate ventilation and oxygenation and effective chest compression.

Pulseless idioventricular rhythm The clinical state in this arrhythmia is one of cardiac arrest with the ECG showing an idioventricular rhythm in the absence of femoral or carotid pulses. Sinus arrest or complete heart block may be present. The etiology of the arrest varies and includes both cardiac and noncardiac causes. Treatment includes the following:

1. The standard resuscitation measures, including those described for cardiac arrest from ventricular asystole.
2. Isoproterenol, 1-2 mg in 250 mL of D5W by intravenous infusion, administered to speed up the rate of a slow idioventricular focus, increase the force of the contractions, and improve AV conduction or sinus rate.
3. Dexamethasone, 1.5 mg/kg by intravenous bolus, which has been reported to be useful in this setting (White, et al., 1979). The drug is presumed to have a rapid action on AV conduction.

Vasoactive Drugs

With the exception of epinephrine, vasoactive drugs generally have no place in the initial resuscitation of cardiac arrest patients unless there is a question of hypovolemia contributing to the absence of a palpable pulse. In such situations a vasoactive drug should be used in addition to intravenous saline or lactated Ringer's solution.

If suspicion exists that full vasoconstriction has not occurred, such as in anaphylaxis, sepsis, or spinal injury, an alpha-adrenergic drug should be used (levarterenol or metaraminol). Their short-term use in this specific setting may be beneficial. Similarly, these vasoconstrictor drugs may sustain the exsanguinating patient until enough intravenous lines can be started and adequate blood replaced.

For all cardiac arrest patients in whom extensive vasoconstriction is evident the vasoactive drug of choice is dopamine. In doses of 2-5 μg/kg/min dopamine produces an increase in cardiac contractility, cardiac output, and renal blood flow, with little change in heart rate and a reduction or no change in peripheral resistance. Less desirable effects are obtained when higher infusion rates are used (5-10 μg/kg/min) because peripheral resistance and heart rate increase and renal blood flow may decline (Braunwald, 1980).

RESULTS OF CARDIAC ARREST RESUSCITATION

The success rate for cardiac arrest resuscitation is directly related to the availability of trained personnel and equipment and to the type of ECG rhythm that is present when resuscitation starts. When one examines the outcomes based on where the patient was at the onset of the cardiac arrest, the best results are obtained in the CCU and ICU, followed by the regular ward, the emergency room, and, finally, the field.

In the critical care areas (CCU and ICU) the survival rates for cardiac arrest vary from 20% to 40%, depending on the cause and excluding those patients for whom cardiac arrest is the terminal event of cardiogenic shock or congestive heart failure (Eliastam, et al., 1977). When primary ventricular fibrillation occurs in the CCU, it has a successful resuscitation rate of about 90%. Late primary ventricular fibrillation (i.e., occurring more than 48 hours after a myocardial infarction) has a successful resuscitation and hospital discharge rate of about 50%, with most of these patients able to function at their precardiac arrest levels (Wilson, 1974). Secondary ventricular fibrillation occurring in the setting of cardiogenic shock has a very poor prognosis.

Cardiac arrest occurring on the regular wards has a successful resuscitation rate of 20%-30% (Eliastam, et al., 1977). The best results appear to come from those institutions that have cardiac arrest teams.

To interpret accurately the overall success rate for emergency department resuscitations, one must recognize two distinct groups of patients. Those patients who suffer cardiac arrest after arrival in the emergency department appear to have success rates similar to patients whose arrests occur in the critical care areas. However, for those patients whose arrests occur in the field and for whom initial field resuscitation is unsuccessful the results are dismal. The outcome depends on the cause of the arrest, the amount of time that elapsed before resuscitation started, the availability of equipment and trained personnel in the community, and the patient's age. For cardiac arrest occurring in the field the results are clearly affected by the availability of an appropriately manned and equipped mobile intensive care unit (Eisenberg, et al., 1979). Communities with such ambulances report survival and hospital discharge rates in the range of 10%-15% in patients with ventricular fibrillation. In communities with extensive citizen CPR training and sophisticated emergency medical service systems the survival rate is approximately 25%. For patients suffering cardiac arrest in the field caused by bradyarrhythmia the survival rates are extremely low, in the range of 0%-5% (Eliastam, et al., 1977).

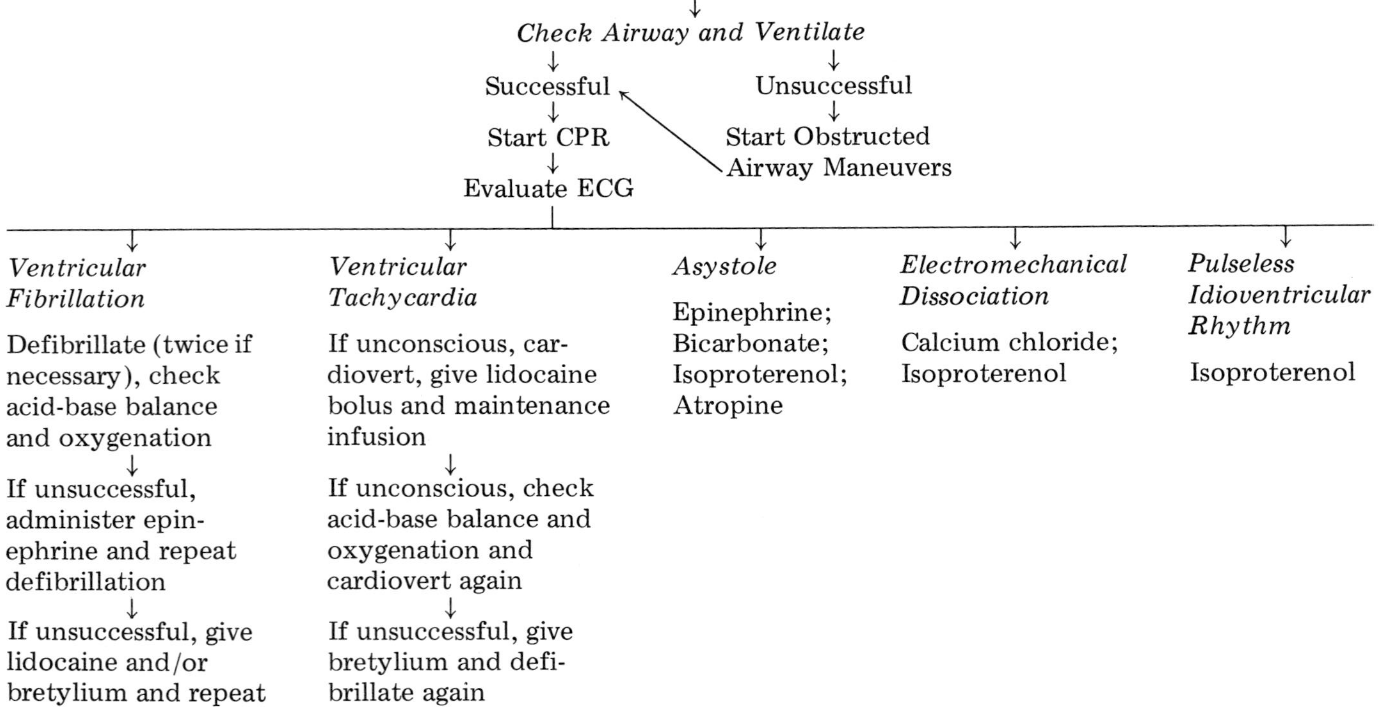

Figure 14-2 Cardiac arrest flow sheet.

REFERENCES

Bander, J. J. 1979. Defibrillation. *Top. Emerg. Med.* 1(no. 2).

Braunwald, E. 1980. *Heart disease: a textbook of cardiovascular medicine.* Philadelphia: W. B. Saunders Co. pp. 553-557.

Brown, D. C.; Lewis, A. J., and Criley, J. M. 1979. Asystole and its treatment: the possible role of the parasympathetic nervous system in cardiac arrests. *J. Am. Coll. Emerg. Phys.* 8:11.

Conn, A. W. 1979. Near-drowning and hypothermia. *Can. Med. Assoc. J.* 120:397-400.

Eisenberg, M. S.; Bergner, L.; and Hallstrom, A. 1979. Epidemiology of cardiac arrest and resuscitation in a suburban community. *J. Am. Coll. Emerg. Phys.* 8:1.

Eliastam, M.; Duralde, T.; Martinez, F., et al. 1977. Cardiac arrest in the emergency medical services system: guidelines for resuscitation. *J. Am. Coll. Emerg. Phys.* 6:12.

Greenberg, M. I.; Roberts, J. R.; Baskin, S. I., et al. 1979. The use of endotracheal medication for cardiac arrest. *Top. Emerg. Med.* 1: - .

Gutgesell, H. P.; Tacker, W. A.; and Geddes, L. A. 1976. Energy dose for ventricular defibrillation of children. *Pediatrics* 58:898-901.

Haynes, R. E.; Chinn, T. L.; Copass, M. K., et al. 1981. Comparison of bretylium tosylate and lidocaine in management of out-of-hospital ventricular fibrillation: a randomized clinical trial. *Am. J. Cardiol.* 48:353-356.

Holder, D. A.; Sniderman, A. D.; Fraser, G., et al. 1977. Experience with bretylium tosylate by a hospital cardiac team. *Circulation* 55:541-544.

Pomeroy, G. L. M.; and Loehr, M. M. 1977. Intralingual injection of lidocaine. *J. Am. Coll. Emerg. Phys.* 6:4.

Reuler, J. B. 1978. Hypothermia: pathophysiology, clinical settings, and management. *Ann. Intern. Med.* 89:519-527.

Rudikoff, M. T.; Maughan, W. L.; Effron, M., et al. 1980. Mechanisms of blood flow during cardiopulmonary resuscitation. *Circulation* 61:345-352.

Weaver, W. D.; Cobb, L. A.; Copass, M. K., et al. 1982. Ventricular defibrillation—a comparative trial using 175-J and 320-J shocks. *N. Engl. J. Med.* 307:1101-1106.

White, B. C.; Petinga, T. J.; Hoehner, P. J., et al. 1979. Incidence, etiology, and outcome of pulseless idioventricular rhythm treated with dexamethasone during advanced CPR. *J. Am. Coll. Emerg. Phys.* 8:5.

Wilson, A. A. 1974. Survival of patients with late ventricular fibrillation after acute myocardial infarction. *Lancet* 2:124-126.

Index